Complete

WOMEN'S HEALTH

ROYAL COLLEGE OF OBSTETRICIANS & GYNAECOLOGISTS

Complete

WOMEN'S HEALTH

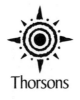
Thorsons

Thorsons
An Imprint of HarperCollins*Publishers*
77–85 Fulham Palace Road
Hammersmith, London W6 8JB

The Thorsons website address is www.thorsons.com

First published by Thorsons 2000

1 3 5 7 9 10 8 6 4 2

© Royal College of Obstetricians and Gynaecologists 2000

A catalogue record of this book is available from the British Library

ISBN 0 7225 3430 2

Printed and bound in Great Britain

This book was created by
SP Creative Design
Editor: Heather Thomas
Art director and production: Rolando Ugolini
Artwork illustrations: Rolando Ugolini and Al Rockall

Contents

CONSULTANT EDITORS

Dr Mary Ann Lumsden FRCOG

Dr Mary Ann Lumsden FRCOG is a Senior Lecturer in the Department of Obstetrics and Gynaecology at the University of Glasgow. As a consultant Gynaecologist and Obstetrician, she runs an antenatal clinic in one of the less affluent areas of Glasgow and has a large gynaecology practice with a particular interest in menstrual problems and the menopause. She has an active research programme in these areas.

Dr Martha Hickey MRCOG

Dr Martha Hickey MRCOG is a Clinical Lecturer and Senior Registrar in Obstetrics and Gynaecology in the Department of Reproductive Science and Medicine at Imperial College School of Medicine, St Mary's Hospital, London. She initially trained and worked in clinical psychology before entering medical training. She works in all areas of clinical obstetrics and gynaecology and her main clinical and research interests are menstrual disorders and the menopause.

CONTRIBUTORS

Hossam Abdalla, Imad Abukhail, Robert Atlay, Philip Baker, Constance Ballinger, Saikat Banerjee, Ros Banks, David Barlow, Lester Barr, Michael Baum, Richard Beard, Alison Bigrigg, Susan Blunt, Peter Bowen-Simpkins, WD Boyd, Michael Brudenell, Geoffrey Chamberlain, Michael Chapman, Oliver Chapatte, Frederick Charnock, Li Chang Cheng, Sarah Chissell, Malcolm Chiswick, Katy Clifford, Ian Cooke, Kevin Cooper, Sarah Creighton, Tom D'Arcy, Alberto de Barros Lopes, Miriam Deeny, James Dornan, Niall Duignan, Ian Duncan, Katrina Erskine, Ian Ferguson, Susan Field, Nicholas Fisk, Diana Fothergill, John Friend, Tham Kok Fun, Kevin Gangar, Ailsa Gebbie, Anna Glasier, Eleanor Goldman, Peter Greenhouse, John Guillebaud, Marion Hall, Shona Hamilton, Joseph Hamlett, Naomi Hampton, Kate Harding, Jonathan Herod, Bryan Hibbard, Paul Hilton, Richard Howard, Pauline Hurley, Julian Jenkins, David James, Colin Jardine-Brown, Richard Johanson, Derek Johnson, Margaret Johnson, David Joyce, David Joynson, Sean Kehoe, Anthony Kenny, Srinivasan Krishnamurthy, Ali Kubba, Geoffrey Lane, William Ledger, Helen Lewison, Brian Lieberman, Richard Lilford, David Luesley, John Malvern, Wendy McCulloughHelen McEwan, Pauline McGough, Heather Mellows, Kenneth Metcalf, Laura Miller, Riva Miller, John Mills, Peter Milton, John Monaghan, John Moore-Gillon, Eleanor Moskovic, Nicholas Naftalin, Catherine Nelson-Piercy, Shaughn O'Brien, Andrew Parfitt, John Parsons, Sara Paterson-Brown, Elizabeth Payne, Roger Peel, David Polson, Elizabeth Poskitt, Andrew Prentice, Fran Reader, Lesley Regan, Brian Reid, Laurence Roberts, Greg Robertson, Charles Rodeck, Sam Rowlands, Janice Rymer, Christobel Saunders, Peter Saunders, Wendy Savage, Margaret Semple, Robert Shaw, John Shepherd, Fiona Sizmur, Chris Spence, John Spencer, Kenneth Stewart, John Studd, Christopher Sutton, Malcolm Symonds, David Taylor, Margaret Thom, Eric Thomas, Meirion Thomas, Margaret Tuck, Ian Vellacott, Eboo Versi, James Walker, Kathleen Waller, Eve Wiltshaw, Laurence Wood and Julian Woolfson.

The writing of Chapter 12 on Infertility, was begun by Mike Hull and completed by David Cahill at short notice after the sudden death of Professor Hull. We would like to especially thank Dr Cahill for undertaking this work.

Alice Murkie, of the Jean Hailes Foundation, Melbourne, Australia, contributed information on complementary therapies and the menopause.

Liz Laverick contributed the sections on antenatal and postnatal physiotherapy.

FOREWORD

I believe that this book will provide a unique resource for women and their partners. It provides information on normal aspects of the reproductive cycle, female genital tract and explains the changes which occur in pregnancy and throughout reproductive life in females. In addition, it provides detailed information on a number of common gynaecological disorders, important aspects of sexual health, information on normal pregnancy, some aspects of complications which may occur in pregnancy and describes a number of gynaecological treatments.

I believe it will provide a wealth of information to readers, to both reassure them regarding common concerns and to help them understand how problems or diseases can occur. It is not meant to replace the need to consult with your general practitioner if and when problems do occur, nor to replace the need for detailed discussion with your obstetrician and gynaecologist when referred for management of specific disorders. General principles are explained within this book and treatment always needs to be individualised to match each patient's specific requirements.

The text has been assembled from contributions from many distinguished and respected obstetricians and gynaecologists, all Members of our College. They have donated freely their time and expertise to ensure we produce an informative and worthwhile book. The final product has resulted from the enormous efforts of the two editors, Dr Lumsden and Dr Hickey, to whom we owe an immense debt of gratitude.

I hope you enjoy reading the book and that it helps you understand the complexities of female reproductive health and disease.

Professor Robert Shaw MD, FRCOG, FRCS
President of the Royal College of Obstetricians & Gynaecologists

PREFACE

Writing a book entitled 'Complete Women's Health' may seem overly ambitious. Our aim is to cover a wide variety of issues that concern women from puberty to older age. A large number of obstetricians and gynaecologists have contributed to this book, as well as midwives and physiotherapists. Inevitably, the emphasis has to be on the sort of concerns that take a women to her doctor, since obstetricians and gynaecologists are principally concerned with helping women who feel that they have a problem that is preventing them from achieving maximum quality of life.

Many of the issues that concern women are not associated with disease as such. Sometimes it is that a normal process is occurring in such a way as to produce inconvenience and diminish quality of life. The issues surrounding these disorders are discussed and the possible ways of dealing with them. Most of the issues that concern women are covered in the book, although some in greater detail than others. Some uncommon conditions are discussed at some length when it is felt that there is little information elsewhere for a woman to draw on.

The aim is to give a balanced view, discussing the possible alternative treatments which are available, and to give facts about them. The purpose of the book is not to give the view of any particular individual or organisation but to try and represent doctors, midwives and the women themselves. It is as up to date as possible, but obviously this is a rapidly moving field and new issues emerge all the time. We hope that these are touched on and will give women ideas about the sort of questions they might pose to their doctors at the time of a consultation.

Mary Ann Lumsden
Martha Hickey

Chapter one

SEE ALSO

HOW THE BODY WORKS

A woman's body has to perform many biological functions throughout her life, as she develops from birth through puberty to pregnancy and the menopause. In order to understand better how the body works, it is necessary to examine the female reproductive organs and how they function within the body.

THE REPRODUCTIVE ORGANS

THE OVARIES

Below: This illustration shows the reproductive organs of a mature woman before the menopause.

The ovaries are two glands that sit inside the cavity of the woman's abdomen. They are almond shaped, solid and greyish-pink in colour. In adulthood they are around 3 cm (1 in) long and 1.5 cm (½ in) wide. The ovaries contain the oocytes, or eggs. There are between one and two million eggs at birth but the number steadily declines thereafter. The ovaries remain dormant during childhood and start to function as puberty ensues. No more than 500 oocytes are destined to mature during a woman's reproductive life (usually one a month) and the rest degenerate. This process is complete by the time of the onset of the menopause when there are no oocytes left and the ovaries again become inactive.

THE FALLOPIAN TUBES

The fallopian tubes arise from the sides of the uterus and are around 10 cm (4 in) in length. The end of each tube is trumpet shaped and sits close to the ovary. When an egg is produced, it is collected by the end of the tube and passes along it, aided by the small hairs, or cilia, it contains and mild muscular contractions. If fertilisation of the egg occurs, it usually does so in the mid portion of the tubes.

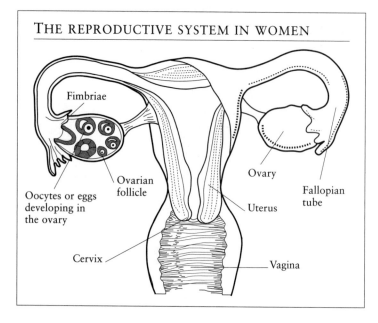

THE REPRODUCTIVE SYSTEM IN WOMEN

Fimbriae

Oocytes or eggs developing in the ovary

Ovarian follicle

Cervix

Ovary

Fallopian tube

Uterus

Vagina

THE UTERUS

The uterus, or womb, is shaped like an inverted pear, tapering down to the cervix, and is situated low in the pelvis. It is hollow with thick muscular walls. It is around 9 cm (3¹/₂ in) long, 6 cm (2¹/₄ in) wide and 4 cm thick. The upper expanded part is called the body of the uterus. In eighty-five per cent of women it is bent forwards at up to ninety degrees to the axis of the vagina (anteversion). In the remainder, it tilts backwards (retroversion). The cavity of the uterus is shaped like an inverted triangle and the fallopian tubes open into it on either side near the top. The uterus has a remarkable ability to stretch and increase in size during pregnancy. By the time the baby is due the uterus fills most of the abdominal cavity.

THE CERVIX

The cervix, or neck of the womb, is the lowest portion of the uterus and is cylindrical in shape, pointing down into the vagina. It contains a narrow canal connecting the vagina to the cavity of the uterus. It is capable of immense stretching during labour to allow the baby to pass through. The cells of the canal of the cervix contain lots of glands producing mucus, forming a clear vaginal discharge. At the opening of the canal into the vagina these cells are replaced by vaginal skin. It is here that the cells can become abnormal or even malignant and therefore this is the area from which cervical smears are taken.

THE VAGINA

The cervix opens into the vagina which is angled somewhat backwards. The front and back walls normally lie against one another

THE REPRODUCTIVE ORGANS

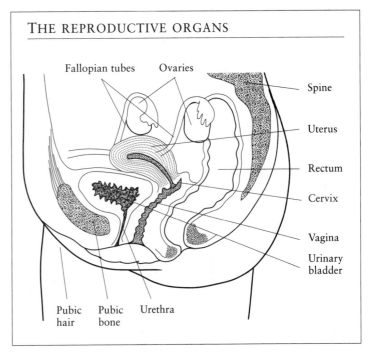

Above: A cross-section of the female external and internal reproductive organs.

but the vagina is very distensible, stretching to allow the baby to pass through during delivery. At the lower end is a thin membrane, the hymen. This normally has holes in it to allow menstrual fluid to pass and tends to be torn at first intercourse or with the use of tampons,

THE EXTERNAL SEXUAL ORGANS (GENITALIA)

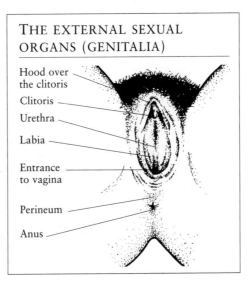

but it may stretch and disappear with normal activity. It is certainly destroyed in childbirth, leaving only small skin tags.

THE VULVA

This is the name used for the external structures and is a vertical cleft bounded at the top by a pad of fat covered with pubic hair, the mons, and at the bottom by the muscles of the perineum. On either side of the vaginal opening are two folds of skin, the labia majora, containing fat and sweat glands corresponding to the scrotum of the male, and the labia minora which are lip-like folds of skin which, at the top, meet at the clitoris. The most sensitive part of the vulva, this contains erectile tissue and is the equivalent of the male penis. The urethra (the tube leading to the bladder) does not, however, run through it but opens instead between the clitoris and the vagina.

MENSTRUATION

The control of a woman's reproductive cycle is complex. The cycle is designed so that a woman produces an egg once each month, allowing her the possibility of becoming pregnant. Each cycle begins with the first day of the period. A number of eggs begin to grow in the ovary until, after fourteen days, one egg is mature enough to be released from the ovary (ovulation).

While developing, the cells around the egg produce the hormone oestrogen. After ovulation these cells produce a second hormone, progesterone, and together the two hormones stimulate the lining of the uterus

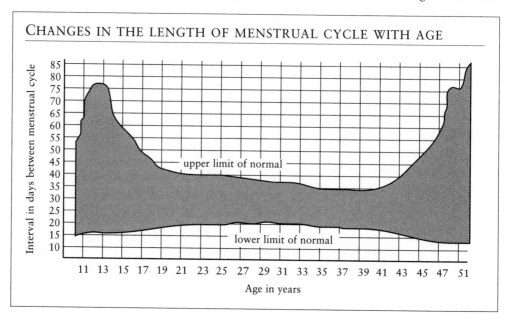

CHANGES IN THE LENGTH OF MENSTRUAL CYCLE WITH AGE

Interval in days between menstrual cycle

upper limit of normal

lower limit of normal

Age in years

(womb) to grow. The ovulated egg enters the fallopian tube and travels towards the womb. If intercourse has taken place and no contraception has been used, the sperm may fertilise the egg while it is in the tube and the resulting embryo will implant into the lining of the womb where it develops into a baby.

The human race is not very fertile and it has been calculated that a woman who is not using contraception has on average only a twenty per cent chance of conception each cycle. If the egg is not fertilised it does not implant and fourteen days after ovulation the lining of the womb, together with some blood, is shed into the vagina and the whole process starts all over again. The shedding of the lining of the uterus is the period, or menstruation. Most women have a period once each month.

THE MENSTRUAL CYCLE

The menstrual cycle is a series of changes that occur at approximately monthly intervals during a woman's childbearing years. This involves cyclical changes in hormones which are preparing the uterus for pregnancy. When pregnancy does not occur, then the lining of the uterus is shed at menstruation. Cycle length (the start of one period to the start of the next) varies among individuals, but anything between twenty-one and thirty-five days is considered normal. Of course, an individual woman's cycle will vary from month to month by two or three days, but this is also normal. Cycle length is constant between the ages of twenty and thirty-five, then gradually becomes shorter.

At the extremes of reproductive life at the start of the periods (menarche) and prior to the cessation of the periods (menopause) the menstrual cycles are often not associated with egg production and may therefore be of irregular length.

The average menstrual blood loss is around 40 ml and the upper limit of normal is usually taken as around 80 ml per period. However, the amount of fluid is very variable. The uterus tends to contract during the menstrual period, especially during the first couple of days of loss, which may account for some of the discomfort felt by many women during this time.

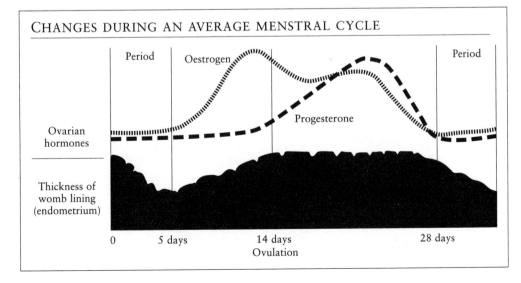

CHANGES DURING AN AVERAGE MENSTRAL CYCLE

Period   Oestrogen

Period

Ovarian hormones

Progesterone

Thickness of womb lining (endometrium)

0   5 days   14 days   28 days
Ovulation

Left: This graph shows the changes in the ovaries and uterine lining (endometrium) during the menstrual cycle. In an average cycle, days 1–5 are the period. The egg develops in the ovary with thickening of the lining of the womb during days 1–14. On day 14 ovulation occurs and the egg is released from the ovary. During days 14–27 the ovary produces hormones which prepare the womb to receive the pregnancy should it occur. If no pregnancy occurs, on days 27–28 the hormone level decreases and the womb lining is shed.

THE EARLY CYCLE
(FOLLICULAR PHASE)

At the beginning of each cycle, small follicles start to develop in the ovary around the eggs and they begin to swell. This occurs under the influence of a chemical messenger or 'hormone' produced by the pituitary gland situated at the base of the brain (follicle stimulating hormone). By around the sixth day, one follicle starts to dominate the others and grow more quickly, whilst the others start to shrink. This follicle produces the principal female hormone oestrogen, which has effects on many tissues within the body and is very important for women's health. One important action is on the lining of the womb which thickens under its influence. Levels of oestrogen in the blood increase up to the time of ovulation (about day fourteen) while the follicle continues to grow. At this point, again in response to a second pituitary hormone (luteinizing hormone), the follicle bursts (ovulation) and the egg is picked up by the fallopian tube which carries it along towards the uterus by the action of small hair-like cilia and muscular contractions. It is in the tube that fertilisation can occur if the egg comes into contact with sperm, the resultant pregnancy usually continuing its passage into the uterus where implantation occurs. However, occasionally, it implants in the tube itself, resulting in an ectopic pregnancy.

AFTER THE EGG'S RELEASE

Once the egg has been released from the ovary, the follicle fills first with blood, then yellow 'luteal' cells which form the corpus luteum. This produces the hormone progesterone which helps to support the pregnancy should implantation have occurred. It also causes changes in the lining of the womb (secretory change) making it ready for the arrival of the fertilised egg.

If the egg does not become fertilised it dies within the next forty-eight hours and the corpus luteum starts to degenerate. The oestrogen and progesterone levels fall and the lining of the womb degenerates, leading to the menstrual period. All but the deepest layers of the lining are shed. Oestrogen secretion from a new developing follicle then encourages it to regrow during the first fourteen days of the next cycle and the process is repeated.

If fertilisation occurs, the levels of oestrogen and progesterone continue to increase, the endometrium (lining of the womb) is not shed and menstruation fails to occur.

CERVICAL MUCUS

The mucus produced by the cervix also changes during the monthly cycle. At the time of ovulation, it becomes watery and stretchy. This change can be used as an indicator of ovulation, albeit a somewhat unreliable one. During the second half of the cycle, under the influence of progesterone, it becomes thicker and more viscous.

REPRODUCTIVE HORMONES

This shows how the brain, ovaries and womb influence each other. The brain influences the production of hormones from the pituitary gland which controls the production of steroid hormones from the ovaries. Oestrogen also affects other tissues, such as the breasts and bones.

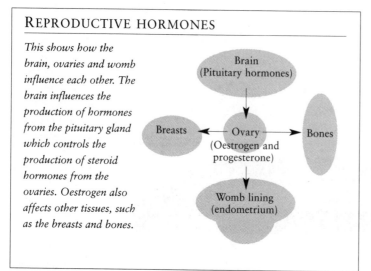

Brain
(Pituitary hormones)

Breasts ← Ovary → Bones
(Oestrogen and progesterone)

Womb lining
(endometrium)

PUBERTY

Puberty is the term used to describe the changes in body, mind and emotions that both girls and boys undergo between the ages of ten and eighteen. During puberty, the child is slowly transformed into a young adult.

The word puberty is derived from the Latin word *pubeltas*, which means adulthood. The main purpose of all the changes of puberty is to enable the individual to produce children and so perpetuate the human race. Girls are born with about one to two million eggs in their ovaries. In childhood, these minute eggs lie dormant. As puberty approaches, the brain starts to send hormones to the ovary via the bloodstream which trigger the development of a few of these eggs. The maturing eggs stimulate the production of other hormones which cause the bodily and psychological changes experienced in puberty.

NORMAL PUBERTY

There is a wide range of ages at which the normal changes of puberty begin and there is no exact order for the development to unfold. The six important bodily changes that occur at puberty are as follows:

- Development of breasts
- Growth of pubic hair
- Growth of underarm hair
- Development of external sex organs
- Increase in height
- Menstruation
- Change in body shape.

BREASTS
The breasts develop in stages. Nipples are the first things to grow, followed by the underlying breast. Breast buds begin any time from nine to fourteen years – usually at around the age of eleven. The full adult breast may take up to nine years to develop, but the average is four years. Breasts are sometimes tender and tingle as this process begins. One breast can be noticeably bigger than the other in ten to fifteen per cent of girls, but this inequality usually disappears by about the age of sixteen.

PUBIC HAIR
Pubic hairs often appear at about the time of the breast buds, but either may precede the other by up to a year. They gradually increase and, after about three years, have produced a fairly thick triangle of curly hair which extends from the junction of the lower groin with the inner thigh, downwards between the legs and covers the external sex organs and genitalia.

UNDERARM HAIR
A year or two after the growth of pubic hair, similar hairs appear in the underarm area. Thicker hairs may also appear on other parts of the body, such as the legs, lower arms, around the nipples and on the upper lip. The amount of this hair growth depends very much on hair colour and genetic make-up, being more obvious in dark-haired girls. Many women may wish to remove the hair from under the arms and on the legs. There is no satisfactory, simple way to do this: shaving, waxing or special hair-removing creams are the most popular treatments. As well as the pubic hair, sweat glands develop.

EXTERNAL SEX ORGANS (GENITALIA)
As puberty progresses, the vagina and vulva

become increasingly moist because of secretions through the vagina and from glands in the vulva and cervix (neck of the womb). These secretions provide a defence against infection and prepare the area for sexual activity.

HEIGHT, WEIGHT AND SHAPE

Children between the ages of four and puberty tend to grow in height at a fairly constant rate of about 5 cm (2 in) per year. Somewhere around the age of ten-and-a-half, girls suddenly begin to grow at 6–12 cm (2½–5 in) per year for about two years. This is called the growth spurt. Thereafter, growth rapidly falls off to only 1–2 cm (½–1 in) a year by the age of fifteen and, shortly after that, to almost nothing. During this time proportions change:
■ Hips widen to help future childbirth
■ Waists slim as fat moves from the tummy to the hips and thighs
■ Buttocks become more prominent
■ Legs lengthen in proportion to the rest of the body.

The growth spurt includes muscle development and, as boys have their growth spurt two years later, this is a time for girls to assert their supremacy! Early 'spurters' tend to worry that they will be too tall, but, in fact, their growth stops earlier, so late 'spurters' may have caught up by the age of sixteen. Faces also alter, with the nose and jaw becoming more prominent, and there is some deepening of the voice, although it is not as marked in girls as it is in boys.

MENARCHE

Starting to have periods is probably the most important event of puberty for girls. It is certainly the most identifiable landmark of puberty, and periods usually start anywhere between the ages of ten and sixteen years. The average age these days is thirteen years. The age of starting periods (menarche) depends to a small extent on race and genetics and, to a much larger extent, on body fat and nutrition. The menarche usually occurs about two-and-a-half years after the appearance of breast buds and pubic hair and as the growth spurt is slowing. The body weight is usually between 42 and 52 kg (92 and 114 lb) and roughly seventeen per cent of this weight is fat. Therefore, very thin girls, such as athletes, ballet dancers and malnourished girls, tend to have a much later menarche.

For the first one or two years after the menarche the periods are usually either pain free or associated with only mild discomfort. They may also be irregular due to immature control mechanisms for the hormone release that governs menstruation. After this initial period they will normally settle down to last between two to seven days with an average inter-menstrual interval of twenty-eight days as described above.
■ Many girls notice a watery vaginal discharge at the time of ovulation and this is entirely normal.
■ Menstrual blood, although clean, may develop an unpleasant smell. It can be absorbed completely by either sanitary towels or tampons. Towels usually have a sticky back to hold them firmly in place, lining the pants. Towels soak up the blood as it leaves the body. Tampons are inserted into the vagina and cannot be felt once correctly positioned. They have the advantage of allowing girls to go swimming and bathing during periods. Towels and tampons should be changed at least every six hours, since this decreases the likelihood of getting toxic shock syndrome. This is where bacteria in the soiled tampon

produce toxins which are absorbed into the body and lead to collapse. This is a very rare condition, which can be avoided by correct use of the tampon.

PSYCHOLOGY OF PUBERTY

In the four to five years of puberty, a child's mentality will become that of a woman. The two are very different and whilst each has its own attractions, the journey between the two is not always easy. Too much emphasis, however, can be placed on hormones. The characteristic difference in adult and child mentality is the appreciation of freedom and choice – small children positively relish being organised and herded, whereas adults need to feel that any decision to co-operate was freely made. This may lead to some of the difficulties with relationships which are discussed on page 18.

MENOPAUSE

The menopause constitutes a time of profound change in a woman's life. It signifies the end of childbearing since the ovaries become devoid of eggs and resistant to control by the pituitary hormones (FSH and LH). Oestrogen is mainly produced by the ovaries. Loss of ovarian function leads to a fall in production of oestrogen. As a result of this, the circulating level of oestrogen in the blood falls. The lining of the womb (endometrium) is no longer stimulated by ovarian hormones and does not thicken. This means that the periods ultimately stop. Lack of oestrogen may also be manifest as hot flushes, vaginal dryness and possibly, in some women, depression. The average age of the last period is fifty-one years, and this has not changed over the centuries (unlike the age of the first period which has slowly been dropping).

The time leading up the menopause when ovarian activity is erratic is known as the perimenopause, or climacteric. It may last as long as four years. As with the earlier periods after the menarche, ovulation is infrequent and therefore periods may be irregular and variable in flow. Since the term menopause is strictly the last period, it can only be made retrospectively after a year free of periods. Any bleeding after this time should be considered abnormal and reported to a medical practitioner.

An interest in women's health has developed over the last few years and this includes the problems of the menopause, which may cause distress in a significant minority of women. These concerns will be discussed in depth later in the book (see page 270).

Chapter two

COMMON CONCERNS AS THE BODY CHANGES

If the onset of puberty is delayed beyond the age of sixteen, particularly if other signs of puberty have failed to occur, then medical advice should be sought. If any secondary signs of puberty occur before the age of eight, or if the menarche occurs before the age of ten, this is generally regarded as early or precocious. It may just be one of those things and may not indicate anything serious, or it may be caused by some other disease that does require investigation and treatment. Therefore, if puberty is precocious, it is wise to seek medical advice.

SKIN PROBLEMS

The circulating hormones of puberty increase the production of grease from the sebaceous glands in the skin of the scalp, face and back. The skin and hair become oily and blackheads can appear which turn into spots if infected. Fortunately for them, girls are less infected in general than boys. Skin tends to be noticeably worse in the week or so before a period. Washing diligently twice a day with a mild antiseptic soap is usually all that is necessary. Cutting out chocolate and other fatty foods in the diet may help. However, severe spots or acne will need medical help and treatment to avoid permanent scarring.

PREMENSTRUAL SYNDROME (PMS)

This condition is fortunately rare in teenagers. The symptoms include mood changes, breast tenderness, bloating and lack of concentration in the two weeks before a period.

PERIOD PAINS

The first few periods are usually not especially painful, but by the time regular ovulation is established, periods are often accompanied by low, crampy pain. Simple painkillers from the chemist are usually effective. Further discussion of period pain (dysmenorrhoea) can be found on page 41.

BODY SHAPE

Body shape is determined principally by the type of body inherited, the amount of exercise taken and the type and quantity of food eaten. Magazines, television and films try to imprint on young minds the role model of an ideal figure. However, it should be remembered that, in reality, different people find different body types attractive and so there is no one type of body that is the most attractive. The body to aim for and to be proud of is the body that is natural – one that is neither overweight nor underweight.

Whilst it is important not to be over-weight, it is of even greater importance not to be severely underweight. Excessive dieting can lead to anorexia nervosa, which is a serious, life-threatening condition causing ill-health and unhappiness.

A healthy diet is one that is low in fat, high in fibre (roughage) and which contains at least five pieces of fruit or portion of fresh vegetables every day. Puberty is a time of rapid body growth and therefore plenty of healthy food is needed.

RELATIONSHIPS

■ **Parents and other adults:** During puberty, the developing feeling of independence and individuality creates potential conflict between the girl and her parents. The adolescent invariably rejects some of her parents' principles as she begins to think more deeply about the basis for them. Similarly, parents find it hard to stop giving well-intentioned advice which is often misinterpreted as interference by the adolescent. In order to get through this very difficult time with the minimum of upset, it helps for both parent and adolescent to respect each other, listen to each other's views and try to avoid angry, confrontational scenes. It is also useful for adolescents to remember that their friends are having similar experiences and moods and that all adults have been through puberty, too. As a girl develops confidence in herself and her own abilities, the moodiness settles. This is a sign that her body has become accustomed to being adult.

■ **Boys:** Along with puberty comes sexual awakening for girls. At first this takes the form of dreams and fantasies about the opposite sex – usually for unobtainable characters, such as film or pop stars. Later this becomes a desire to touch and be touched physically. Such touching does not have to lead to sex – not just because of the danger of pregnancy or catching AIDS or other infectious diseases (although these are very real risks indeed), but because sex provokes very strong emotions and establishes a deep psychological bond which, if broken, will cause pain and disturbance of emotions.

ANOREXIA NERVOSA

'You can never be too rich, or too thin.' Sadly, Wallis Simpson's words of wisdom were misguided. Anorexia nervosa has become one of the major illnesses of adolescence in the West, affecting an increasing number of people, mostly young women. The gynaecological implications of anorexia are stark.

■ Excessive weight loss is interpreted by the brain as starvation.

■ In response, the hypothalamus, situated at the base of the brain, ceases to secrete regular pulses of the hormone GnRH.

■ This, in turn, stops release of a follicle stimulating hormone (FSH) from the pituitary gland and, as a consequence, the ovaries stop producing eggs (see page 14).

■ Dangerous osteoporosis due to a prolonged lack of oestrogen then occurs.

This mechanism exists within the body to prevent a woman becoming pregnant in adverse

19

STAYING HEALTHY DURING PUBERTY

SMOKING

Both smoking and alcohol are addictive and can cause health and social problems. A third of all cancers are thought to be directly related to smoking, which also causes bronchitis, heart attacks and strokes. Very few adults take up smoking, but persuading teenagers that it is more mature not to smoke can be difficult.

ALCOHOL

Small doses of alcohol make people feel relaxed and confident. However, larger doses affect judgement and often make the drinker sick, dizzy and do all sorts of things that they wished they had not! Alcohol is invariably served at most social occasions, so the most important thing is for young adults to learn how to drink sensibly. Either diluting alcoholic drinks or alternating an alcoholic with a non-alcoholic drink may prevent any serious regret in the morning.

PERSONAL HYGIENE

The glands that develop under the arms and in the pubic area produce sweat and other secretions which, when stale, develop an unpleasant smell. It is therefore important to wash these areas as frequently as necessary, normally daily. An underarm antiperspirant will reduce sweating which, as well as smelling offensive to most people, can stain and ruin clothes.

EXERCISE

Regular exercise is essential for good health. Not only does it avoid the build-up of fat, but it improves the circulation of the blood, promotes sound sleeping and produces a sense of well-being.

times – pregnancy during extreme starvation would result in harm to the growing baby and also to the mother. The ovaries therefore 'shut down' until food supplies improve.

REASONS FOR ANOREXIA

Although this strategy made sense thousands of years ago, the modern anorectic form of starvation has nothing to do with lack of food. Anorexia nervosa results from an altered perception of self, a sense of appearing obese and unattractive despite extreme thinness. It can also be a consequence of a desire to remain a 'little girl' in those girls who have not yet gone through puberty. As weight continues to be lost, a self-reinforcing spiral of increasing lethargy, disconnection with reality and further weight loss emerges. Leptin levels fall and the woman's reproductive cycle ceases. Menstrual periods become erratic, then stop altogether. As ovulation shuts down, the amount of oestrogen hormone in the body falls to levels usually seen only after the menopause.

The anorectic patient develops a coat of fine 'peach-fluff' lanugo hair. Her nails become brittle and her hair thins and is lost. Internally, the uterus and ovaries shrink to pre-pubertal size. Most significantly, the loss of oestrogen hormone leads to the onset of osteoporosis, the loss of bone from the skeleton. In young women, this can also result in permanent stunting in growth. These effects are made worse by cigarette smoking, a habit that many anorectic women find hard to break.

WEIGHT DISORDERS AND STRESS

Anorexia nervosa is not uncommon and has a mortality of over five per cent. It represents one end of a spectrum of disorders involving permanent dieting, obsession with weight, bulimia (vomiting) and abuse of laxatives. Many will come close to true anorexia in times of stress, but will recover when their quality of life improves. Indeed, many young women suffering from anorexia have retreated into their disease as a means of escaping from intolerable stresses, often resulting from their personal relationships or in their home situation.

EXCESSIVE EXERCISE

In the 1960s and 1970s, enhancing physical attractiveness by losing weight was achieved almost entirely by dieting. More recently, physical fitness has been seen as an important goal in life, not only for health benefit, but also to improve appearance. Ironically, excessive exercise, with loss of body fat and conversion to a more muscular physique, can also have an adverse effect on women's health. Athlete's amenorrhoea – a total lack of periods in otherwise fit young women – is frequently seen among marathon runners, and devotees of other high-energy sports. The phenomenon also appears in ballet dancers, who combine high physical fitness levels with constant attention to body weight, bringing together the two main causes of anorectic damage to health.

CONSEQUENCES OF ANOREXIA

Prolonged lack of oestrogen will result in permanent damage to the skeleton, problems with growth and increased risk of fracture after relatively minor injury. While the anorexia continues, the woman will be infertile, as she is not producing eggs. Sadly, some women will not resume ovulation even after they recover and gain weight, and will still need drug treatment if they wish to conceive.

OTHER CAUSES OF WEIGHT LOSS

Many women want to be thinner than they are, and yet are not anorectic. Irregular or absent periods are an unmistakable warning sign from the body that the quest for perfection has become excessive. Conversely, regular periods are a sign of good health and well-being. If excessive exercise or weight loss cannot be avoided, then it is sensible to protect the skeleton by replacing the lost oestrogen hormone with oestrogen-containing drugs, such as the contraceptive pill or hormone replacement tablets or patches. This will avoid the worst of the long-term effects of bone loss, and should be used by amenorrhoeic athletes even though they see themselves as very fit people. However, the best solution to this self-induced health problem is to reverse the weight loss or reduce the level of exercising until periods return.

Chapter three

COMMON GYNAECOLOGICAL PROBLEMS

Attitudes towards women and their role in society have changed greatly during the twentieth century. This has, however, been a slow process, but at last, problems of a gynaecological nature can be discussed openly without the furtive glances and embarrassed nudges that formerly would have accompanied such topics. These attitudes caused great harm to women who would often be reluctant to discuss their concerns and relied on rumour, old-wives' tales and misinformation in place of education and informed advice.

Even in the new millennium, it is sad that so many women still understand little about their bodies and find it difficult to seek advice about gynaecological problems. Thus, the discussion of these problems, which is now found regularly in magazines and newspapers, is to be welcomed. The fact that an advertisement for a sanitary towel on the television can still provoke outrage in a small-minded minority shows that there is still some way to go.

The term 'gynaecological problems' encompasses a wide variety of complaints, some common examples of which will be discussed in this book. What is certain is that there will be almost no woman who will live her life without being troubled by a gynaecological problem at some time or another.

The effects of what may appear to be relatively minor problems have often been underestimated since, in addition to any physical discomfort or pain, there is often considerable psychological concern. Anxiety regarding the possibility of, for example, cancer, infertility or sexually transmitted diseases may often lurk deep in the minds of women with benign, self-limiting conditions. In such circumstances, reassurance and advice may be of much greater benefit than any treatment that is prescribed.

Indeed, the provision of a welcoming and relaxed environment in which time constraints are not a constant pressure during a consultation is very important in providing a situation where women can talk about their problems and receive appropriate and high-quality advice. The development of the 'Well Woman' clinics and independent organisations, such as the Brook Advisory Centres, are examples of attempts to provide such an environment.

In addition, the growth of self-help groups encourages women to discuss their concerns with others who directly understand their predicament. The word 'problem' is used here to describe an issue that causes worry to a woman or leads to inconvenience. Frequently, problems do not result from serious disease as such, and what is a 'problem' to one woman may not be of significance to another. However, the problems described in this chapter are common reasons why women go to their family doctors or gynaecologists asking for help.

HORMONAL IMBALANCE

MENSTRUAL DISTURBANCE

Most women experience periods during the 'reproductive years'. For a majority of women these are a fact of life which must be accepted even if there is some mild discomfort or premenstrual irritability. Periods may have some nuisance value but do not interfere with the quality of life. However, one of the most common gynaecological problems is that of menstrual disturbance. Periods may be:
- Too heavy (menorrhagia)
- Too long or frequent (polymenorrhoea)
- Too infrequent (oligomenorrhoea)
- Or they may be accompanied by pain (dysmenorrhoea).

All these problems will now be considered in some depth. Up until recently, women were expected to put up with their menstrual problems as part of their lot in life. However, things are changing. Since women now have fewer children and often only breastfeed for a short time, if at all, they have many more periods than their Victorian counterparts. Also, those involved in exacting jobs are not able to be incapacitated on a regular basis and so many doctors have become much more interested in solving menstrual problems.

INFREQUENT PERIODS

Periods often occur infrequently at the beginning and at the end of a woman's reproductive life, but this is quite normal. Many girls have infrequent periods for the first two or three years. Even though puberty has started, the ovaries take some time to mature and adolescent girls may have spells of infrequent and/or irregular periods. This is nothing to worry about unless they are

particularly heavy, and there is nothing wrong with a girl who takes a few years to establish a regular cycle.

Periods may also become infrequent after giving birth. It may be three or four months before a woman starts to have regular periods again and if she chooses to breastfeed her baby it may be even longer than that, depending on how often the baby suckles.

INFREQUENT PERIODS WHICH MAY BE ABNORMAL

Irregularity of the menstrual cycle may also occur at the time of the approaching menopause. However, should it occur earlier and the periods come less often than once every five weeks then it may mean there is some abnormality. It should also be emphasised that the menstrual cycle may be affected by environmental factors, such as stress, and so most women will experience irregularity from time to time. In addition, some women never develop a regular cycle, since the monthly development of the egg followed by the shedding of the lining of the womb which leads to a menstrual cycle does not occur, and the irregularity is a consequence of irregular egg production. This may be associated with the polycystic ovarian syndrome (see page 49).

Since the control of the menstrual cycle involves a complex series of events, even a minor hormone imbalance can cause infrequent periods or can switch them off altogether. The control of regular ovulation and periods is a particularly sensitive bodily function, and it is quite possible that this is an environmental safeguard to ensure that women do not become pregnant unless they are in good health.

THE BALANCE OF HORMONES

Many events can upset the balance of hormones. Conditions that are known to affect the reproductive cycle and result in infrequent periods include the following:

■ **Stress:** The reproductive system is very sensitive to stress and you may find that your periods become infrequent if life is particularly difficult – while working for exams, for example, or while caring for a sick or dying relative. When life settles down again, your periods usually return to normal.

■ **Weight change:** The loss or gain of more than half a stone in weight may affect the regularity of your periods and you may take some time to get back to normal even after you have regained your ideal body weight.

■ **Diet:** For reasons that we do not understand, making a major dietary change such as becoming a vegetarian is sometimes associated with the cessation of periods. Provided the diet is a balanced one this usually resolves and returns to regular periods.

■ **Exercise:** Taking regular strenuous exercise can affect regular menstruation, and many female athletes have irregular periods.

■ **Chronic ill health:** Women who already suffer from chronic diseases, such as Crohn's disease, and especially those who have hormonal problems, such as diabetes or thyroid disease, may have infrequent or absent periods often improved by effective treatment.

■ **Drugs:** Some drugs can interfere with regular menstruation – for example, anti-depressants. This may be by effects on hormones in some cases.

■ **Contraceptives:** Some contraceptives, particularly the progestogen-only or mini-pill and the injection (Depo-provera), may cause infrequent or absent periods.

SPECIFIC DISORDERS OF OVULATION

Some women have infrequent periods because of a specific imbalance of reproductive hormones which is not associated with stress, weight loss or any of the other conditions listed above.

1 Polycystic ovary syndrome (PCOS)

Some women are unable to develop eggs in a synchronised manner each month because of a hormonal imbalance. An ultrasound picture of the ovary often shows a number of small, immature follicles developing at different rates and it may be difficult for the ovary to develop any single egg to the point where it is mature enough to ovulate. These follicles or 'cysts' are numerous and form a ring around the ovary which appears 'polycystic'. The irregular growth of eggs in women with PCOS results in irregular and usually infrequent periods. Some women with PCOS may tend to be overweight and troubled with acne and hirsutism (excess hair growth, see page 51). This is due to an abnormal balance of the hormones produced by the ovaries. For more information, see page 49.

2 Hyperprolactinaemia

Prolactin is a hormone produced by the pituitary gland to stimulate milk production after childbirth (postpartum). Since, in evolutionary terms, pregnancy would not be appropriate while an infant is breastfed, high levels switch off ovarian function. Some women produce high levels at other times which lead to infrequent or absent periods, possibly associated with milk production from the breast. Some of these women may have a small benign tumour in the pituitary gland which is causing the over-production of the hormone.

3 Premature menopause

Although the average age for women reaching

the menopause in Britain is fifty-one, some women (about one per cent) can develop a premature menopause. It is possible for this to happen as early as twenty years of age, but this is most unusual.

WHEN TO SEE YOUR DOCTOR

Infrequent periods during adolescence or approaching the menopause are normal and are nothing to worry about. If your periods are infrequent but not causing any inconvenience and you are either an adolescent or in your forties, then reassurance can be given that there is nothing wrong and there is no need for you to see your doctor.

■ **Heavy periods:** If, as occasionally happens during adolescence and around the menopause, the period when it does come is particularly heavy and troublesome, then it may be advisable to consult your doctor.

■ **Change in menstrual rhythm:** If periods become infrequent, stop altogether or if regular periods have never been established, then consultation with your doctor may be worthwhile. However, one of the first signs of pregnancy is an absence of periods, so if pregnancy is a possibility it is important to have a pregnancy test. It will be helpful to the doctor if you keep a record of your menstrual cycle so that any pattern may be obvious.

■ **Women wanting a family:** If you are trying to start a family and have irregular or absent periods, it is important to seek medical advice, as there may be difficulty getting pregnant compared with women who have periods once each month.

■ **Women requiring contraception:** If you do not wish to have a baby, it is important not to rely on the absence of periods, because the system could correct itself at any time. Therefore an appropriate method of contraception, which is most suited to you as an individual, should be used. If you have any anxiety, visit your family doctor.

WHAT WILL YOUR DOCTOR DO?

After asking some questions, performing an examination and possibly taking some blood or urine for tests, it may be possible for your doctor to reassure you that there is nothing fundamentally wrong and that your periods will normalise given time. Some women, particularly those who are trying to get pregnant, may need further investigations and treatment. Their family doctor may make a referral to a specialist who will undertake some more investigations in order to determine if treatment is required.

DON'T WORRY

Absence of periods does not mean that large amounts of blood are being 'stored up' in the body. When the cycle is not functioning properly it often means that the lining of the uterus does not thicken during the month and there is little tissue to be shed during the period except under particular circumstances as described below.

HEAVY PERIODS (MENORRHAGIA)

Menorrhagia is the term that doctors use for periods that are heavier and often more frequent than what is acceptable to a woman. Most girls nowadays start menstruating between eleven and thirteen years of age and their periods may take a little while to settle into a regular pattern, which should continue through their reproductive lives. Although most women have few problems, a number will find that they need to consult their doctor because their periods are unacceptably heavy. The average period lasts for three to five days and will occur approximately every twenty-eight days as described on page 13.

THE MENSTRUAL CYCLE

The way in which this works has already been explained (see page 00). We know that the remarkably complex hormone system takes time to settle down at puberty and some girls may have rather heavy periods then; similarly, it may become rather unreliable prior to the menopause (change of life). If anything happens to disturb the activity of the glands in a woman's body, or indeed the womb itself, then her periods may become heavier than normal. In some cases, the causes of heavy periods is never established.

COMMON CAUSES OF TOO MUCH MENSTRUAL BLEEDING

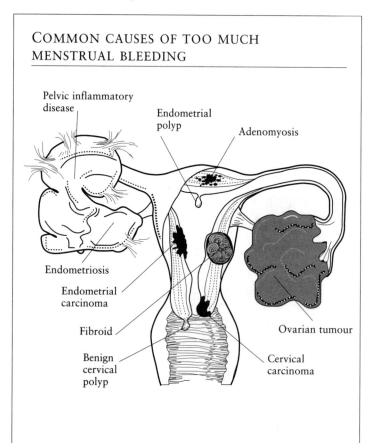

Pelvic inflammatory disease

Endometrial polyp

Adenomyosis

Endometriosis

Endometrial carcinoma

Fibroid

Benign cervical polyp

Ovarian tumour

Cervical carcinoma

HOW MANY WOMEN GET HEAVY PERIODS?

Approximately five to ten per cent of women in general get prolonged or heavy periods or both. This is one of the commonest complaints for which women are seen in their doctors' surgeries or in hospital gynaecological clinics each year.

SEEKING HELP

Any persistent change in the pattern of periods should be discussed with a doctor. The periods may be heavier or longer than normal, resulting in an increased amount of sanitary protection required. There may be some pain with the bleeding and frequently clots of blood are passed rather than the usual menstrual flow. This may get to the stage where clothes are soiled which restricts usual activities during a period.

When the periods are heavy, more blood than normal will be lost and this may result in anaemia which, in turn, may increase the feeling of tiredness or can even lead to fainting episodes.

Not uncommonly, women find that their periods become heavier after they have been sterilised. The main reason for this is that many women choose to have this operation in their mid-thirties because they have decided to stop taking the contraceptive pill. The pill, in fact, makes the 'periods' very light by inhibiting ovulation so when the sterilisation is carried out and the woman stops the pill, the periods seem to be much heavier. However, in reality they are as they would have been had she never been on the pill. Periods do tend to get heavier anyway with the passage of years and with having a family.

WHAT WILL YOUR DOCTOR DO?

Your doctor will ask about any other change

in the pattern of your periods, which may be significant, such as bleeding between periods or after intercourse. You will also be asked about other illnesses, about the possibility of pregnancy (because some heavy periods may in fact be a miscarriage), and about contraception. For instance, the intrauterine device may lead to heavy periods in some women.

Your doctor may carry out an examination of your abdomen and also a vaginal examination to see if the womb is enlarged or is involved in any other associated disease. This may be an opportunity for a cervical smear, if one is due.

Finally, your doctor may take a blood sample and send it off to check the level of haemoglobin to see if you are anaemic. Many women will benefit from taking a course of iron tablets, but there is clearly a

significant problem if this has to be repeated or prolonged treatment is required.

Your doctor may give you a tablet to help make the periods lighter immediately, or may decide to seek advice from a gynaecologist at a hospital out-patient clinic.

At the hospital it is likely that many of the same questions will be asked again and a vaginal examination will usually be done. Further tests may also be arranged, including the following, although not all women require these tests.

■ **Endometrial biopsy** (a scraping of the lining of the womb) will exclude abnormalities of the endometrium. This may be carried out at the out-patient department without the need for anaesthetic.

■ **Ultrasound examinations** are a painless way of looking at the womb as well as the

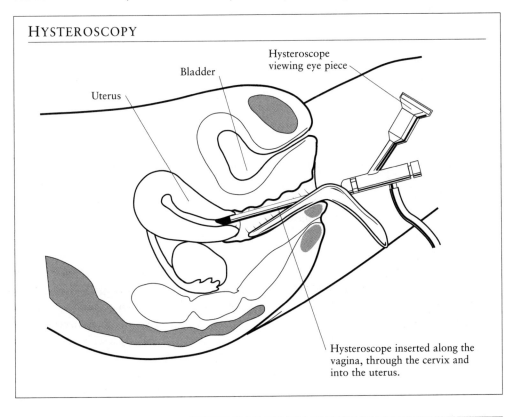

HYSTEROSCOPY

Bladder

Hysteroscope viewing eye piece

Uterus

Hysteroscope inserted along the vagina, through the cervix and into the uterus.

ovaries, rather like an X-ray but with no risks at all. They might show a fibroid or an ovarian cyst (see pages 28 and 62).

■ **Telescopic examination (hysteroscopy)** of the womb has been introduced in recent years to get accurate information from within the womb. Sometimes the cause of the problem, namely a polyp or fibroid, can be seen, and biopsies (samples) can be taken from the exact areas of abnormality.

WHY DO YOUR PERIODS GET HEAVIER?
There are many reasons for heavy periods including the following:
■ Alteration of the hormone balance
■ Benign diseases (not cancerous) of the uterus (womb)
■ Cancer – a rare cause
■ Dysfunctional uterine bleeding.

1 Alteration of the hormone balance
This is a common cause of heavy periods. It may be temporary, owing to excessive stress, anxiety or grief, in which case the periods are likely to settle in a short period of time. For example, it is not uncommon for teenage girls to experience heavy periods, generally due to immature glands (both pituitary and ovary) causing irregular and unreliable ovulation.

Hormone balance can also be affected by some benign (innocent) problems of the ovary, thyroid or adrenal glands.

2 Benign diseases of the uterus
These include polyps, fibroids, endometriosis, long-standing pelvic infection and the intrauterine coil.
■ **Polyps** may form in the lining of the womb and can be removed easily.
■ **Fibroids** are benign or innocent lumps which occur in twenty per cent of women, but cause

problems only in a smaller number. These are discussed in more detail later in this chapter.
■ **Endometriosis** may occur when the lining of the womb (endometrium) may lie outside it within the pelvis. These bits of tissue also bleed when a woman has her period. It may increase blood flow and alter hormone balance, thereby affecting the periods, and may also cause pain (see page 58).
■ **Long-standing pelvic infection** affects periods in the same way as endometriosis. Thorough treatment of pelvic infections initially is essential to get a reasonable cure. Otherwise it becomes difficult to eradicate infection.
■ **Intrauterine devices** may affect the internal environment of the womb and thereby the heaviness of the periods. In the majority of cases, the womb adjusts itself to the presence of the coil and the periods get back to normal.

3 Cancer of the lining of the endometrium
This is very rare in women before the menopause but is very occasionally seen in younger women with irregular or heavy bleeding. If detected early, a complete cure can be expected.

4 Dysfunctional uterine bleeding
In a majority of women with heavy periods, there are no abnormalities demonstrated, either in the structure of the womb or in the production of hormones. It is likely that the problem lies within the womb itself where abnormal amounts of chemicals which control blood loss are produced. This is known as dysfunctional uterine bleeding (DUB), a term often used by gynaecologists.

FIBROIDS

These are benign smooth muscle tumours

arising from the uterine wall, also known as leiomyomas or fibroleiomyomas. They are the most common tumour found in the uterus, genital tract or, indeed, the human body and it has been estimated that twenty per cent of women will develop them at some stage.

Their cause is uncertain but there is a strong genetic or racial predisposition. Women of Afro-Caribbean descent are much more likely to develop fibroids. They require the presence of the hormone oestrogen and therefore tend to shrink after the menopause.

APPEARANCE AND STRUCTURE

Fibroids appear as firm, round, pale tumours which vary greatly in size, from pea-sized nodules to large masses filling the abdomen. Most are situated wholly or partially within the wall of the uterus. Some project into the uterine cavity or from the outer, peritoneal surface of the uterus. When this occurs, fibroids may develop a stalk or pedicle and are described as pedunculated or polypoid. Occasionally a fibroid may develop from muscular fibres present in the cervix.

SYMPTOMS

In many cases, fibroids will cause no symptoms and exist undetected. Associated symptoms frequently include menstrual problems and pelvic pain. In the case of large fibroids, abdominal swelling or pressure effects are noticed. It has been suggested that fibroids may cause either infertility or recurrent miscarriage although the evidence for this is not strong in most instances. When pregnancy does occur, fibroids occasionally undergo degeneration which is associated with severe pain. This complication can be managed with strong painkillers and is unlikely to threaten the pregnancy. Rarely, a large cervical fibroid can cause obstruction of labour.

A common association in a woman's later reproductive life is heavy and/or painful periods, particularly when the fibroids are situated in the endometrial cavity.

DIAGNOSIS AND INVESTIGATION

If a fibroid is suspected, investigations should aim to exclude the possibility of other pelvic masses or causes of the symptoms present.

FIBROIDS

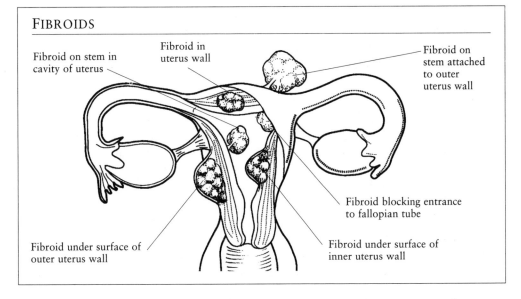

Fibroid on stem in cavity of uterus

Fibroid in uterus wall

Fibroid on stem attached to outer uterus wall

Fibroid blocking entrance to fallopian tube

Fibroid under surface of outer uterus wall

Fibroid under surface of inner uterus wall

Left: The illustration shows fibroids in the cavity of the uterus which often produce symptoms, and also in the wall which commonly do not produce many problems, depending on their size.

> DRUGS USED IN THE
> TREATMENT OF MENSTRUAL
> PROBLEMS
>
> ■ Non-steroidal anti-inflammatory
> agents
> ■ Anti-fibrinolytic agents
> ■ Oral contraceptive pill
> ■ Progestogens
> – oral – depot injection – intrauterine

Many women will be concerned that they have a cancer but whilst a fibroid occasionally turns into cancer, this is a very rare event. Most of these rare cancers are diagnosed as a chance finding at histological (laboratory) examination of a hysterectomy specimen.

TREATMENT

This will be determined by the symptoms experienced and will be influenced by the age, reproductive intentions and wishes of an individual woman. Sometimes reassurance and observation are all that is required. Medical treatments may include drugs used to combat symptoms, while there are others that attempt to prevent further growth or even cause shrinkage of a fibroid. Surgical treatments commonly involve total hysterectomy, although in some circumstances removal of one or more fibroids (myomectomy) with preservation of the uterus is possible. Newer techniques to remove or destroy fibroids employing 'keyhole' surgery techniques or by cutting off their blood supply (embolisation) are currently being developed.

MAKING PERIODS LIGHTER

The method chosen will depend upon age,

desire to have further children, effect on normal life and, of course, the cause of the problem. However, not all women need anything since, once reassured that there is no sinister cause for the change in their periods, they are able to cope.

DRUG THERAPY

Drug therapy may be the first line of help and may offer reasonable relief. The advantages of drugs are that they are taken generally during the periods on a regular basis and have few side effects. Some of the preparations are used as painkillers, e.g. ibuprofen, but they work against some of the local hormones produced in the womb which cause heavy and painful periods.

There are other drugs available that affect the bleeding mechanism in general and thus are effective in reducing the amount of bleeding – these are taken daily during the period. Iron tablets may also be required to improve anaemia due to blood loss.

The former group is known as the non-steroidal anti-inflammatory agents (NSAIDs). These tablets are often taken for conditions such as arthritis, but studies have shown that when taken during the period they are very successful in relieving period pain in a majority of women and decreasing bleeding in about forty per cent of women. Although this may not seem a very high proportion, the tablets can be extremely successful and since they are very safe when administered only during the period they are often worth a trial as a first line of therapy.

The second group of drugs affect the way the blood clots and are known as anti-fibrinolytic agents. These have been shown to be effective in about sixty per cent of women and, again, serious side effects are very unusual. They are not widely used in the UK but large trials have been carried out in Scandinavian countries where they are the first therapy that women are given when they visit their doctor complaining of heavy menstrual bleeding. However, they do not seem to be as successful in treating period-associated pain as the NSAIDs.

HORMONAL PREPARATIONS

There are many ways of giving hormonal preparations which must be taken for at least two weeks each month to be at all effective. Many women in the UK are given hormonal treatment (a progestogen) to take for two weeks each month. This is effective in regulating the periods but does not decrease the amount of blood that is actually lost. If the same tablet is given for three weeks each month when it alters the way the ovaries function, then it is likely that the blood lost during the period will be decreased.

An alternative to taking a progestogen is the oral contraceptive pill, which is extremely effective in treating menstrual problems. However, many women complaining of these problems have already been sterilised and do not wish to return to taking this particular preparation.

New methods of administering progestogens have been developed. One that is proving to be very useful for many women is the levonorgestrel secreting intrauterine system (Mirena). This is inserted into the womb like a contraceptive coil and it produces a very small amount of hormone each day. It is a very successful method of decreasing menstrual blood loss although the chance of having irregular bleeding for many months is very high. It appears that this device is also good for treating period pain and it is an excellent contraceptive which makes it a valuable alternative for many women. Some women have hormonal side effects (sore breasts, bloating and irritability). However, it is likely that these side effects will improve with time.

OPERATIVE TREATMENT

Operative treatment no longer means only hysterectomy since new alternatives have been developed as will be described. In many cases operative treatment is used after medical treatment has failed, although in certain instances it may be appropriate to carry out a surgical procedure immediately. One example of this would be when the menstrual problems are associated with other problems in the womb, such as fibroids, since medical treatments are less likely to be effective. The following section will describe hysterectomy and the newer technique of endometrial ablation in some detail.

ENDOMETRIAL ABLATION FOR
HEAVY PERIODS

Endometrial ablation is an operation to remove the lining of the uterus or womb. The main reason for the operation is to deal with the discomfort and the inconvenience of heavy periods. It means the problem can be treated without resorting to a hysterectomy, which is the removal of the uterus and perhaps the ovaries.

Below: The border between the endometrium and the myometrium is not smooth and some myometrium must be removed or destroyed.

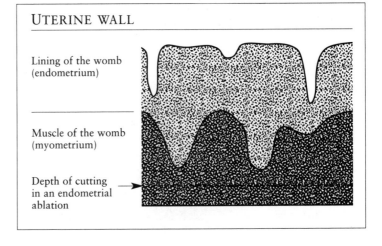

UTERINE WALL

Lining of the womb (endometrium)

Muscle of the womb (myometrium)

Depth of cutting in an endometrial ablation

Endometrial ablation takes away the lining of the uterus completely, or virtually completely, and a new lining doesn't form in its place, so periods are either reduced or stopped entirely. This effect in many cases is permanent, or at least lasts for many years because the layer of the lining of the womb which regenerates every month is actually removed or destroyed. This means that a new endometrium does not grow each month.

WHICH METHODS ARE USED?

There are a number of different techniques most widely used in the UK:

■ **Transcervical resection** of the endometrium (TCRE), which is sometimes used with a technique known as rollerball ablation
■ **Hysteroscopic endometrial ablation** by laser (HEAL)
■ **Microwave coagulation** uses microwaves to destroy the endometrium
■ **Thermal balloons.**
Note: Other methods are also being developed.

One technique might be more suitable for some women than for others. Also, some surgeons are more experienced in one technique than another. The gynaecologist will discuss with you which method he/she is using, and why this is preferred.

ENDOMETRIAL RESECTION

The lining of the womb is cut away along with some underlying muscle so there are no lining (endometrial) cells remaining to regrow. Alternatively, the tissue can be destroyed using laser, heat or microwaves.

Cutting loop

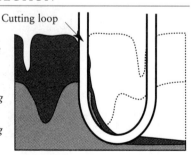

WHAT ARE THE DIFFERENCES?

■ **TCRE**, or transcervical resection of the endometrium, is the most common method and is used in most parts of the UK. It uses a hysteroscope, a special telescope that looks inside the uterus. It is placed in the uterus through the vagina and the cervix (the neck of the uterus). Then another instrument is inserted, called a resectoscope. It has a small wire loop on the end, connected to a high frequency electrical energy source. When the loop is activated, the surgeon can cut away the endometrium in strips. At the same time it seals off the inside wall of the uterus, and prevents too much bleeding.

■ **Rollerball ablation** uses a small rotating metal ball or bar at the end of the resectoscope, rather than a loop. The surgeon rolls it over the whole inner surface of the uterus, rather like using a paint roller. The heat applied to the surface burns the endometrium. The tissue doesn't actually come away, so there's nothing to send off for laboratory analysis. This might be a disadvantage compared with the loop, if the surgeon needs to rule out any abnormality – but this can be overcome by taking a sample of tissue before the ablation. The rollerball is probably safer than the loop because it doesn't actually involve cutting, so there is less likelihood of accidentally perforating the uterus. The choice between the loop and the rollerball depends on what your surgeon feels he/she is most used to working with.

■ **Hysteroscopic endometrial ablation** by laser (HEAL) is the longest established technique. It uses laser energy, which causes destruction of the tissue by burning. As before, the surgeon introduces a hysteroscope into the vagina to allow a clear view of the inside of the uterus. Then, a fibre optic cable on the end of the hysteroscope delivers the laser beam, which vaporises the endometrium.

METHODS OF ENDOMETRIAL ABLATION

Different methods of removing the endometrium to reduce bleeding.

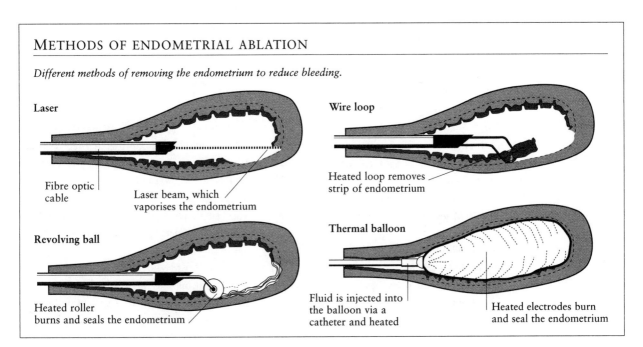

Laser

Fibre optic cable

Laser beam, which vaporises the endometrium

Revolving ball

Heated roller burns and seals the endometrium

Wire loop

Heated loop removes strip of endometrium

Thermal balloon

Fluid is injected into the balloon via a catheter and heated

Heated electrodes burn and seal the endometrium

OTHER TECHNIQUES

■ **Microwaves** can be applied to the endometrium after inserting a small probe into the uterus through the vagina, using microwave energy. This destroys the endometrium very effectively. This technique is not widely used in the UK, but has gained popularity in many other countries in Europe and further afield in the world. It is particularly useful for patients where there is a worry about excessive fluid being absorbed into the bloodstream which can happen with other forms of endometrial ablation. Usually, this isn't a problem, but some women with heart disease or kidney disease are not suitable for other methods of endometrial ablation, and may be more suitable for microwave ablation. It can also be carried out under local anaesthetic.

■ **Thermal balloons** are placed in the uterus via the cervix, inflated, and electrodes activated which coagulate the endometrium. These methods are particularly successful in those with a normal-sized uterus.

ARE THERE ANY COMPLICATIONS?

Very occasionally, in the techniques using a hysteroscope, the body can be overloaded with the fluid solution used to distend the uterine cavity and to flush out the uterus during the operation. If too much is absorbed into the bloodstream, it can lead to problems arising from fluid in the lungs and the heart. These need urgent treatment. Microwave and thermal balloons do not use any flushing fluid and therefore avoid this problem, but other risks are present with these techniques. Accidental heating of the tissue between the uterus and the bladder can cause small burns in the bladder, which can be a problem if the instrument is not placed correctly in the uterine cavity.

There is also a very small risk of accidental penetration of the uterine wall, leading to damage to the bladder and blood vessels and internal bleeding.

These problems are rare and if they do arise, they can be dealt with on the spot, even if this means that the abdomen has to be opened and an operation performed.

WHAT ANAESTHETIC IS USED?

Usually, these procedures are performed under a general anaesthetic, regardless of which method of endometrial ablation is used. However, it is perfectly possible to have any method with just a local anaesthetic, or a regional anaesthetic, such as an epidural. This can be discussed with the surgeon and anaesthetist before the operation is performed.

IS ABLATION ALWAYS A CURE?

On average, seventy-five per cent of women who have one of these operations are cured. About one-third don't experience any periods afterwards. This proportion rises with increasing age.

Research shows that some women start to have problems again after a while, and they need further treatment. One option is for the endometrial ablation to be repeated, and another is to have a hysterectomy which removes the uterus. It is important to realise that a hysterectomy, although a bigger operation with a longer recovery period, does guarantee the end of periods.

WHAT ABOUT CONTRACEPTION AFTERWARDS?

Endometrial ablation is an option only for women who have completed their families. In most cases, it results in sterilisation, which means that conception will no longer be possible. However, since there is still a very small chance of pregnancy it may be worth considering being sterilised at the same time.

For those who are not sterilised, other contraception will be required because pregnancy is associated with a very poor outcome and miscarriage is likely. This happens because the walls of the uterus can't stretch properly after ablation, because they are scarred.

HORMONE REPLACEMENT THERAPY?

You will not need, necessarily, to take HRT after having endometrial ablation. As long as your hormones are normal, and you haven't reached the age of menopause, then, of course, your hormones will be unaffected and it will not be necessary.

When HRT is prescribed, it will be a combined preparation – one containing oestrogen and progestogen. This is because it is possible that some of the endometrium cells are still left behind after ablation even in the absence of periods.

An oestrogen-only preparation may increase the chances of getting a cancer which begins in the endometrium so those cells that may remain could turn malignant under the effect of oestrogen-only HRT. Giving progestogen as well as oestrogen prevents this happening.

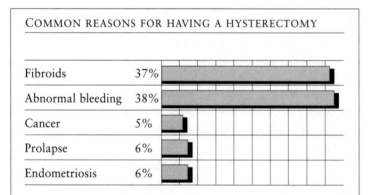

COMMON REASONS FOR HAVING A HYSTERECTOMY

Fibroids	37%	
Abnormal bleeding	38%	
Cancer	5%	
Prolapse	6%	
Endometriosis	6%	

Above are the common reasons for having a hysterectomy. It is likely that there is some overlap between 'fibroids' and 'abnormal bleeding'. Note how rare cancer is compared to other problems.

RECOVERY TIME AND SEX LIFE
Most women will only need two or three days off normal duties or work to recover after this operation. Endometrial ablation has no effect whatsoever on a women's sexual activity or on libido (sex drive) or on orgasm. Some months may be needed before the periods decrease in volume.

HYSTERECTOMY

Hysterectomy is the removal of the uterus (womb), and, in most cases, the cervix (neck of the uterus). In the UK, about 75,000 hysterectomies are done each year, making it one of the most common operations. There are many reasons why a hysterectomy might be performed and these include the following:
■ Cancer
■ Endometriosis
■ Fibroids
■ Heavy menstrual bleeding
■ Severe premenstrual syndrome and/or period problems.

WHY A HYSTERECTOMY?

In a few cases, a hysterectomy is a life-saving measure. The reasons for this would include cancer, or a massive haemorrhage (bleeding) from the uterus. Most of the time, though, a hysterectomy is done to relieve heavy, painful or irregular periods, or if there are large fibroids present. Because a hysterectomy means there will be no more periods and no more children, it is a particularly major step for women to take.

1 Heavy menstrual bleeding
This is one of the most common reasons for a hysterectomy. Extremely heavy, possibly painful, long-lasting periods can be a very distressing and disabling condition. They can happen even though there is nothing wrong with the uterus itself. As described previously, menorrhagia may also be associated with uterine fibroids or endometriosis.

2 Prolapse
Sometimes the muscles and ligaments supporting the uterus have become so weak that the uterus cannot stay in place and it slides down into the vagina.

3 Severe premenstrual syndrome
Together with period problems, this is a further possible reason for hysterectomy.

HOW IS IT DONE?

There are three ways of doing a hysterectomy:
■ Abdominal hysterectomy
■ Vaginal hysterectomy
■ Laparoscopic hysterectomy.
In a majority of cases these operations will be carried out following general anaesthetic.

1 Abdominal hysterectomy
An incision is made in the abdomen, usually below the bikini line, which allows the surgeon to free the uterus, and to take it out through the same incision.

2 Vaginal hysterectomy
This is done through the vagina. The cut is

Right: This is the scar you can expect after having an abdominal hysterectomy.

Right: The two small scars after a laparoscopic hysterectomy.

Right: If the uterus is very large, an 'up and down' cut may be needed.

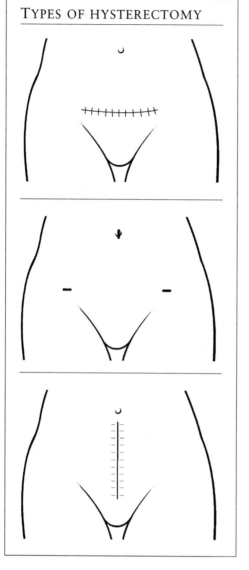

TYPES OF HYSTERECTOMY

has a tiny video camera in the end of it. After pumping up the abdomen with carbon dioxide gas, to make more room inside, the surgeon uses the laparoscope to get a close-up, detailed view, as he/she watches a screen which shows the area visualised by the laparoscope.

Two or three further small cuts are made in the abdomen, and fine tubes are inserted into them. They provide narrow channels for other surgical instruments, such as a laser, scissors and forceps, used in the actual operation itself.

After the uterus has been separated from the body it is removed through the vagina and the incision in the vagina closed.

WHICH IS THE BEST SORT OF OPERATION?

Some conditions are more suited to one procedure than another. For example, vaginal hysterectomy is often done in cases of prolapse, because the supporting tissues of the vagina, which are probably weakened, can be repaired more easily at the same time. If the ovaries are being removed at the same time as the uterus, then it may be easier to have an abdominal or laparoscopically-assisted vaginal hysterectomy. An abdominal hysterectomy will also be done if there are very large fibroids or advanced cancer.

In some cases, removing the ovaries as well as the uterus is the best option. This might be the case for a woman over fifty, if cysts are found at the time the operation is done, or if a woman suffers from severe pelvic pain linked with the menstrual cycle. However, removing the ovaries will be discussed with each woman before the operation, and it will only be done with her consent.

Recovery time differs according to how the hysterectomy is done but not on whether the ovaries are removed. It may take less time

made inside the body at the top of the vagina, and so there is no visible scar. The uterus then comes out through the vagina.

3 Laparoscopic hysterectomy

This uses a very fine telescope, called a laparoscope, which is inserted into the abdomen through a very small cut in the navel (the technique is sometimes called keyhole surgery). It to recover from a laparoscopic or vaginal hysterectomy and, once home, full recovery may only take about four weeks. After abdominal hysterectomy, recovery time may be longer with women ready to return to a normal life after two to three months.

BEFORE THE OPERATION

Emotional and physical preparation is important before going into hospital for the hysterectomy.

BE EMOTIONALLY PREPARED

It is important to focus on the reasons for the operation, particularly when the hysterectomy is to treat menstrual problems, and the impact these have on daily life. This may include being unable to swim or even leave the house for a few days each month. The priority will no longer be the bearing of children as after a hysterectomy this will no longer be possible. However, a woman's role as mother, wife or partner need not change.

Discussing the problem with the appropriate people should lead to more understanding and help during the post-operative period. The most appropriate time to discuss the effect of hysterectomy on your sex life is usually before the operation.

BE PHYSICALLY PREPARED

Stop smoking or, at least, cut down eight to twelve weeks in advance of the operation. Don't leave it until the last minute.

Try to get your body used to a more healthy style of eating. If it has been suggested that you should lose some weight before the operation, leave plenty of time and aim for no more than two to three pounds per week. Crash diets may slow down the healing process so avoid the latest fad diet. Concentrate on reducing your fat intake and eating at least five portions of fruit or vegetables per day, and drinking lots of water. Some constipation is common after a hysterectomy, but if you already eat a healthy diet, which is high in fibre, it will be easier to overcome this after the operation. Diuretics must be avoided.

Try to take some form of exercise, such as a brisk walk or some swimming, a few times a week. This improves the circulation and your general level of fitness and will help the body get fit for what will be a major operation. Set aside some time from your daily routine to do this; it will make it easier to

TYPES OF HYSTERECTOMY

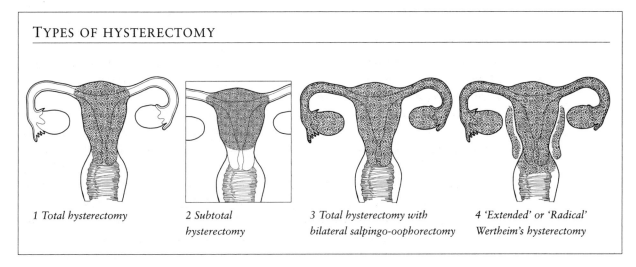

1 Total hysterectomy

2 Subtotal hysterectomy

3 Total hysterectomy with bilateral salpingo-oophorectomy

4 'Extended' or 'Radical' Wertheim's hysterectomy

continue with a gentle exercise programme after the operation.

THE OPERATION

Do ask your doctor about what happens before the operation, as hospital procedures and routines are different from place to place. However, you'll probably be asked to come in the day before your operation, and you will be asked not to eat or drink anything for some hours before your operation is due. This is because a general anaesthetic is unsafe otherwise.

You will meet a number of medical and nursing staff, who will ask you questions and give you the chance to ask them anything about which you are not clear. You may need to have your pubic hair shaved or clipped – you can do this yourself if you prefer. Your general health will be checked, and you will have a blood test, and a blood pressure check. You will also meet the anaesthetist who will be responsible for anaesthesia during the operation.

An hour or two before your operation, you may be given a pre-med. This is a drug you take by mouth, or in an injection, which relaxes and calms you. Not everyone needs one – your anaesthetist will discuss it with you beforehand.

QUESTIONS YOU MAY ASK

How long does the operation take?

On average, the operation takes about an hour. It will take longer if you are also having a repair operation or if it is a laparoscopic hysterectomy.

What lies in the place of the uterus when it's no longer there?

The uterus is not very big, and as all the abdominal organs lie quite closely together anyway, once it is gone, the bowel tends to move over slightly and occupy the space. You do not have any space inside you.

What can you expect straight after the operation?

You will have been given a strong painkiller before you recover consciousness, plus something to prevent sickness. You will wake up feeling drowsy, and you shouldn't be in any pain. As after any operation, you will have a drip in your arm at first, and maybe a catheter to remove urine from your bladder. These will probably be removed the next day. You may also have a drain from the wound, to take fluid away. Again, this is usually removed the next day. None of these procedures is painful.

When can you get up?

The next day. It is important to get moving, to encourage the circulation of the blood. You can have a bath or a shower as soon as you want one, and go to the toilet. It is normal to take a few days before your bowels start functioning properly. You may be given advice on gentle leg exercise, to prevent thrombosis (blood clotting), and you may be asked to wear special stockings.

What about eating and drinking?

You will probably find that your appetite takes a day to return, but you can eat and drink normally as soon as you wish.

Will you be in any pain after the operation?

You may find that you suffer from discomfort because of wind trapped in your abdomen – ask the nurse for medication, and any pain relief you need. Don't worry about sneezing, coughing or laughing. They will not affect your scar.

You may be given injections of heparin to help prevent the formation of blood clots in the deep veins of the legs. These will continue until you go home. Also, antibiotics are now given routinely immediately prior to the operation in most units.

GOING HOME

You can go home when you are ready. Often this is three days or so after a laparoscopic or vaginal hysterectomy; perhaps five to seven days after an abdominal one. Try to have some help at home for at least the first week, or perhaps arrange to stay with a friend for that time. You'll feel the need to rest, and you should avoid doing any heavy housework for the first few weeks. Gentle exercise every day is important, and you should practise the exercises the physiotherapist will have shown you in hospital. When your vaginal discharge has ceased, you can go swimming. You'll be advised to avoid standing for long periods, and not to do any heavy lifting for at least three months.

HELPING YOUR RECOVERY

You can help your recovery by doing the following:

1 For the first seven to ten days:
■ Arrange for help in the home after your return
■ Avoid any heavy housework for the first few weeks
■ Do some form of gentle exercise every day, e.g. walking a short distance
■ Do the exercises you have been shown by the physiotherapist.

2 After three to four weeks:
■ Do some exercise – swimming is beneficial
■ Avoid standing for long periods
■ Avoid lifting anything heavy.

VAGINAL DISCHARGE

The discharge you'll experience is rather like the end of a period, and lasts about three or four weeks. It may be red or brown and it may have threads from dissolving stitches. Don't worry about it unless it becomes heavy or smelly, which might indicate an infection – in which case, see your doctor. Use sanitary towels rather than tampons, to reduce the risk of infection.

WHAT WILL YOU FEEL LIKE?

Feeling low and tearful after any operation is normal, and this may happen to you. But there's no reason to expect any longer term feelings of depression. In spite of newspaper beliefs that depression frequently follows hysterectomy and lasts for many months, the reality is that depression is less common when the heavy painful periods and symptoms related to the periods have been treated by hysterectomy.

GOING BACK TO WORK AND DRIVING

Talk to your doctor about this, as advice will differ according to the sort of job you have. It is usually okay to drive when you feel you could do an emergency stop but check first with your insurance company.

WHAT ABOUT SEX?

Many women who are considering having a hysterectomy are concerned that this will alter their sex life and feelings of sexuality. This may occur for two reasons:
■ Firstly, the act of sexual intercourse is associated with fertility and, therefore, removal of the womb obviously removes that aspect of it
■ Secondly, the womb or the neck of the womb (cervix) are associated and important for the sexual response.

There is little scientific evidence to confirm or refute this since it is a very difficult subject to study and much of the discussion rests on very small surveys. It would appear that some of the women who do experience sexual dysfunction after hysterectomy have actually had this problem for a long time and that it is exacerbated by hysterectomy. When women are asked whether they are satisfied with the operation, over ninety per cent report that it has made no difference to either their interest in sex or their ability to attain orgasm which would strongly suggest that the uterus is not necessary for enjoyment and that other factors are more important.

Recently there has been a school of thought that has suggested that the cervix is an important part of achieving orgasm and that sexual problems are less likely to occur if the cervix is left behind – a sub-total hysterectomy. This may occur for two reasons:

■ Removing the cervix is the most difficult part of a hysterectomy.

■ It may be associated with bleeding, which can cause a large 'bruise' at the top of the front passage after the operation. This may take a long time to resolve and is likely to be associated with pain on intercourse for some time.

However, there are no good data to suggest that leaving the cervix behind is important if complications are avoided. Again, it must be emphasised that women who have no problems before the operation are unlikely to have problems after it.

Feelings of femininity related to the presence of the womb vary very much with the ethnic origin of the woman. There are some groups who will avoid hysterectomy at all costs for this reason and this must be taken into account in the counselling before an operation. It should be possible for most women, unless they have had a malignant dis-

ADVANTAGES AND DISADVANTAGES OF DIFFERENT TREATMENTS FOR HEAVY MENSTRUAL BLEEDING

Treatment	Advantages	Disadvantages
Non-hormonal drug treatment	Taken only during the period. Short courses only required. Will relieve any associated period pain. Avoids operation. Effective control in some. Fertility is not removed.	May not be effective.
Hormone treatment	Avoids operation. Effective control in some. Fertility is not removed.	Must be taken throughout the whole cycle. Side effects may be a nuisance. Contraindicated in some women. Prolonged courses may be necessary. May lose effect in time.
Hysterectomy	Periods stop altogether.	Risks of any major operation — bleeding, infection, blood clots. Temporary discomfort and up to a week in hospital. Off work for 4–8 weeks.
Endometrial ablation	Smaller operation. No cuts involved. Fast recovery: 2–3 weeks. Short hospital stay: 1–2 days.	May well not stop periods. May still require hysterectomy. later. Long-term problems not yet known.

ease to avoid hysterectomy and find a satisfactory alternative. It is unlikely that an alternative will be as successful as hysterectomy in terms of efficacy since removal of the womb will lead to cessation of bleeding. However, a lighter period may be perfectly acceptable provided that you know what to expect from your treatment.

Sex should not feel any different either for you or for your partner. It is usually all right to start having sex again after your six-week check following the operation.

FURTHER TREATMENT

You may be given an appointment to come back to an outpatients' clinic in six weeks' time, so the doctors can check you have fully recovered. This is also a chance for you to ask any questions. If you have had your ovaries removed you have now 'gone through the menopause', you'll be given a hormone replacement medication. Ask your doctor about whether you still need to have routine cervical smear tests.

Your doctor will talk to you about whether you need any hormone treatment if you have had your ovaries removed, or if you have been through the menopause. Hormone replacement therapy (HRT) may be one option, or oestrogen can be prescribed immediately after the operation. It can also be given to you in the form of oestradiol, perhaps with testosterone, inserted as a pellet as the surgeon is stitching up the incision.

It is important that all options are carefully considered. A brief outline of advantages and disadvantages of the different treatment options is given in the table.

PAINFUL PERIODS (DYSMENORRHOEA)

Period pain is now well understood and, for many women, successful treatment can be achieved by taking tablets rather than resorting to a major operation.

WHAT IS DYSMENORRHOEA?

Dysmenorrhoea means pain associated with the periods. It is usually like a 'cramp' in the lower part of the abdomen and may start either some days before the period or with the onset of bleeding. Young women tend to experience it mainly on the first two days, whereas some, particularly older women, may find it gets worse as the period progresses. It may be associated with other problems, including the following:

- Sickness and diarrhoea
- Headache
- Pain going down the legs
- Tiredness
- Mood changes.

WHO GETS IT?

A majority of women occasionally get some dysmenorrhoea. However, about seven per cent of women are so badly affected that they need to take time off work or school on a regular basis.

WHAT CAUSES IT?

There are two sorts of dysmenorrhoea, which are known as 'primary' and 'secondary'. Essentially, primary means that the cause is unknown, whereas secondary dysmenorrhoea has a recognisable cause.

■ **Primary 'spasmodic' dysmenorrhoea**

This classically occurs in girls in their teens. It usually starts within a year of the first period and will continue intermittently. It is a cramping pain often likened to the contractions of labour. The uterus is a muscular organ and the contractions occur because of increased activity in the muscle. This means that the pressure inside the uterus increases, the blood vessels supplying the womb are compressed and less blood is able to pass along them. The blood carries oxygen and other nutrients to all the tissues in the body and if, for any reason, not enough gets through, then pain occurs. A similar thing happens in the heart when people get pain in their chests during exercise (angina).

The pain may be caused by the release of some chemicals within the uterus called prostaglandins. These are found in large amounts in the uterus and some of them cause an increase in the activity of the womb muscle as well as a decrease in blood flow which leads to the pain. There are more of these prostaglandins in the uteruses of women with dysmenorrhoea than those without, which confirms the opinion of most of today's gynaecologists that dysmenorrhoea is not all in the mind. Prostaglandins are not the cause in everybody and it is likely that in some women other substances are involved.

■ **Secondary dysmenorrhoea**

This is period-associated pain in the presence of recognised disease. Here are some of the common causes:

■ Congenital abnormalities
■ Uterine fibroids
■ Pelvic infection
■ Cervical stenosis (narrowing)
■ Intrauterine coil devices
■ Endometriosis.

■ **Congenital abnormalities** are defects in the structure of the womb which are present at birth. If the outflow of menstrual blood is blocked in any way, then the womb works very hard to overcome this blockage and this can give rise to pain. A similar problem may occur when there is narrowing of the cervix (cervical stenosis) which may occur after surgery and can be a cause of dysmenorrhoea.

■ **Uterine fibroids** are benign (non-cancerous) lumps which appear in the womb muscle and probably alter the way it contracts. The exact cause is not certain because many women with fibroids do not have any period pain.

■ **Pelvic infection:** Infections generally cause an increase in the amount of prostaglandins (pain-producing chemicals found in the womb) produced as well as other chemicals which may cause pain, and this is probably why people with pelvic infection often have period pain. This may also be true for women who have endometriosis and partly explains why many women who have a contraceptive intrauterine coil often have pain although it is possible that the presence of a foreign body is an irritant to the uterus.

WHAT SHOULD YOUR DOCTOR DO?

If your doctor is sure that the pain is dysmenorrhoea, he/she may do no special investigations before starting treatment. The diagnosis can be established by asking questions concerning the relationship of the pain to the period and about other associated symptoms, such as premenstrual tension, nausea, headaches or backache. A pelvic examination, which involves examining the uterus and ovaries through the front passage, may be performed, although obviously not in young girls.

However, if your GP is unhappy for any reason, then referral to a gynaecologist may be recommended. This occurs if:

■ Standard treatment fails (see below)
■ An associated disease is suspected.

The gynaecologist will ask questions, perform an examination and may organise an ultrasound scan or a laparoscopy.

■ An **ultrasound** scan is a simple procedure which involves the moving of a rounded probe over the tummy or inside the front passage. It is painless and does no harm and enables the gynaecologist to identify abnormalities in the shape or size of the uterus and ovaries. It does not require admission to hospital. Uterine fibroids are often discovered in this way.

■ A **laparoscopy** does require hospital admission although usually only for a day. The patient is usually given a general anaesthetic and a special telescope is inserted into the abdomen. It is then possible to see the uterus, the ovaries, the fallopian tubes and the surrounding tissues. Any disease present, such as infection or endometriosis, can then be identified easily and it may be possible to treat at the same time. This can be discussed with the gynaecologist. For a diagram, see page 63.

TREATMENTS
Self help
Women have been using menstrual remedies for centuries. It is often worth trying simple remedies before starting drug treatment. General methods include:

■ **Heat,** perhaps either a hot bath or application of a hot water bottle to the lower part of the abdomen
■ **Exercise** is often very helpful, e.g. cycling, swimming or fast walking
■ **Diet:** There is no particular dietary advice although some women may find that reducing their intake of salt, sugar, alcohol and caffeine may help. Vitamin B6 may help the mood changes as well as easing sore breasts
■ **Painkillers:** If the above measures fail, many women find that their pain is helped by ordinary painkillers, such as paracetamol, which they are likely to have in the home.

Specific treatments
The following treatments may also be useful in treating women with menstrual problems other than pain.

■ Prostaglandin synthetase inhibitors stop the production of the chemicals that are believed to cause dysmenorrhoea. They are successful in about eighty per cent of young women although they are less successful in the presence of recognisable disease, such as infection, endometriosis or fibroids.

The most commonly used in the UK are mefanamic acid (Ponstan®) and ibuprofen (Brufen®, Nurofen®) although in other countries other similar drugs may be used. Sometimes one tablet may suit a patient better than another and so it may be necessary to try more than one member of this group to find the most effective one.

They need only be started with the onset of the pain or the period, whichever comes first, and should be taken only while the period lasts. They are very safe when taken this way, the commonest side effect being a stomach upset or acid indigestion, which will be less if the tablets are taken with food.

■ **The oral contraceptive pill** is a very effective treatment and is particularly useful for those women who wish to avoid pregnancy. The period tends to be lighter and virtually pain-free. If necessary, it can be used in combination with the tablets described above.

■ **Danazol** is a hormonal preparation which has a structure similar to the male hormone testosterone. It causes the endometrium (lining of the womb) to become thin and also alters female hormone release. A moderate dosage will cause the period to stop altogether, whereas smaller dosages will make it lighter. There are side effects associated with these tablets although they are not usually very significant unless higher doses are used. However, their use is not recommended for more than a few months at a time.

■ **Progestogens** are a group of drugs that are similar in structure to the female hormone progesterone which is produced in the second part of the monthly cycle. They include norethisterone (Primulot ®), dydrogesterone (Duphaston ®) and medroxyprogesterone acetate (Provera ®) which can be given for between ten and twenty-one days each month and are successful in a certain proportion of cases. There are no serious side effects although some women may get breast pain, water retention or other minor problems, such as headaches.

The new hormone-secreting intrauterine systems are also successful after the first few months of treatment. Side effects appear to be less than with the oral route in the long term.

TREATING DISEASE

Pelvic infection may be treated with antibiotics, an **intrauterine coil device** can be removed and alternative contraception employed, and **structural problems** of the uterus, such as fibroids, can be treated surgically. The medical treatments described above are often much less successful in the presence of disease, such as endometriosis, with the exception of those that stop the periods altogether. These include danazol and a group of drugs similar in structure to a hormone released from the pituitary gland which is found underlying the brain and controls the hormone output from the ovaries – gonadotrophin releasing hormone agonists. (see page 60).

These drugs are also widely used to treat endometriosis and the menstrual problems associated with this disease. Since they stop periods, they are very effective but may not be suitable for long-term use and the 'carry over' effect once treatment is stopped is variable.

SURGICAL TREATMENT

When medical treatment fails, or in older women who have finished having their families, surgical treatment may be more appropriate. It is possible to interrupt the nerves supplying the uterus which leads to relief in some women. It used to be done as part of a major operation but now laser energy can be used to divide the nerves, or they can be divided using 'keyhole' surgery. It is possible to have children after this treatment as it does not alter the way in which the uterus functions.

■ **Endometrial ablation** will help dysmenorrhoea in about forty per cent of women. However, there is a small proportion (twelve per cent) who actually will have a new problem after the operation. This may be due to small pockets of endometrium bleeding at the time of menstruation and the scarring resulting from the endometrial ablation preventing the loss of the menstrual fluid. Overall, if dysmenorrhoea is the main problem and not associated with heavy periods, then endometrial ablation is not felt to be the treatment of choice.

■ **Hysterectomy:** As with menorrhagia, hysterectomy is an extremely successful treatment, but, as has already been discussed, it is a major operation. Hysterectomy will relieve menstrual associated pain in all cases and is the best option for some women.

POSTMENOPAUSAL BLEEDING

This term refers to vaginal bleeding which occurs more than twelve months after the last menstrual period (the menopause: see Chapter 14) in women who are not taking HRT. This symptom should always be reported to the doctor, and the GP will usually then make a specialist referral.

The most common cause of postmenopausal bleeding is thinning or 'atrophy' of the uterus (womb) and vaginal tissues associated with the normal hormonal changes of the menopause. Benign (non-cancerous) polyps of the uterus can also cause bleeding. However, this symptom is also a feature of cancer of the lining of the uterus (endometrium) or of the cervix. Approximately ten to twenty per cent of women with postmenopausal bleeding have a cancer of the uterus. Often, early diagnosis and treatment of these cancers has excellent results, so investigation with a cervical smear, ultrasound scan, hysteroscopy (direct inspection of the uterine lining using a magnifying telescope) and biopsy of the endometrium is usually advised. At hysteroscopy, polyps can be identified and removed. If the uterine cavity and cervix are normal, and atrophy is thought to be the cause HRT (tablets, patches or cream) may be offered in order to strengthen the uterine tissues and make bleeding less likely.

PREMENSTRUAL SYNDROME

Many women know when their period is due because of regular changes in their body such as breast tenderness or mood changes. For a majority this is a normal, physiological response to the changing hormone environment and does not cause problems. However, the extent of these changes can vary and some women find they begin to affect the quality of life.

Premenstrual symptoms have been recognised since the days of Hippocrates, but it was only in 1831 that an American doctor, Robert Frank, described women who complained of a 'feeling of indescribable tension', 'unrest',

'irritability', 'like jumping' out of their skin' and 'a desire to find relief by foolish and ill-considered actions'. Since that time these symptoms were referred to as 'premenstrual tension' (PMT). As tension is only one of many other symptoms, a new name emerged to describe the condition – premenstrual syndrome (PMS).

WHAT IS PMS?

PMS is a group of physical and psychological symptoms; they start anything between two and fourteen days before menstruation, and they are relieved with, or soon after, the onset of menstruation. In many women, mood changes and swings are the most prominent features, sometimes to a state of extreme irritability which shows as irrational anger, impatience and snappiness. However, in some women, their lifestyle, work and material life are affected. A severely affected woman with PMS may describe her life as a 'Jekyll and Hyde' existence, where one part feels deranged and the other part appalled by what her premenstrual self is doing and saying. PMS is even reputed to cause baby battering, arson, inability to work, examination failure, marital disharmony and even murder and suicide in some cases.

HOW COMMON IS PMS?

It is difficult to say exactly how common PMS is. Many women experience premenstrual 'awareness' without recognising it as a problem. Many sufferers will never complain and never seek any help because of lack of knowledge and also embarrassment. About ten per cent of women have no physical or psychological symptoms before their periods. Five per cent of women have very severe symptoms, enough that they need to see a specialist, usually a psychiatrist. The remaining women will have symptoms between the above two extremes.

PMS occurs between the ages of thirteen and fifty when the ovaries are producing hormones, and studies have shown that it is more common between the ages of thirty and forty.

It appears that PMS is commoner in the daughters of affected mothers than those whose mothers did not suffer with it. In addition, it appears to occur in all races and cultures and in all social classes.

WHAT CAUSES PMS?

Many theories have been proposed for the cause of PMS, but no one theory has strong scientific support. Some researchers have suggested that PMS is caused by a lack of some hormones produced by the ovaries, while others have talked about a deficiency of vitamins or essential fatty acids as the cause but none of the above has proved to be the only cause. PMS might represent an exaggerated response to the normal rising and falling levels of the hormones produced by the ovaries in normal cycles. It is well known that when the ovaries are removed surgically or when they are suppressed by some specific medication, the PMS symptoms disappear.

WHAT SYMPTOMS MAY OCCUR?

Over 150 symptoms have been reported, and the most common and typical ones are usually as follows:

PHYSICAL SYMPTOMS
- Bloatedness
- Breast swelling/pain
- Headaches, migraine
- Constipation/diarrhoea
- Abdominal pains
- Tiredness/lethargy
- Joint and muscle pains
- Dizziness
- Nausea

PSYCHOLOGICAL SYMPTOMS
- Tension
- Irritability
- Aggression
- Anxiety
- Depression

- Crying bouts
- Diminished self-esteem
- Food craving, e.g. for chocolate
- Insomnia (inability to sleep)
- Loss of sexual desire
- Accident proneness
- Loss of confidence
- Mood swings
- Social isolation
- Violence

A PMS sufferer can complain of one or more of these symptoms. The severity of symptoms might vary from one cycle to another although the character of symptoms appears to remain constant in a particular woman.

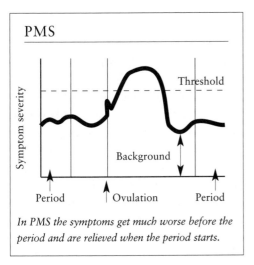

PMS

In PMS the symptoms get much worse before the period and are relieved when the period starts.

HOW TO RECOGNISE PMS

There is no specific medical test to show whether a woman has PMS or not and the similarity of symptoms with other psychological disorders makes the differentiation between these disorders and PMS difficult. The best available way to find out if a woman is really suffering with PMS is to record her symptoms on a chart or diary every day for a period of at least two months; if they occur in a regular pattern each month in the two weeks before the period and disappear or improve after a period, then the problem is more likely than not to be PMS.

WHO CAN HELP

PMS sufferers should talk to their partners or a close friend. Physical exercise reduces stress and enhances a feeling of well-being so that a regular programme of exercise should be encouraged. Increasing dietary fibre helps regulate the bowel habit and possibly relieves symptoms of distention. It is important for the woman to know that she is not becoming mentally ill and that some sort of treatment is available.

TREATMENTS

The treatment of PMS is not easy and the best approach is to start with very simple methods and then work gradually through the rest. Often, simply talking about your concerns with someone who takes you seriously can help considerably.

FOR MILD SYMPTOMS

If you have mild PMS symptoms, the following treatments may help:
- Counselling
- Education
- Reassurance
- Stress management
- Relaxation techniques
- Vitamin B6
- Evening primrose oil
- Exercise, gym, yoga, etc.

You can obtain help and advice from self-help groups, well woman clinics, family planning clinics and general practitioners.

FOR MODERATE SYMPTOMS

With moderate symptoms, some sort of **hormonal treatment** similar to the steriods produced by the ovaries may help, provided there are no medical reasons against this. If contraception is also required, the oral **contraceptive pill** seems a good choice but it is important to know that although the effect could be beneficial in some women, in others it could make their symptoms worse.

The use of pure **progesterone hormone pessaries** or **suppositories** or even **injections** has been advocated for a number of years, although again the response varies from one woman to another. Another option is the use of **progestogens** (synthetic progesterone hormones).

The use of **diuretics** (water losing drugs) for treating PMS has been advised without any evidence that PMS sufferers retain water in their bodies before periods or actually put on weight during that time. If you have weight increase and swelling prior to the periods, your general practitioner can prescribe a diuretic called spironolactone. True weight gain and swelling occur in only a small number of PMS sufferers.

When breast pain and tenderness are most prominent then it is advisable to have a formal **breast examination** by a medical practitioner and, provided it is normal, the use of some medications can be helpful. These include: evening primrose oil, bromocriptine and danazol.

FOR SEVERE SYMPTOMS

When PMS symptoms are very severe and not responding to the measures mentioned above, then you should be referred to see a specialist who has particular interest in PMS; this could be a psychiatrist or a gynaecologist.

The options open at this stage can include approaches such as oestrogen therapy in a dose which stops ovulation and decreases hormone production from the ovary. An alternative is to give an antidepressant such as the serotonin reuptake inhibitors (SRIs), which can be taken just during the bad weeks.

The **gonadotrophin releasing hormone (GnRH) analogues** can suppress the function of the ovaries and decrease hormone production. This will lead to cessation of menstruation as well as PMS symptoms, and during the treatment course the woman might experience hot flushes and night sweats. The treatment has to be stopped after a period of six months, otherwise it is associated with a tendency for bones to become thinner which may lead to osteoporosis.

The only totally reliable and effective cure for PMS would be to remove the uterus (hysterectomy) and the ovaries and to give the woman HRT. However, very few specialists would recommend this approach to treatment and, of course, it is only used as a last resort. Most often it is performed when the woman has another reason to have an hysterectomy and her ovaries removed – for example, heavy periods or fibroids, as well as PMS – or when the woman has completed her family.

It is important to know that when the uterus is removed but not the ovaries, some women will notice an improvement in their symptoms, possibly because problems with the period itself are removed. However, in others, PMS may remain because the ovaries will continue to produce hormones in a cyclical pattern until the woman reaches the menopause.

RELAXATION

This is a technique that is learned quite easily, and many women are given relaxation classes before the birth of a baby. If you need help in learning relaxation techniques contact your health visitor or enquire at your local clinic or health centre, consult your doctor or ask about classes at your local Health Education Department, College of Further Education or Night School Institute. Relaxation may also take the form of yoga, hypnosis, acupuncture, aromatherapy or any other technique or method that suits an individual.

■ Be aware of the areas of your body where you feel tension, e.g. shoulders. jaws, fists, etc.

■ Avoid constipation: eat a high-fibre diet, especially for breakfast, e.g. Wheat Bran, All Bran, Oat Bran, brown wholemeal bread, etc.

■ Increase the fibre in all meals, e.g. eat jacket potatoes, raw vegetables and wholemeal bread, and cook with wholemeal flour.

Always remember: if your symptoms do not improve, see your doctor.

OTHER TIPS

■ Increase exercise very gradually. Try walking or running on the spot in the privacy of your own home. Increase the time given for exercise very gradually until you reach a level you feel good with. Try punching the air, arms above your head as you jog.

■ Never get too out of breath.

■ STOP for breath and rest whenever you need to do so or if you have pain.

POLYCYSTIC OVARY SYNDROME

A polycystic ovary contains a collection of small fluid-filled cysts (less than 5 mm/^{1}/$_8$ in in diameter). Polycystic ovaries are common and benign, with no association with ovarian cancer or with a risk of forming large, medically significant cysts. However, some, but not all, women who have polycystic ovaries will encounter a variety of hormone problems which, in some cases, can have a profound effect on their lives.

Some women with polycystic ovaries are **anovular** – they do not make and release eggs on a regular monthly basis. This is a fairly common cause of infertility and, since the production and release of eggs sets the biological clock that regularises the menstrual cycle, these women can have irregular and often infrequent periods.

Some women with polycystic ovaries have an excess of the hormone **testosterone** in the bloodstream. They may find that they are troubled by acne, particularly in their teens and twenties, and that they have excess hair growth on the face, abdomen and around the areola of the breasts.

Some women with polycystic ovaries develop metabolic problems and are prone to **obesity**. Those who do lose control of their body weight can find it hard to return their weight to normal, and their weight gain can worsen other difficulties with anovulation and infertility, excess hair growth and period irregularity. Weight loss is often recommended as a means of treating these problems.

Polycystic ovary syndrome describes the collection of symptoms listed above. We now know that many women will have a milder variant of the syndrome, perhaps with irregular periods and subfertility but without excess hair growth and obesity, while others will have problems with hair growth, obesity and acne but remain fertile. There is a tendency for the condition to run in families and it is probable that it has a genetic basis. Recent research has identified clear long-term risks to health, particularly in those who gain excess weight. Overweight women with polycystic ovary syndrome are at excess risk of developing diabetes and of early problems with heart disease and high blood pressure. Doctors will advise weight loss and exercise, and set up a programme of regular health screening for diabetes and high blood pressure.

TREATMENT

Women with polycystic ovary syndrome are treated according to their particular problem. Those who wish fertility may be given tablets of clomiphene citrate which can induce ovulation, or be treated with hormone injections or surgery. Newer drug treatments with metformin may also be tried.

Those who have difficulty with excess hair growth or acne may need testosterone-lowering drugs such as certain brands of the oral contraceptive pill, e.g. Dianette® or spironolactone, whilst also using physical therapies, such as electrolysis, waxing or bleaching under professional supervision.

Those with weight-related problems and polycystic ovaries should try to reduce their weight and be aware of the long-term health implications of their condition.

As one of the most common conditions to affect young and otherwise healthy women, polycystic ovary syndrome is beginning to attract considerable research interest and new information and treatments are beginning to appear. The most promising is the puncture and cauterisation of the ovaries using a needle at the time of laparoscopy. It is as yet unclear how this procedure works but it causes some women to start ovulating regularly, which means that they can become pregnant more easily.

WEIGHT CONTROL

Women with polycystic ovary syndrome often tend to be overweight. Weight control is very important as increases in body fat can cause a lowering of the protein that binds androgen hormone in the blood. If the level of this protein called sex hormone binding globulin (SHBG) is low, then there will be a higher level of free testosterone to stimulate the hair follicles and cause hirsutism. Of course, weight control is also very important for being healthy in general. Exercise is useful for the following reasons:
■ To help maintain the correct weight
■ To help keep the heart and circulation in good order
■ To help keep bones sturdy and strong.

One hour of swimming, jogging, dancing or tennis three times a week is sufficient to keep the body healthy. Any amount of exercise is better than none at all. Even walking to work and using the stairs rather than the lift will help.

A balanced diet is also very important for weight control and good health in general. Avoid too much red meat and eggs and use low-fat cheese and dairy products. A good intake of dietary fibre is vital, so make sure you eat plenty of whole-grain cereals, beans, pulses and fresh vegetables and fruit.

Vitamin supplements are not necessary if you eat a balanced diet. It is better to get vitamins and minerals from fresh food rather than from a tablet.

HIRSUTISM

This is the presence of excessive coarse body hair, which a woman finds socially unacceptable. The areas of the body that may be involved include the chin, upper lip, sideburn areas, chest, thighs and lower abdomen. There is great variation in the amount of body hair that is normal in women of different races. Also, hirsutism can run in families. In one study, fourteen per cent of hirsute women had another female family member with the same problem. It is estimated that as many as one-third of women have some hair growth on the upper lip and sides of the face. Many women will be tolerant of a moderate degree of hirsutism whereas others will become very concerned when there is only a slight variation from normal.

Hair growth will vary greatly at different times in a woman's life – for example, hair in the armpits will appear at puberty. After the menopause, when the body's hormonal environment has markedly changed, excess facial hair growth can occasionally become troublesome for the first time.

Other abnormalities can be associated with hirsutism, including an increased tendency to acne. It is also important to tell your doctor if you have irregular periods as well as hirsutism.

TYPES OF HAIR

There are two different types of hair. At birth the body is covered with fine, short, unpigmented hair called **vellous hair**. The hair of the scalp, eyebrows and eyelashes is, however, longer, coarser and often pigmented – this is called **terminal hair**. At the beginning of puberty in the female, hormones called androgens, are produced and these are responsible for the change from vellous into terminal hair in the pubic and axillary regions (armpits). Hair in these regions is termed ambosexual, as these changes occur in both men and women.

TESTOSTERONE AND OESTROGEN LEVELS

Androgens are a group of sex hormones, which include testosterone. If androgen levels increase further, as they normally do in the male at puberty, then male sexual hair will grow. Terminal hair growth will then appear in areas such as the chin, chest, and lower abdomen. Androgens act to increase the growth rate of hair, and increase the diameter and pigmentation of the keratin column of the hair. After puberty, androgens are normally present in small amounts in women. These hormones are secreted by the adrenal gland above the kidneys and by the ovaries in equal amounts. In the male, however, these hormones are secreted by the testes at much higher levels. They are responsible for producing male-type hair pattern and other male characteristics – for example, increased muscle mass and strength.

Testosterone is carried in the bloodstream attached to a protein from the liver called sex hormone binding globulin SHBG. Almost all the hormone is attached to this protein, but about one per cent is free in the bloodstream. This free hormone is available to act on the hair follicle.

The amount of SHBG present in the bloodstream determines the amount of active free testosterone. Oestrogen from the ovary acts to increase the amount of SHBG and testosterone acts to decrease it. Therefore oestrogen decreases free testosterone levels. The balance between testosterone and oestrogen hormone levels is very important. Small alterations in hormone levels can upset that balance, even though the total testosterone levels may only become slightly raised.

WHAT CAUSES HIRSUTISM?

There are many different reasons why hirsutism can occur. For example, it can occasionally affect women taking drugs to control **epilepsy**, or women taking **steroids**. However, for many women, the cause of their hirsutism is not known and this condition is known as **idiopathic hirsutism.**

Several different types of hormone imbalance can cause hirsutism – a deficiency of **thyroid hormone** or an excess of **growth hormone**, for example. Hirsutism can also be associated with an excess of **prolactin**, which, like growth hormone, is produced by the pituitary gland at the base of the brain. Prolactin is the hormone concerned with milk production. An excess of **androgen hormone**, can have other effects in addition to increased hair growth, including increased secretion of sebum from the glands in the skin, resulting in acne, a greasy skin and scalp.

■ **Androgen** (male hormone) excess can be caused by an extremely rare condition called **congenital adrenal hyperplasia** where there is a programmed inherited disorder of hormone production in the adrenal gland. Small benign growths of the adrenal gland and the ovary itself can also cause disordered and excessive hormone production, but this is very rare.

■ **Polycystic ovary syndrome** is the most common cause of androgen excess. This condition is discussed in more detail earlier in this chapter.

WHAT TESTS WILL THE DOCTOR DO?

Women worried about excess hair growth should consult their doctor. Many women can often be reassured that their pattern of hair growth is not abnormal, and that they are not developing male characteristics. However, some routine tests may be necessary, which can be performed by the general practitioner or hospital gynaecologist. These tests usually consist of:
■ Blood tests to measure hormone levels
■ An ultrasound scan of the ovaries.

If polycystic ovary syndrome is present there is usually a raised level of a hormone called **luteinising hormone** (see page 14). This is released from the pituitary gland. There may also be raised levels of testosterone or other hormones in the androgen group. An ultrasound scan commonly shows that both ovaries have multiple small cysts.

Other causes of hirsutism are rare, and it is only occasionally that more specialised tests need to be done to exclude abnormally functioning adrenal glands, and to exclude benign growths which may be producing excess androgens.

TREATMENT OF EXCESSIVE HAIR GROWTH

If a specific cause is found for hirsutism, such as a benign growth, then this needs to be treated. In the majority of cases, however, this is not the case. Treatment can be difficult, and there is often no cure – just temporary control.
■ **Removal of unwanted hair** is the main method of treatment.
■ **Drugs** are used only in persistent or severe cases. Many drugs have side effects and

patients are unable to conceive whilst taking them. Some can be taken only for specified periods of time, as they are unsuitable for long-term use. There are three main ways to treat excess hair growth:

1 Removal of unwanted hair
2 Control of androgen hormone excess in the form of drugs
3 Weight control.

REMOVAL OF UNWANTED HAIR

Physical removal of hair can be accomplished using many different methods. Shaving, depilatory creams, bleaching and plucking can all be used. These methods do, however, have to be repeated frequently as the hair will soon grow again.

■ Waxing

This method of hair removal is very satisfactory and lasts for four to six weeks. Waxing can be done at home or professionally at a salon. It can be used to remove hair on the legs, thighs and lower abdomen. Hot wax therapy is commonly used; the wax is applied to the skin when warm to form a thin coating and strips are applied. These are rapidly removed, taking the whole hair shaft, which has embedded in the wax. Large areas of unwanted hair can be removed at once and hair regrowth is fine-ended and feels soft in texture. The procedure itself, however, can cause temporary discomfort.

■ Electrolysis

This is the only permanent method of hair removal. The hair follicle is destroyed using an electric current. The disadvantages of electrolysis are that it has to be performed by a specially trained electrologist and the treatment can be expensive. Only small areas of hair can be removed at one time. A temporary stinging or pricking sensation can be felt during the process. It is hoped that once the hair follicle has been destroyed by the electrolysis it cannot return to producing hair growth again. In addition laser treatment is becoming available in some centres.

CONTROL OF ANDROGEN HORMONE EXCESS

The combined oral contraceptive pill

Certain oral contraceptive pills are very useful in this respect, because the pill acts to suppress ovarian function which decreases the production of androgens. The therapy needs to be continued for six to nine months before there is an observable diminution of hair growth. The contraceptive pill is a particularly useful therapy for those who also require a method of birth control. The side effects of the contraceptive pill are usually minor, and include slight weight gain and breast tenderness. Blood pressure needs to be checked regularly for all women on the contraceptive pill.

Cyproterone acetate

There is one particular oral contraceptive pill which contains the anti androgen cyproterone acetate which directly opposes the action of androgens, and thus it is called an anti-androgen. It acts at the level of the hair follicle as well as having other actions which combine to lower androgen levels.

Other medications

Hormone replacement therapy can be helpful for women who develop hirsutism at around the time of the menopause. Other, non-hormonal types of medication are occasionally used for the treatment of hirsutism. These include the drugs called spironolactone and cimetidine, which are useful for some women with hirsutism.

PELVIC PAIN

Pain or discomfort in the pelvis or lower abdomen is a problem familiar to most women at some time in their lives. Although for many this may be tolerated as 'normal', it is for others a distressing and often incapacitating problem with seemingly little advice or help available.

Pain may occur suddenly and unexpectedly (acute pelvic pain) or it may be chronic and occur either intermittently or continuously over months or years. The pain may be made worse by many physical factors, such as straining, crouching, walking or prolonged standing. Sexual intercourse (or even the thought of it) may cause pain. Stress and worry can also lead to pelvic pain, making matters worse still.

While there are many different conditions that may cause pelvic pain, there are some women who have no obvious 'medical' cause for their pain. This can lead to the suggestion of psychiatric disturbance, malingering or simply time-wasting by doctors, leaving many women profoundly unhappy and demoralised – and still in pain.

THE PELVIS

The pelvis is much more than a bony cage which transmits body weight from the spine to the legs. Within the ring of bone that protects the pelvis is a complex yet delicate lattice of muscles and ligaments to support the organs of reproduction (the uterus, tubes and ovaries), and the bladder and lower bowel. There is both a rich blood supply and intricate network of tiny nerves which provide the control, co-ordination and sensitivity essential to the pelvis. It is not surprising that a wide variety of physical and emotional influences can precipitate pelvic pain.

THE PAIN

Pain is often accompanied by great fear: the fear of serious and life-threatening disease, such as cancer. There may be fear of incapacitation or even the fear that the pain may be a punishment for wrongdoing – engendering considerable guilt for some women.

The assumption that pain is caused by 'signals' sent via the nervous system to the brain from an injured or diseased part of the body is an oversimplification which is not altogether valid. Pain may be influenced by a wide range of different factors, no matter what actually 'causes' the pain. The way the pain is felt can vary depending on such factors as childhood experiences, social, cultural and family influences, emotional state and general well-being. Gauging the severity of pain is difficult and possibly fruitless. The real issue is to what extent the pain interferes with daily life and affects the quality of that life. Pelvic pain may prevent a woman from carrying out her job, fulfilling domestic commitments, caring for her children or family, and participating in sporting, recreational and other social activities. Pelvic pain may also interfere with or totally prevent sexual intercourse with all the attendant anxiety, disharmony, mistrust and guilt that may then be engendered in a relationship.

COMMON CAUSES OF PAIN

PROBLEMS DURING THE MENSTRUAL CYCLE

Many women experience pain regularly – as part of their monthly menstrual cycle. This may be accepted as normal or may interfere with everyday life to such an extent that medical advice is sought. There are two common sorts of pain that may occur on a regular, cyclical basis:

■ Ovulatory pain

This is associated with ovulation, when the egg is released from an ovary with a small amount of fluid. The pain is a dull ache, occasionally rather a sharp pain, which usually develops mid cycle when ovulation occurs. Sexual intercourse may be uncomfortable at that time. Pain rarely lasts more than twenty-four hours. Sometimes this particular pain is called 'mittelschmerz', from the German, meaning 'middle pain'.

■ Menstrual pain

Commonly called dysmenorrhoea, this may start either before or with the onset of menstrual bleeding. The latter is often known as spasmodic dysmenorrhoea – 'cramp-like' pain which may be sufficiently severe to make the sufferer go to bed (see page 41).

PREGNANCY PROBLEMS

Pelvic pain is common, occurring in fifty per cent of pregnant women. This often provokes a great deal of anxiety but is rarely serious. Occasionally, however, the pain may be due to something more worrying.

■ Early pregnancy

In the first few weeks of a pregnancy, the presence of pain in the lower abdomen or pelvis brings the fear of miscarriage, or even of an ectopic pregnancy (pregnancy developing in the wrong place, such as in the fallopian tube) which can cause serious internal bleeding (see below). Both of these problems may be accompanied by vaginal bleeding and the advice of a doctor should be sought as a matter of urgency.

■ Later pregnancy

In the later stages of pregnancy it is common to experience pelvic discomfort. The softening of ligaments which normally hold the bones of the pelvis firmly together may provoke unpleasant discomfort in the pubic bone at the front of the pelvis and in the lower back. It can be brought on by prolonged standing or walking and is cleared by lying down.

GYNAECOLOGICAL CONDITIONS

Doctors tend to divide those patients who have pelvic pain into two groups: namely those women who have acute pain which is often of short duration (less than twenty-four hours) but severe; and chronic pain which is usually of more than six months' duration and predominantly not severe. It is useful to consider both groups separately as they are generally due to very different problems.

ACUTE PELVIC PAIN

The sudden onset of pain may be both frightening and incapacitating. When this happens, women are strongly advised to see a doctor as soon as possible. Some of the more common causes of this type of pain are as follows:

■ Ectopic pregnancy

This is a pregnancy growing outside the uterus (womb), most commonly in one of the fallopian tubes. The pain may be mild to begin with and is in the lower abdomen, but is often quite severe, sometimes like colic. It may be associated with some scanty vaginal bleeding. If there is sufficient internal bleeding from the ectopic pregnancy it may cause lightheadedness and a sensation of dizziness. Any woman with a sudden onset of pain should see a doctor immediately, even if she does not think that she could be pregnant. An operation is almost always necessary to deal with this problem. It is discussed in depth in the section on Sexual Awareness.

■ Torsion of an ovarian cyst

The development of an ovarian cyst is usually due to the accumulation of fluid within the ovary creating a large bubble on the surface of the ovary. Less commonly, cysts can arise from the overgrowth of normal ovarian tissue. Most such cysts are painless but occasionally can cause pain in several ways. If the cyst is very large indeed it may press on other organs and cause discomfort – a feeling of bladder pressure or the need to empty the bowel, for example. Smaller ovarian cysts can twist creating a tight knot of tissue which cuts off the blood flow to the ovary causing severe pain. While it is important to seek medical advice for this, nowadays it is by no means certain that an operation is necessary. We are able to identify ovarian cysts with an ultrasound scan. However, if the ovary is twisted or a cyst is quite large, it must be dealt with surgically.

■ Infection in the pelvis

This presents classically with lower abdominal pain, fever and often an unpleasant vaginal discharge. The cause is an infection, usually acquired during sexual contact. This causes inflammation of the lining of the cervix, uterus and fallopian tubes, depending on the severity of the infection. The diagnosis is often self-evident if there is a high temperature and an offensive vaginal discharge. However, if doubt exists, it may be wise to have a laparoscopy (inspection of the pelvis with a fine telescope) to make a firm diagnosis.

The patient's general practitioner should first carry out tests to exclude urinary infection or an unexpected pregnancy with complications and then immediately proceed with appropriate antibiotic treatment. A swab specimen is usually taken from the vagina, before treatment with antibiotics is started, to identify the particular infection – there are several possible types. If a woman is particularly unwell, hospital admission may be required for further investigation and treatment. It is also advised that the sexual partner be examined and treated if necessary.

CHRONIC PELVIC PAIN

This type of pain is one of the most common reasons for a woman to seek the advice of a gynaecologist. Unfortunately, only in about half of these women are there any signs of disease to explain the pain when investigated by conventional methods.

Pelvic infection was looked at above as a cause of acute pain. Occasionally, it can also give rise to chronic pain although the reason for this is not clearly understood. Some unfortunate women progress from one acute

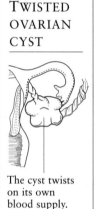

TWISTED OVARIAN CYST

The cyst twists on its own blood supply.

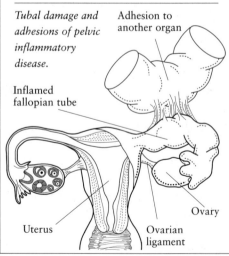

PELVIC INFLAMMATORY DISEASE

Tubal damage and adhesions of pelvic inflammatory disease.

Adhesion to another organ

Inflamed fallopian tube

Uterus

Ovary

Ovarian ligament

attack to another and end up with pain that is present most, or all, of the time. Repeated infection may lead to scar tissue (adhesions) forming between the delicate tissues which cover the pelvic organs and line the pelvis and lower abdomen itself (the peritoneum). Repeated courses of antibiotics are generally not helpful because the transitory improvement that follows their use is not sustained and further investigation is necessary to clarify the diagnosis. Uncommonly there are extensive adhesions following infection when the only long-term cure may be complete removal of the uterus, tubes and ovaries. However, there is no good evidence that repeated episodes of infection result in the condition generally referred to as chronic PID (pelvic inflammatory disease). In most cases, no obvious abnormality is found on laparoscopy.

ENDOMETRIOSIS

This is a common disease of otherwise healthy women in their reproductive years. It is caused by the implantation of tissue lining the uterus (endometrium) in other sites. The tissue responds to the hormones of the menstrual cycle and in about fifty per cent of women this can cause pain, which may be cyclical or present most of the time. Endometriosis is discussed in detail below.

It often has a negative influence on the quality of a woman's life, leading to painful intercourse and pain around the time of menstruation. The diagnosis is usually made by inspecting the pelvis with a laparoscope and looking for the characteristic deposits within the pelvis. Treatment may consist of hormonal treatment or surgery. Recent interest in using the laser to destroy abnormal areas shows promise. Some affected women will even be offered hysterectomy as the most effective

method of relieving the pain of endometriosis.

Chronic pain may be associated with congested pelvic veins in some women. These have been demonstrated using ultrasound or a special X-ray known as a venegram. Treatment is by giving a synthetic form of the hormone progesterone for some months. However not all gynaecologists believe that this is an important cause as dilated veins can occur in women without pain.

Sympathy and understanding is an important part of treatment to help women come to terms with the pain, particularly if there is no obvious underlying cause. Some women may be offered hysterectomy with removal of the ovaries, but this may not be effective for all women. A trial with a drug to stop the ovaries functioning maybe useful. If this helps the pain then removing the ovaries is more likely to be an effective treatment.

OTHER CAUSES

There are, of course, other rarer gynaecological conditions which may lead to chronic pelvic pain. Some women may already have had pelvic surgery and the onset of pain may develop after it. For those women who have had a hysterectomy, it is possible that the ovaries have become trapped in scar tissue formed around the ovaries after operation, and causing painful small tension cysts to develop. Occasionally, when the ovaries have been removed, for whatever reason, a fragment (or 'remnant') is left behind and this may cause considerable pain which can be recognised because it is usually cyclical.

The **older woman** is particularly liable to suffer from pain around the vulva and anus, or in the vagina. Undoubtedly, this is a most distressing and real pain but, unfortunately, little is known about this and no effective treatment for it is, as yet, available.

The possibility of **cancer** is often foremost in the minds of a great many women who have long-standing pelvic pain; its exclusion is, in itself, a source of great relief. It is now possible to make a diagnosis without resorting to major operative procedures. The advent of ultrasound scans, endometrial aspiration (sucking out the lining of the uterus for testing), and the use of the laparoscope to inspect the pelvis and the hysteroscope to inspect inside the uterus are major advances. Most of these can be carried out as an out-patient procedure or during a single day on the ward and exclude the possibility of pelvic cancer much more securely than was possible in the past.

NON-GYNAECOLOGICAL CAUSES OF PAIN

In addition to the many gynaecological causes of pelvic pain, there are abnormalities or disease in other organs that create pain or discomfort felt in the pelvic region. Such conditions can include the following:
- Myofascial or 'trigger point' pain, caused by torn fibres in the abdominal muscles
- Irritable bowel syndrome – pain accompanied by alternating constipation and loose stools

- Cystitis
- Diverticulitis
- Crohn's disease
- Kidney or bladder stones.

Very occasionally, disease affecting the lower spine, pelvic bones or the muscles in that region may lead to pain in the pelvic area.

SUMMARY

Acute and chronic pelvic pain commonly leads a woman to seek advice from her doctor. This may, in turn, lead to a referral to hospital for a gynaecological opinion. When the pain is severe and of recent onset, it is wise to seek urgent advice. If, on the other hand, the pain is of longer duration, it may be less urgent to seek help but no less important as chronic pain can seriously interfere with quality of life and emotional stability. The general practitioner is often the best person to deal with the condition but will need a diagnosis from the gynaecologist.

There is much that can be done to reach a diagnosis. Treatment may be with drug therapy, surgical procedures and counselling in an attempt to cure or alleviate the underlying problem leading to pain relief. Self-help groups can also play an important role.

ENDOMETRIOSIS

Endometriosis has been recognised for over 130 years but recently it appears to be diagnosed more frequently in women of all ages. It is a difficult disease for doctors to explain easily.

Endometriosis is the presence of endometrium (the lining of the womb) outside the cavity of the uterus (womb). It is commonly found on the ovaries and tubes and also on the peritoneum, the lining which covers the tubes, womb and supporting ligaments. In response to the hormones made by the ovary during the menstrual cycle, endometriosis will grow and bleed, just like the endometrium.

Endometriosis is a benign (non-malignant) condition which does not lead to cancer.

Another condition, called adenomyosis, is the presence of endometrium in the muscle of the uterus. This should not be confused with endometriosis as the mechanisms which cause the conditions are different.

HOW DOES ENDOMETRIOSIS OCCUR?

During menstruation the endometrium not only flows from the womb down the vagina but also back along the fallopian tubes and out over the ovaries, tubes, uterus and peritoneum. This is normal and it is now thought that for reasons not fully understood some of that endometrium sticks to the structures in the pelvis and grows as a new tissue that is stimulated by the hormones from the ovary – endometriosis. In most women this only happens to a mild degree and it is possible that endometriosis comes and goes throughout a woman's reproductive life. In some women, however, the endometriosis continues to grow, while the chemicals that it secretes cause inflammation which, in turn, creates pain and can lead to damage of the tubes, ovaries and peritoneum. It is not known why this should occur in some women and not in others, but current theories are that the endometriosis may be more sensitive to the ovarian hormones and can grow more easily, or that the body's defence mechanisms cannot stop the endometriosis growing.

WHAT PROBLEMS DOES IT CAUSE?

The chemicals that endometriosis secretes can cause pain. This pain may be constant, but more commonly occurs just before or during

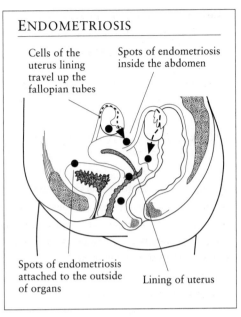

ENDOMETRIOSIS

Cells of the uterus lining travel up the fallopian tubes

Spots of endometriosis inside the abdomen

Spots of endometriosis attached to the outside of organs

Lining of uterus

Left: Endometriosis of the ovaries, the pelvic peritoneum and the back of the womb.

a period because the endometriosis is most active then and may be bleeding. Some women also experience severe pain in the middle of the menstrual cycle when the endometriosis is stimulated by the fluid that is released with the egg at ovulation. Pain during sexual intercourse is also a common symptom because the endometriosis grows on the uterosacral ligaments which are behind the womb and are knocked by the penis.

Sometimes the endometriosis forms fluid-filled cysts and these can twist or burst and cause pain. Lastly, the endometriosis may not cause any pain, but slowly grows until a mass is found in the pelvis incidentally during an abdominal or vaginal examination. One of the major problems that endometriosis causes is where the body tries to protect itself and covers the area of inflammation with scar tissue. This will often heal the endometriosis, but unfortunately the tubes and ovaries can become part of that process. As a result, the tubes can be blocked or become stuck to the ovaries, womb or walls of the pelvis. The ovaries can also become stuck to the womb or the pelvic walls. This means that the tubes cannot pick up the egg from the ovaries and so the woman becomes infertile. Often the woman will have no symptoms at all to tell her what is happening.

HOW IS IT DIAGNOSED?

Firstly, if any of the above symptoms are present, or the doctor finds that there is tenderness within the pelvis during a vaginal examination, endometriosis might be the cause. Unfortunately, there is no blood, ultrasound or X-ray test that can accurately diagnose endometriosis, and the only effective technique is to look inside the abdominal cavity and pelvis. This is most commonly done with a laparoscope, an instrument that is inserted just below the navel and allows the doctor to see the whole of the pelvis. This is usually done under a general anaesthetic and can nowadays be regarded as a common and safe technique. The endometriosis appears as white, red or black spots. It can also appear as cysts which contain a thick, dark brown fluid and are known as chocolate cysts. It is very important that the endometriosis is visualised before a diagnosis is accepted, as there can be other causes for pain and masses in the pelvis.

TREATMENTS

When considering the treatment of endometriosis, we need to look at how the problem it is causing influences treatment and then how the treatment itself works. Basically, endometriosis can be treated either by:

■ The prescription of drugs that stop it growing and allow healing to occur

■ The removal of the disease surgically, either by cutting it out or destroying it with heat (cautery) or laser.

SYMPTOMS

■ **Pain:** Endometriosis that causes pain can be treated either by drugs or by surgery. Which method is used will depend upon the severity of the symptoms, the amount and position of the endometriosis and your desires for future fertility. Therefore, each decision is an individual one and you should expect to be involved in this. For example, it may be better to recommend the removal of the uterus and ovaries for the treatment of endometriosis in a forty-year-old woman with severe disease who has had three children, whilst this would be completely inappropriate in a twenty-five-year-old woman with small amounts of endometriosis who has not yet had children.

■ **Infertility:** Endometriosis can cause damage to the tubes and ovaries, leading to infertility. This problem can be treated by surgery to remove the damaged areas and reconstruct the ovaries and tubes so that they are as normal as possible. All endometriosis identified at laparoscopy, even when very mild, should be destroyed as this has been shown to improve fertility rates. Endometriosis has minimal effect on the success of IVF and in some women is the favoured option. However, most drug therapy is contraceptive, and therefore not desirable for an infertile couple.

■ **Pelvic mass:** Even though a pelvic mass may not be causing symptoms, the doctor cannot be sure what the mass is. It may be endometriosis, but it is also possible that it is another type of cyst. In view of that lack of certainty, the doctor will usually recommend the removal of the mass by surgery.

TREATMENTS

DRUGS

There are several drugs that are effective in the treatment of endometriosis. Because endometriosis depends upon hormones for its survival, these drugs are hormonal in nature. This means that some women will experience hormonal side effects.

GnRH agonists

These drugs stop the stimulation of the ovary by the pituitary gland. The ovary does not, therefore, produce the hormone oestrogen which is essential for the continued growth of endometriosis. As a result, the endometriosis shrinks and healing takes place. These drugs are effective in endometriosis but because there is a decrease in oestrogen secretion, menopausal side effects, such as hot flushes, can be experienced and there is also a loss of bone strength as happens in post-menopausal osteoporosis. It is not suitable for long-term treatment unless a small amount of oestrogen is 'added back' which will relieve the side effects without reducing efficacy.

Progestogens

These are compounds that are similar to the natural hormone progesterone. When given continually, they change the endometriosis, as during pregnancy, making it soft and it is then absorbed. Possible side effects are fluid retention, breast tenderness, weight gain and prolonged vaginal bleeding.

Danazol

This drug is similar to male reproductive hormones and causes the endometriosis to shrink and be absorbed. It is a very effective treatment, but some women experience side effects, such as weight gain, greasy skin and spots because of male hormonal effects.

Gestrinone

This drug has male hormonal activity and works against the hormone progesterone. It has similar efficacy to danazol and similar side effects.

SURGERY

There are two main surgical approaches: laparoscopy or laparotomy.

Laparoscopy

This was used principally for the diagnosis of endometriosis but now many surgeons have become skilled in destroying the endometriosis with either the laser or cautery during a laparoscopy. Surgeons are also able to remove endometriotic cysts and divide fibrous adhesions at laparoscopy.

Laparotomy

This is a traditional method of performing abdominal or pelvic surgery through an

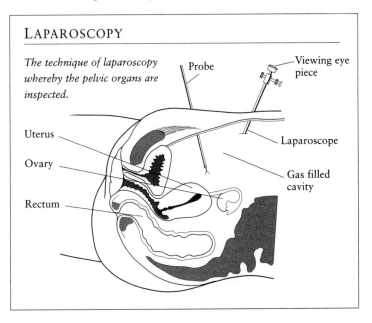

LAPAROSCOPY

The technique of laparoscopy whereby the pelvic organs are inspected.

Probe

Viewing eye piece

Laparoscope

Gas filled cavity

Uterus

Ovary

Rectum

abdominal incision. All gynaecological surgeons are trained in laparotomy whereas at the moment not all are trained in laparoscopic surgery.

HOW LONG SHOULD MEDICAL THERAPY LAST?

Traditionally medical therapy has been prescribed for six months. This is currently being reviewed. You should expect some effect on your symptoms within three months if the drug is working.

WILL THE ENDOMETRIOSIS RETURN?

There is evidence that endometriosis will eventually return in most women. However, it may take up to ten or twelve years to reoccur. It is not possible to predict how quickly the disease will return in a single individual.

CAN IT BE PREVENTED?

There are few definite ways of preventing endometriosis. There is evidence that it can occur in families. If your sister or mother has endometriosis it may be sensible to consider using the pill as a contraceptive, as that will decrease the menstrual flow in most women which, in turn, may decrease the potential for endometriosis. There is less evidence that pregnancy will treat established endometriosis but you are less likely to get the disease in the four years after a pregnancy.

HRT AND HYSTERECTOMY

The evidence suggests that there may be a higher chance of endometriosis returning if the ovaries are left behind at a hysterectomy rather than removed. Therefore, you should discuss in detail with your surgeon whether the ovaries should be removed at a hysterectomy for endometriosis remembering that if the ovaries are left behind, there is the possibility of re-operation for pain. This is not to suggest that the ovaries should be removed in all women, simply that you need to discuss the risk of recurrent symptoms if they remain. Although there are very few published data in this area, what evidence there is suggests that if the ovaries are removed, then the use of low dose HRT will not restimulate the endometriosis in a majority of women.

For women who have had a natural menopause and have had endometriosis there are some reports that HRT can stimulate the disease. However, it appears that the large majority of women can take HRT without endometriosis returning and they should only consider that possibility if they experience a return of the symptoms that were associated with endometriosis before the operation.

ENDOMETRIOSIS OUTSIDE THE PELVIS

Endometriosis can occur away from the pelvic structures. Most commonly it is found in the bowel and can lead to disturbances of bowel function or bleeding from the rectum. Rarely, it appears in sites such as the lung and can present with coughing up blood during a period. As a general rule, the same considerations about treatment of the disease in the pelvis are relevant when considering distant sites.

OVARIAN CYSTS

Many women become very worried when told that they have an ovarian cyst and think that they must have a serious condition. Fortunately, however, this is usually not the case.

A cyst is a collection of fluid in a sac-like structure. It may be only a few millimetres in diameter, like a blister on the surface of the ovary, or it may grow to a very large size indeed, weighing up to several kilograms. The fluid within it can be of different types, including clear fluid akin to water, blood, thick mucous or sebaceous material.

WHEN CAN CYSTS OCCUR?

Ovarian cysts can occur throughout your life. During the time in the womb a female fetus can develop ovarian cysts; a baby or child may be affected before the start of periods. A woman may get them during the years of having periods and in the post-menopausal years after her periods have stopped. The most common time for cysts to occur is when the ovary is most active producing hormones which lead to periods (approximately from fifteen to fifty-one years old). The next most common time is after the menopause when the ovary is inactive. Usually only one ovary will develop a cyst at any one time.

SYMPTOMS OF CYSTS

Cysts often cause no symptoms and are discovered only by accident – for example, when having a routine cervical smear and check-up, your family doctor may detect a swelling in your pelvis. To confirm whether it is a cyst, you would be asked to have one or more ultrasound scans of the area if needed.

If you have experienced pain or problems with your periods or fertility, then your doctor may diagnose a cyst on internal vaginal examination, or with the help of an ultrasound scan.

TYPES OF CYST

Cysts are described according to the microscopic appearance of the tissue in and around the cyst. Some technical terms that are used to describe cysts include:
- Physiological
- Corpus luteum
- Polycystic ovaries
- Endometriosis
- Dermoid cysts.

Less common types of cysts include epithelial cells, stromal and germ cells. While most cysts are innocent, a very small percentage can be cancerous.

PHYSIOLOGICAL OVARIAN CYSTS
In a menstrual cycle of about twenty-eight days, an egg is released from the ovary on about the fourteenth day (ovulation). The eggs inside the ovary are in small fluid-filled spaces called follicles, which look like small blisters on the surface of the ovary. The mature follicles are two to three centimetres in diameter, whereas the other follicles which do not mature fully, usually resolve and cause no problems. Functional cysts arise from an exaggeration of this process, with either the follicle becoming larger than usual and/or persisting for longer than the usual ten to fourteen days.

CORPUS LUTEAL CYSTS

After the mature follicle ruptures and the egg is released, the follicle reseals to form a corpus luteal cyst (a yellow body or structure). This produces hormones to prepare the lining of the womb for pregnancy. However, if you do not become pregnant, this type of cyst usually starts to shrink within two weeks. Very infrequently, it does not and slowly enlarges to possibly cause problems in the future.

If pregnancy occurs, the corpus luteal cyst persists, producing essential hormones to support the pregnancy for the first eight to ten weeks. It then usually resolves naturally without symptoms. However, occasionally it may enlarge and although this will not harm or affect the pregnancy directly, it may need treatment. This treatment usually does not cause problems to the pregnancy.

POLYCYSTIC OVARIES

In this very common condition, the ovaries have several small cysts of less than one centimetre on their surface. This condition occurs in twenty-five to thirty per cent of normal women. While many of these women have no symptoms, polycystic ovaries can be associated with fertility problems, obesity, period upset, and skin and hair growth disturbances. These symptoms may require treatment, but usually not of a surgical nature. These small cysts do not cause pain.

ENDOMETRIOSIS

When this condition is present on the ovary, it can form cysts which are filled with old blood. This is dark brown or black in colour, and hence they are often referred to as 'chocolate cysts'. Ovarian endometriotic cysts can cause severe pain and problems with fertility.

DERMOID CYSTS

These cysts are more common in adolescents and young women. They occur in both ovaries in ten to fifteen per cent of cases, and can contain many different substances, such as mucus, hair and even teeth. The risk of cancer is extremely rare in this type of cyst. If a dermoid cyst is diagnosed, then surgery is the standard treatment to remove it and to check the other ovary to see if it also contains a small dermoid cyst.

LESS COMMON TYPES OF CYSTS

There are many other types of cysts of the ovary. These can be lined with epithelial cells, and may be simple cysts filled only with fluid or more complex cysts with solid areas within them. These complex cysts have the potential to be cancerous. However, the risk of simple cysts being cancerous is remote in women before the menopause.

ULTRASOUND SCAN FINDINGS

A scan can tell you the number of cysts you have, but usually there is only one significant one. It can also tell you whether the cyst is filled with clear fluid, rather like a blister, or if it has thicker contents such as mucus or hair. Finally, it may tell you if there are any solid areas or swellings inside the cyst. This is important as these solid swellings may be cancerous and would warrant further investigation. However, most cysts with solid tissue are benign.

SYMPTOMS OR PROBLEMS ARISING FROM CYSTS

When a cyst forms on one of the ovaries, a number of things can happen:

■ It may resolve spontaneously

- It may reform
- It may bleed into itself (haemorrhage)
- It may twist (torsion)
- It may enlarge
- It may cause pain.

The majority of cysts resolve themselves with no treatment. However, if a cyst twists, bleeds into itself or suddenly enlarges, then this can give rise to pain. If the pain is severe and an ultrasound scan confirms an ovarian cyst, then it is most likely that emergency treatment will have to be carried out. If the pain is mild, often observation will suffice and if the pain improves then surgery will be avoided. Usually when a cyst resolves itself, it does not reform. However, a separate new cyst may reform instead.

PREGNANT WOMEN

Doctors try to avoid surgery during pregnancy, but it may be necessary to remove a cyst if it is causing severe pain. If a cyst is causing mild pain or there are no symptoms, it is usually rescanned when the pregnancy is twelve to fourteen weeks. It is usually found to have resolved. If, however, the cyst is still present and over five centimetres in size, then it is removed when the pregnancy is between twelve and sixteen weeks, which is the safest time for performing surgery. This is because the risk of miscarriage is low and the uterus has not become too big so as to make surgery difficult.

CANCEROUS CYSTS

In women who have had the menopause, approximately twenty-five to thirty per cent of ovarian cysts are malignant or cancerous. This risk is remote in women who have not had the menopause. However, cancer of the ovary is most common in older women and the risk increases with advancing age.

If you have a family history of cancer of the ovary (or of cancer of the uterus, breast or bowel), then you are at a higher risk of developing cancer of the ovary itself. Therefore if you are a younger woman with ovarian cysts and with a positive cancer family history, this would be an indication to remove the cyst or ovary at a younger age than usual.

IS AGE IMPORTANT?

Age is a very important factor when considering treatment of an ovarian cyst. The ovaries have two main functions: one is to produce an egg (ovulation) so that you can become pregnant; and the second is to produce female hormones (oestrogen and progesterone). If you are a younger woman (in your twenties or thirties) both of these functions are important. Surgical intervention may cause adhesions and scarring of the ovary, which may hinder fertility. If you are in your forties but still before the menopause, the main function of the ovaries is to produce female hormones. Therefore surgery on the ovary to remove a cyst with the possibility of causing scarring is not so important. Finally, if you have had the menopause (have stopped having periods), the ovaries produce very small amounts of hormones and do not produce any eggs at all, and therefore surgery on the ovary is not a problem.

TREATMENTS FOR OVARIAN CYSTS

Treatments for ovarian cysts are as follows:
- **Conservative:** Observe, rescan in three months, and report any symptoms
- **Medical:** Oral contraceptive pill, GnRH analogues, e.g. Zoladex®
- **Surgical:** Aspiration (drainage), remove the cyst (cystectomy), remove the ovary.

TREATMENT WITH MEDICINE

If a cyst is not causing any pain and is five centimetres or less, then waiting and repeating an ultrasound in approximately two to three months is the standard treatment if you have not had the menopause yet. If on rescanning, the cyst is still present but less than five centimetres, then a three to six month course of the contraceptive pill will stop ovulation and thereby stop the stimulation of the cyst and hopefully help spontaneous resolution.

If the pill does not work, then a group of other drugs called GnRH analogues are very potent in suppressing ovarian activity and thus help spontaneous resolution.

If a woman has had her menopause, then removing the cyst and possibly both of the ovaries would be advisable.

SURGERY

If the medicines do not work and the cyst continues to grow in size or starts to cause prob-lems, then surgery of some sort will have to be considered. If the cyst is larger than five centimetres or, if on repeating the ultrasound, it has enlarged and is now greater than five centimetres or is causing considerably pain, there are a number of options for treatment.

1 The cyst can be drained using a long fine needle. This procedure can be performed under local anaesthetic. The needle can be inserted into the cyst either through the abdominal wall (tummy) or through the top of the vagina (birth canal) using an ultrasound machine to guide the needle. Approximately forty to fifty per cent of cysts will reform.

2 Another way to aspirate or drain the fluid from a cyst is to introduce a laparoscope (a modified telescope) into the abdomen through the umbilicus (navel) under general anaesthetic. The abdomen is filled up with special gas and the cyst seen directly. The cyst can then be drained with a needle. Several small perforations or holes can be made in the cyst wall to try and prevent it reforming.

3 Alternatively, the cyst can be removed either through the laparoscope or by making a small cut in the abdominal wall – usually in the bikini line with good cosmetic results. The advantage of using the laparoscope is that usually you can go home the following day. When the cyst is removed, the remaining part of the ovary is then sewn back together and will still function.

If the cyst has solid areas within it (a complex cyst) then removal may be advisable. However, further tests, such as blood tests and detailed ultrasounds, may need to be performed first to gain more information.

Finally, the ovary with its cysts can be removed completely in some cases – for example, in women in their late forties or past menopause. It might be necessary also if for technical reasons the cyst could not be

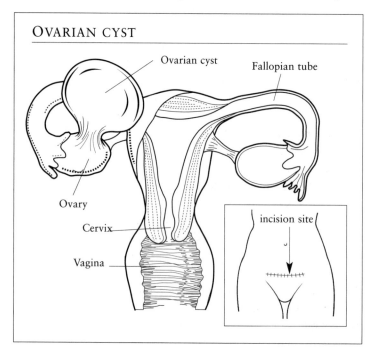

OVARIAN CYST

Ovarian cyst
Fallopian tube
Ovary
Cervix
Vagina
incision site

removed without damaging the remaining ovarian tissue.

PREVENTION OF CYSTS

While you are pregnant or on the combined contraceptive pill, you do not ovulate, and the risk of developing a simple cyst of the ovary is therefore significantly reduced. It has also been shown that if you have been on the pill, even for a short time, or have had children that you have a significantly lower risk of developing cancer of the ovary. Nobody knows what causes this and there is ongoing research to find an accurate screening method for ovarian cancer so that if you have a cyst on one of your ovaries it can be assessed more accurately. With more accurate information in the future, doctors will be able to avoid performing unnecessary surgery with its complications, and they will not miss a cancer. However, this research has still got a long way to go.

VULVAL PAIN

Pain in the vulva can be distressing and, if prolonged, may have a profound effect on a woman's lifestyle. Pain may be due to a variety of causes, most of which can be treated with relief of symptoms.

The vulval region is the area of skin between the legs around the vagina. The area includes two labia on either side and the clitoris at the front. The skin is hair bearing and may be affected by symptoms such as itching or burning, but we will concentrate on the conditions causing pain. The causes of the pain may range from infective causes, such as thrush or herpes virus, through to more sinister but much less common causes as found with vulval cancer. Most importantly, it is vital to advise women not to ignore symptoms but seek advice from their doctor, however embarrassing it may seem.

INFECTIONS

The most common cause of vulval pain is due to infection, either bacterial, fungal, viral or other causes that are rarely seen in the UK.

■ **Bacterial infections** can affect the hair follicles or glands, causing abscess formation, which are similar to small boils. These may resolve spontaneously or, if they worsen, may require antibiotics or even lancing of the abscess under an anaesthetic. Recurrent infections should be investigated to exclude diabetes and other rare problems. The most commonly affected gland is the Bartholin's gland which is situated just inside the lower vagina. When infected, it causes a painful swelling on the lower aspect of the vulva bulging into the vagina. If not treated early with antibiotics, it may spontaneously burst or require drainage under anaesthetic. There are other less common causes of vulval pain caused by bacteria which tend to occur more frequently in tropical countries, such as 'chancroid'.

■ **Viral infections** have become increasingly common in the last two decades, both in frequency and in public awareness. Without doubt, **herpes simplex virus** (HSV) is prominent, of which Type II affects the vulva although Type I, usually associated with 'cold sores', can also affect it. Without realising it, as they have no symptoms, thirty to fifty per cent of the population are infected. Asymptomatic infection at the time of intercourse is the major reason for its continued spread. Equally it may occur when one partner has only a mild attack. Recurrent attacks occur in about eighty per cent of women within the first year, often prompted by stress, ultra-violet light, emotional trauma or even sex or menstruation.

However, recurrent attacks are usually shorter and the interval between each attack longer. Herpes is further discussed in the section on Sexual Awareness.

■ **Shingles,** known as herpes zoster, can also cause painful vulval ulceration, especially in women who are immunosuppressed (such as kidney transplant patients) or the elderly. 'Vesicles' or blisters form, usually on one side only, then burst and crust over, healing without scarring. Pain may persist at the site for some months but the overall disease is much more mild than HSV II infections.

■ **Wart virus infection,** or human papillomavirus (HPV), can involve the vulval region as genital warts. These usually occur at or around the base of the vagina with an incubation time of about three weeks to nine months. If these warts become very large or infected, then pain can result.

However, sub-clinical (infection not able to be seen with the naked eye) wart virus infection can also cause pain, especially with attempted vaginal entry or local pressure. This is thought to be one of the causes of a syndrome called vulval vestibulitis.

Whereas treatment for obvious warts is by destroying them (such as with laser, diathermy or chemicals like podophyllin),

treatment for vestibulitis is much less certain.

■ **Fungal infections** are usually no strangers to many women, as the genital region has a very delicately balanced environment whose acidity can be upset by such things as antibiotics, sexual intercourse or even menstrual periods. This can result in an overgrowth of Candida, a fungus normally present in the vagina, commonly known as thrush. While it often is noticed as itching around the opening to the vagina (i.e. the vulva), the irritation is caused by by-products of the thrush infection in the vagina.

However, the vulval skin can also be the site of candida infection, often deep within the hair follicles. This is thought to be responsible, in chronic cases, for causing severe pain on touching the vulva or attempting to enter the vagina. Unfortunately, diagnosis is often made only after excluding other conditions first, based on cure of symptoms by prescription of antifungal medication. For further information, see page 134.

TRAUMA

Local trauma to the vulva can certainly cause pain, either due to the force itself or due to swelling or haematoma formation (collection of blood beneath the skin). If a haematoma does form, then management is usually conservative, unless the size of the blood collection makes movement intolerable or infection supervenes. Treatment is by drainage of the contents if required. Of course, the most common cause of trauma is the cutting of an episiotomy or spontaneous perineal tear associated with childbirth.

VULVAL CANCER

This is very uncommon, representing only

about five per cent of all cancers of the genital tract. Whilst it is mainly a disease that affects women in their sixties, it can also affect much younger women, as early as their teens. Pain can be a feature but it is more common for women to experience symptoms of irritation, itching or a lump.

If the tumour is detected early, then the prospects for survival are extremely good when treated by surgery. The surgery involved depends on how advanced the cancer is, ranging from removing the local area of skin to also taking the lymph nodes from the groin. Modern surgery practice now results in very rapid healing and minimal time in hospital although it is important to be referred to a team who specialise in management of this disease. Although the clitoris is sometimes removed, some women report no loss of sexual pleasure as the nerve endings are still present.

VULVODYNIA (PAINFUL VULVA)

This term is used to classify symptoms of vulval pain which are of a chronic nature, described as burning, stinging, irritation or rawness, with a range of causes. The reason that this group is identified is because treatment response is often poor and it is best to be referred by your doctor to a specialist who has a special interest in the management of such conditions.

The 'burning vulva' syndrome is part of the spectrum of vulvodynia. Women have symptoms of burning, but not itching, which are often worse on sitting. While it may be possible to find a cause for vulvodynia, such as thrush or wart virus infection, in some cases it may be triggered by the nerve fibres around the area or even by a psychological response to stress. An allergic response to clothing, deodorants or powders can also be a cause.

Treatment therefore involves meticulous examination, including skin scrapings and the use of vulvoscopy, a technique to look at the vulva with a magnifying instrument. Treatment may well be by using antifungals and mild steroid creams. Sometimes surgery has been used successfully in selected cases but results cannot be guaranteed.

The symptoms of vulval pain can have a variety of causes, but it is not uncommon for one not to be found. This represents a difficult dilemma for the patient and the doctor. It is important that involvement is sought with an interested doctor as frustration will be compounded by multiple opinions and lack of continuity in care. Often these facilities exist within special Vulva Clinics, which combine interested and specialist skills with equipment dedicated to caring for women afflicted by these problems.

COMMON QUESTIONS ABOUT VULVAL PAIN

WHAT SHOULD I DO IF I AM ITCHY OR SORE?

There are several simple causes of irritation which are worth excluding before consulting your doctor. A change of clothing or detergent may be a factor or the use of vaginal deodorant sprays or scented soaps to which you are sensitive. These can contain chemicals that may irritate the skin. Avoidance of tight-fitting clothing or synthetics may also be of value. If you have recently altered any of these and now notice symptoms it may be worth reverting back to your normal routine to see if it helps. Also, rather than using scented soap to wash, use either just water, aqueous cream or simple soap. Try wearing cotton underwear for a time.

WHO SHOULD I CONSULT?

Your family doctor is the best person to contact initially if you are experiencing itchiness or soreness down below. Often your doctor will be able to quickly reassure you that the cause of your discomfort is readily treatable. If there is anything your doctor is unsure about, he/she will arrange for a specialist to review your case. It is best to be seen by a specialist who has an interest in dealing with cases such as yours.

WHY DOES IT HAPPEN?

Many women cannot understand why vulval pain, itchiness or soreness affects them, especially if they are very clean and bathe regularly. However, such distressing symptoms are rarely related to hygiene. There are many factors often beyond your control that can be the cause of your problem. By seeking help you give yourself a chance to identify any of the causes. In younger women, pain is often associated with infections of the vulva, including yeast infections, such as thrush, infections of the gland that produce secretions (Bartholin's) or infections of hair follicles causing boils. Herpes infections can also cause severe pain. In the more mature woman, particularly after the menopause, the vulval skin becomes thin due to lack of hormones. Pain can be due to trauma associated with intercourse or the use of tampons. There are some other conditions which a specialist may diagnose using a small sample of skin taken from the vulva.

WHAT CAUSES THE PAIN?

Pain in the vulval region usually has several causes. Local inflammation due to infection resulting in swelling, irritation of the nerve supply by viruses or even rarely by growths or changes in the skin structure can all contribute to the pain.

WHAT WILL THE DOCTOR DO?

Most importantly, the doctor will look at the area. He/she may take a swab from the vulva or inside the vagina. Occasionally, a small sample of skin may be taken, first by using a little local anaesthetic to numb the area and pinching off a small fragment of skin. This will be looked at under a microscope to try to find a cause for your discomfort. If there are any blisters there, such as with herpes infections, the doctor may release the fluid in the blister to take a sample.

URINARY INCONTINENCE

Urinary incontinence is a common problem and can affect women of all ages. It is most common in older women, particularly those approaching or past the menopause. Approximately twenty per cent of women in their fifties are thought to suffer from urinary incontinence. Women who have delivered babies vaginally may be more prone to urinary incontinence in later life, but incontinence can also occur in those who have not had children, or women whose babies were delivered by caesarean section.

For many years incontinence was considered a 'taboo' subject, and many women had little support or advice about how to improve their symptoms. Now that medical understanding of urinary incontinence has greatly advanced and specialist physiotherapists exist to treat incontinence, there is a wide range of measures available to prevent and manage this condition.

THE RIGHT TREATMENT

Conservative treatment of incontinence means treatment without involving a surgical operation. It may involve drug therapy, exercises and other techniques. Conservative treatment can be very successful if used correctly; indeed, in some cases it is the only appropriate treatment, while in other cases it may allow you to defer or even completely avoid an operation. It is important, however, to have the right type of treatment for your condition.

There are several different causes of incontinence, and their treatments are different. Firstly, it is important to establish which type of incontinence you have before deciding upon treatment. Your family doctor may have some idea of this from your symptoms. Usually, however, you will be referred to a gynaecologist for further investigations. You will have full details taken of your bladder problem and will have a vaginal examination. You may then need some bladder tests (urodynamic studies) to find out exactly how your bladder is functioning. There are two main causes for incontinence in women and these are:

■ Stress incontinence
■ Detrusor instability.

These are by far the commonest causes and have entirely different treatments.

STRESS INCONTINENCE

If you have stress incontinence you will often notice that you leak urine on physical effort, such as coughing, laughing, sneezing and running. Stress incontinence is more common in women who have had children due to damage to the pelvic floor causing weakness. Stress incontinence responds well to conservative treatments. Treatment is geared to strengthening the muscles of the pelvic floor and improving the support of the bladder.

PELVIC FLOOR EXERCISES

These exercises are usually taught by a physiotherapist and involve repeated contractions of the pelvic floor muscles. The muscles that must be contracted are those that would be used to stop passing urine midstream. Some women, however, are unable to isolate and contract these muscles. This may be overcome by the physiotherapist performing a vaginal examination and instructing the patient how to contract the pelvic floor muscles around the examining finger. The standard instruction would be to hold the squeeze for four to five seconds and perform five squeezes in a row. Once the woman has learnt how to contract her pelvic floor, she needs to perform several series of pelvic squeezes every day throughout the day. These can be done at any time during normal daily tasks, particularly when standing or waiting – for example, when queuing for public transport.

Pelvic floor exercises are very effective for treating mild stress incontinence and may allow a complete cure. If the leakage is severe, however, exercises may improve it but not cure it completely. Unfortunately, pelvic floor exercises are like any other exercise in that you only remain fit for as long as you exercise regularly. The exercises can be boring and eventually many women give up. Once the exercises stop, the muscle tone will deteriorate and the symptoms return. Exercises are more likely to be effective in a motivated woman who is regularly supervised by a trained physiotherapist or medical practitioner. Some women may wish for a permanent cure and this is best achieved with surgery. Surgery is not advisable if more children are planned as giving birth may destroy the effects of the operation and so pelvic floor exercises may provide temporary help for these women.

VAGINAL CONES

These have been introduced recently to make pelvic floor exercises more acceptable and effective. They are small conical weighted cones, approximately the size of a tampon, with a fine nylon string attached for easy removal. They are of increasing weight, starting from 20 g to the heaviest cone weighing 100 g. The cones are produced in sets of five or three. They can be purchased without a prescription and are easy to use.

When a cone is inserted into the vagina, the pelvic muscles are made to work to keep the cone in place. The woman is asked to insert the cone into the vagina for fifteen minutes twice a day. If this is done regularly, the pelvic floor muscles become stronger. The lightest cone is used first. When a woman can hold this in place comfortably, the next weight of cone is used. This is gradually increased until she can hold the heaviest cone with ease.

Cones work in the same way as conventional pelvic floor exercises. Some women prefer this method as they can exercise at home. Some initial muscle soreness is often noticed. This is similar to the soreness experienced after exercising any muscle which has been under used. As when starting any exercise programme, the soreness disappears with continued exercise as the muscles become stronger.

Cones only work for stress incontinence and thus you should consult your doctor before using them to confirm that they will be of benefit. Vaginal cones have been shown to be effective in treating mild stress incontinence. They are no better in terms of cure than conventional exercises, although some women find them easier to use, convenient and more acceptable.

ELECTRICAL STIMULATION

Various electrical treatments have been designed to contract the pelvic floor and thus strengthen it. These treatments may be useful in women who are unable to contract their pelvic floor. They can be used alone or with ordinary pelvic floor exercises and treatment is given by the physiotherapist. The most commonly used form of electrical stimulation used nowadays is called interferential therapy. This is pain free and has been shown to he effective.

This treatment involves placing two plastic electrodes (flat plastic stickers) on the lower part of the abdomen and another electrode on the inner aspect of each thigh. A small electrical current is applied and contracts the pelvic floor, thereby strengthening it. Interferential therapy has been used successfully to cure and improve stress incontinence. It does not, however, seem to be any better than ordinary exercises of cones. It also does not confer any extra benefit when used in combination with exercises or cones.

SURGERY

Women with stress incontinence leak urine because the pressure inside the abdomen is greater than that in the urethra when a woman coughs or sneezes. This forces urine to pass from the bladder into the urethra and out of the body. Surgery is designed to lift the tissue around the junction between the bladder and the urethra so that more pressure is required to force urine out of the bladder.

The tissues surrounding the bladder neck can be lifted from above or pushed up from below. If there is a major degree of prolapse, pushing up is preferred. One method of lifting the tissues is a 'colposuspension' where stitches are placed through the vagina and inserted through a ligament on the back of the pubic bone. Some gynaecologists achieve the same end with a slightly different operation.

New methods are being developed which use substances such as collagen to support the tissues around the urethra.

URGE INCONTINENCE

If you have urge incontinence (detrusor instability), you will find that you have to pass urine very frequently throughout the day and often also during the night. When you need to pass urine you will have to reach the toilet in a rush. In severe cases, you may begin to pass urine before reaching the toilet. Urge incontinence is caused by an overactive bladder muscle or detrusor. The detrusor muscle squeezes to increase your bladder pressure and make you have the urge to pass urine when your bladder may only contain a small amount of urine. This kind of incontinence may worsen during the menopause, although it occurs most commonly in the elderly.

BLADDER RETRAINING

The simplest and most effective way to help treat urge incontinence is by retraining the bladder to hold a normal amount of urine without contracting too soon. This is called 'bladder drill' and very good results can be achieved. Some gynaecologists admit their patients to hospital for bladder drill. Alternatively, this can be co-ordinated as an out-patient with close support from the continence advisor.

The patient is initially asked to keep a record of the number of times she usually pass urine each day. The shortest time interval she can last before passing urine is taken as a starting point. Fifteen minutes is then added to that time and the patient is not allowed to empty her bladder until then. For example, if the patient normally passes urine every thirty minutes, she is asked not to empty her bladder at any time less than forty-five minutes. She is not allowed to pass urine even if it is painful or she wets herself. This sounds cruel but allows the patient to exert her own will power over her bladder instead of letting her bladder dictate when to pass urine. After a certain time period, between two and four days, it becomes much easier for the patient to last the allotted time. The time limit is then increased for a further fifteen minutes and the same process followed. This is gradually increased over several days until the patient can last for three to four hours before having to pass urine. A time of four hours before passing urine will allow most normal activities to be performed without undue interruption to go to the toilet.

Bladder drill is very successful in about ninety per cent of cases. Once the technique is learnt, the patient can retrain herself in the same way if her symptoms start to come back.

DRUG TREATMENT

This is probably the most common form of treatment for this condition. The drugs are usually given as tablets and are designed to reduce the pressure of the overactive bladder muscle. This will allow the bladder to hold a larger amount of urine and reduce the urgent desire to pass urine.

The most commonly used drug at present is oxybutynin (trade names: Ditropan®, Cystrin®). Oxybutynin works very well and is effective in reducing both the frequency of passing urine and the urgency. It is usually taken as a tablet twice a day although the dose can be decreased or increased for individual patients. The main disadvantage of oxybutynin is the side effects. These occur in most cases with varying severity. Oxybutynin causes dry mouth, blurring of eyes and constipation. The dry mouth in particular may be difficult to tolerate, and the usual response of patients is to drink more which obviously exacerbates the bladder problem. The dose of the tablets can be reduced to balance the best effects on the bladder with the least side effects. However, all of the side effects are temporary and disappear on stopping the tablets.

Other commonly prescribed drugs include propantheline bromide (trade name Pro-Banthine®) and imipramine (trade name Tofranil®). Propantheline works in the same way as oxybutynin. Unfortunately, to achieve a beneficial effect on the bladder, high doses need to be taken. These can also cause the same unpleasant side effects of dry mouth, blurred vision and constipation. Some patients find propantheline more helpful than oxybutynin with fewer side effects. The only way to know which one is preferable is to try the tablets out. Imipramine also works to reduce bladder over-activity. It is more commonly used as a treatment for depression but has the useful added effect of treating the overactive bladder. It is particularly useful in treating a small group of women who find their incontinence is worst during orgasm at intercourse.

OTHER METHODS
Detrusor instability is made worse by anxiety and stress. Patients may notice that their symptoms are much worse when they are under family or job stress. Therapies that relieve stress such as yoga, psychotherapy and hypnosis have all been used to good effect in the treatment of detrusor instability.

GENERAL ADVICE
The above treatments are specific to the type of incontinence. There are, however, some general pieces of advice applicable to all sufferers.

■ A slight reduction in your usual intake may improve symptoms. Fluid intake should be about 1-1.5 litres per day. If your main problem is getting up at night, have your last drink early in the evening.

■ Constipation may aggravate bladder symptoms, and changing to a diet including more fibre should help this.

A chronic cough can make symptoms of stress incontinence worse. Giving up smoking is, of course, important in relieving a chronic cough.

Losing weight may help alleviate symptoms of stress incontinence. It will certainly make any surgery that is needed easier to perform and therefore more likely to be successful.

A bladder infection or cystitis can give symptoms of frequency and urgency and your doctor should check a specimen of your urine. If an infection is present, it can be treated with a course of antibiotic tablets.

SEEKING HELP

All of the above methods can be very helpful and, if used appropriately, may help to avoid or delay surgery. Most people, however, find incontinence a very embarrassing condition and are reluctant to seek medical advice. Your doctor can start simple treatments and can also refer you to a specialist if necessary.

Life can be miserable for women with incontinence and the sooner advice is sought, the quicker the condition can be helped.

Chapter four

SCREENING AND HEALTH CHECKS

Health screening involves testing a healthy person to try to detect a disease in its early stages. Screening is important because disease that is detected in its early stages is usually easier to treat and is less likely to lead to significant problems or death. There is a great deal to be optimistic about since the introduction of screening programmes in the National Health Service. Over the last decade the cervical screening programme has led to a reduction in the number of women with cervical cancer and reduced the number of deaths from this disease in Britain. The breast screening programme seems to be having a similar positive effect on the incidence of breast cancer in women.

There are several very important screening checks for cancer available throughout the United Kingdom. However, not all women choose to have them done, sometimes out of fear or lack of knowledge. It is vitally important that women are aware of these screening tests and take up the opportunity to have them performed regularly. Cancer is a common disease and nearly one-third of all women will get cancer at some time in their life. Prevention is always better than cure.

There are several screening tests that are widely available to women. These include the following, which will be discussed in more detail in this section:

■ Breast screening
■ Cervical smear screening
■ Other health checks, e.g. blood pressure, rubella screening, weight or cholesterol.

BREAST SCREENING

One in twelve women in the UK will develop breast cancer at some time in their lives, and women fear it more than any other disease. There is good evidence that the earlier breast cancer is detected and treated, the longer a woman will survive. Screening for breast cancer is therefore most important.

Sometimes breast cancer runs in families which is particularly worrying for some women. For those with close relatives with breast cancer, breast screening is particularly important and it may also be possible to attend a special breast cancer screening clinic for extra advice.

SELF EXAMINATION OF THE BREASTS

All women, especially those who are over the age of thirty-five, should regularly examine their own breasts. By doing this, any change in the breasts will be detected quickly, and advice from a doctor can be obtained immediately. The breasts should be checked about once every month, usually just after a menstrual period when the breasts are softer and less likely to be tender and swollen. Many women prefer to do this with a soapy hand while they are in the bath or a shower. The breasts should be examined in a mirror to detect any irregularities of the skin or nipples. Some women's breasts do feel lumpy naturally so it is important to look for any changes to the norm. It is important to examine them for puckering or dimpling of the skin or a discharge from the nipples as well as lumps.

HOW TO EXAMINE YOUR BREASTS

1 Stand or sit up straight in front of a mirror with the arms loosely by the sides.

2 Look at the size, shape and appearance of the breasts. They should look similar to one another. Note any changes in the size of the breasts and the nipples as well as colour or shape.

3 Lift up one arm and look for any dimpled skin or swelling under the armpit, then raise the other arm and check the other breast in the same way.

4 Lie back on some pillows in a comfortable, relaxed position and put the left hand behind the head. Move the right hand gently but firmly from below the left armpit under the left breast to the middle of the chest and then around the top of the breast and down to the nipple. Press gently, looking for any lumps or lumpy areas.

5 Repeat the process with the left hand, examining the right breast in the same way.

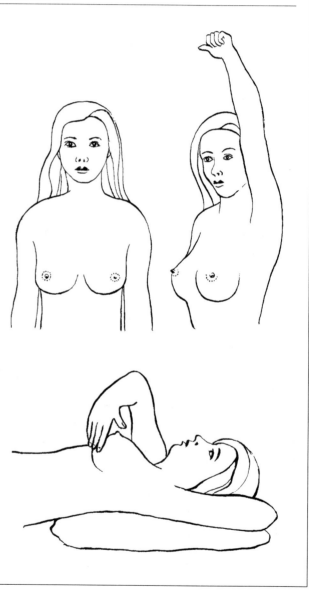

Normal breast tissue can often feel quite lumpy but both breasts will generally feel similar to each other. A serious lump is noticeably harder than the surrounding breast tissue and is obviously not symmetrical with the other breast. Breast cancer can also cause symptoms such as bleeding or discharge from the nipple, skin puckering or indrawing of the nipples. If you are worried about any breast changes, you should consult your GP or local Well Woman Clinic without delay.

BENIGN BREAST DISEASE

Of course, not all breast tenderness, pain or even lumps are indicative of cancer. There is a whole range of symptoms and non-malignant conditions in the breast which are not breast cancer, and can therefore be managed by simple treatments and reassurance. There are four main types of benign breast disease:

■ **Fibrocystic disease**, including fibro adenomas, cysts and nodularity of the breasts
■ **Duct ectasia** or **periductal mastitis**, which leads to inflammation in the breast ducts, nipple discharge and sometimes abscess formation
■ **Pregnancy-related conditions**, including infections and milk cysts
■ **Congenital disorders**.

Over ninety per cent of breast complaints are due to benign breast disease, and some studies have shown that up to thirty per cent of women are treated for this at some point in their lives. Most women with benign breast disease are not at risk of developing breast cancer. However, if cells that do not appear normal and may be pre-cancerous (atypia) are found, there is a significant increased risk.

Simple measures, such as weight loss on a healthy diet, a well-fitting bra, simple analgesia if appropriate, or oil of evening primrose, will often help.

For those unsure whether there is a discrete lump or simply nodularity, it is best to talk to the GP who may wisely advise a return visit at a different part of your menstrual cycle. However, if the abnormality persists, a consultation at the hospital breasts clinic will be arranged. Delay may result in unnecessary anxiety as the majority of 'lumps' in the breasts of young women are completely benign.

BREAST EXAMINATION BY A DOCTOR

Some women feel reassured by having their breasts checked regularly by a doctor. There are no fixed rules as to when or how often to have this done but many well woman clinics will offer this annually to women over thirty-five years old. It is often offered to women taking the contraceptive pill or hormone replacement therapy when they attend to renew their prescription.

MAMMOGRAPHY

In the UK women between the ages of fifty and sixty-four years are automatically invited once every three years for a breast X-ray (mammogram) as part of a national screening programme. These appointments are sent in rotation depending on the location of the GP's surgery so the invitation to attend for screening may not arrive until a year or so after a woman's fiftieth birthday.

Recent research has found that regular mammography performed in women over the age of fifty can detect changes in breast tissue caused by a developing breast cancer long before a woman can feel or notice anything unusual herself. This allows a much earlier diagnosis. Treating breast cancer at this early stage means that the chances of cure are much higher than if it is more advanced.

WHAT IS A MAMMOGRAM?

A mammogram is an X-ray examination of each breast, usually involving two 'pictures' of the breasts showing their internal structure. Its purpose is to detect any abnormalities within the breasts that are too small to be felt on examination. A mammogram can give information to decide whether the lump is simply one of the common benign (non-malignant) conditions, or a more serious condition, such as breast cancer (malignant). If any signs of cancer are seen on the mammogram, then the lump will need to be removed.

The radiologist may ask if previous mammograms have been performed and will wish to obtain those X-rays for comparison. The reason for this is that the appearance of breast tissue on a mammogram is almost as unique to any individual as a fingerprint, and therefore a mammographic abnormality that has not changed over several years is likely to be benign rather than a cancer.

■ **A benign tumour** or a cyst will usually be round with a very well-defined border, like a pea, a marble or even a golf ball, depending on its size.

■ **A malignant tumour** will again vary in size but typically has a border which is irregular. Doctors often use the words 'stellate' or 'spiculated' to describe this irregular border.

■ **Microcalcification** can take many forms and may be difficult to interpret. It is usually benign, its appearance being part of the natural ageing process, and it is caused by tiny amounts of calcium (the same material that is found in teeth and bones) being laid down in breast tissue. Benign microcalcification is often found in both breasts, although the amount in different parts of each breast may vary. However, some breast cancers also contain deposits of calcium, so that when microcalcification is localised to one small area of one breast, the abnormality may be regarded with suspicion.

The result of the mammogram X-ray will be sent to the woman and to her doctor and, if anything unusual has been discovered, an appointment will be made to attend an assessment clinic for further examination.

If the mammogram is normal a letter of recall for further screening will be sent every three years. Women over the age of sixty-four may also attend for screening mammography by making an appointment directly through their doctor or through their local breast screening centre.

For various reasons, screening mammography has not been shown to be of benefit in women under the age of fifty (premenopausal) and it is therefore not currently recommended in the UK. For those under fifty, there is little advantage in having mammography performed unless there is a definite lump in the breast, in which case a mammogram may give some useful information about the nature of that lump. However, it may be offered to young women with a particularly strong family history of breast cancer.

Although the actual X-rays are entirely painless, quite a few women find the positioning of the breast within the X-ray machine uncomfortable. The amount of X-rays used to produce these pictures is very small.

Once the X-rays have been taken, a senior doctor inspects the films. If there is any doubt about a possible abnormality, a further examination may be required. Any serious abnormality will be discussed with the woman, and a plan for treatment made. The result will not be available immediately, but of course the report will be conveyed as soon as possible, either through the referring doctor (to whom the report will be sent) or through the post (as part of the National Breast Screening Programme).

An abnormal mammogram does not necessarily mean that the diagnosis is breast cancer. Sometimes the abnormality is caused by a technical problem with the X-ray picture and further X-rays may be needed. Sometimes the abnormalities are caused by a benign lump, such as a cyst, which is very common and not at all serious.

OTHER TESTS

These may add extra information.

■ **Ultrasound** of the breast uses sound waves to build up a picture of the breast tissue.

■ **Aspiration cytology** involves the removal of cells from the lump using a fine needle (aspiration), and the sample is then analysed in the laboratory using a microscope (cytology).

Sometimes a combination of these tests will be sufficient to make a diagnosis of the cause of the abnormal mammogram, but if there is any doubt, a biopsy (sample of tissue) from the abnormal area will be taken.

■ **A biopsy** is an operation to remove a piece of breast tissue so that it can be analysed in the laboratory by the pathologist who examines it under a microscope and can tell exactly whether it is benign or malignant. It is usually performed under a general anaesthetic, but can sometimes be done just with local anaesthetic to freeze the skin, particularly if the lump is lying close to the surface of the breast.

If the abnormal area to be biopsied has been picked up on the mammogram and cannot be felt by the woman herself or the surgeon, then she may be asked to have a

'localisation biopsy'. This involves further mammography performed immediately before the biopsy and, using a thin needle, a fine wire is positioned with its tip in the abnormal area, which allows the surgeon to remove the correct spot. The result of this biopsy is usually available within a few days.

For every 1,000 women attending their first screening mammogram, about seventy will be recalled to an Assessment Clinic for further examination and tests, of whom only ten will go on to have a biopsy performed and, of these, about seven will be found to have a breast cancer. You can thus see that sixty-three out of those seventy women recalled for further tests after their initial mammogram will have no reason to worry. Furthermore, a high proportion of the cancers found by screening mammography are caught at an early stage before the cancer cells have had a chance to spread. Treatment at this early stage gives a high chance of cure.

RELIABILITY OF SCREENING MAMMOGRAPHY

As a general rule, mammography in the over-fifties seems to be a reliable means of picking up early breast cancers and only a very small number of women will go on to develop a breast cancer following a negative screening mammogram. If a breast lump is found, or a significant alteration in the breasts between visits for screening mammography, then this should be discussed with the doctor.

SUMMARY

Mammograms are an important weapon in the fight against breast cancer. Some women are reluctant to undergo screening mammography because they fear that breast cancer may be detected, or because they believe that they will risk losing a breast if the result of the tests is positive.

For the small number of women who are found to have breast cancer by mammography this is, of course, a frightening prospect. However, for the one out of twelve women destined to develop breast cancer at some time during their lifetime, its detection by screening mammography offers the best chance of cure.

Breast cancers detected in this way rarely recur after treatment and usually that treatment does not involve a mastectomy.

It is not necessarily disastrous news to be told that your mammogram is suspicious or even positive for breast cancer. Women have nothing to lose and everything to gain by having regular screening mammography.

CERVICAL SMEAR TESTING

The cervical smear test is one of the most important screening procedures available to women. Cervical smears can detect abnormal cells present on the cervix (neck of the womb) which are pre-cancerous and treatment can be given to prevent cancer developing. Since cervical screening programmes have been introduced in the UK, the number of women dying from cervical cancer has fallen.

Cancer can develop in the cervix but fortunately most cervical cancers can be prevented. This is because doctors can recognise abnormalities in the cells of the cervix before they become cancerous. These abnormalities are called CIN (which stands for cervical intraepithelial neoplasia). This is not cancer, but contains cells which have the potential to develop into cancer.

Many more women develop CIN than will ever develop cancer. In most instances the CIN disappears and the cervix returns entirely to normal. In others, the CIN persists but does not cause the woman any problems and does not develop into cancer.

In some instances, however, the CIN gradually gets worse and sooner or later turns into cancer. Unfortunately it is not possible to predict with complete accuracy whether pro-

gression will occur. It is important, therefore, to identify those women who have CIN and treat the worst grades of CIN (CIN 2 and CIN 3). CIN 1 may either be treated or followed up at the discretion of the woman and her doctor. The majority of CIN 1 will return to normal, and so may not need treatment.

CIN does not give rise to any symptoms whatsoever. The usual way that CIN is suspected is by the presence of abnormal cells in a small sample taken from the cervix during a smear test.

THE SMEAR TEST

Cervical smear tests are taken at the family doctor's surgery or a Well Woman Clinic by the GP or a specially trained nurse. Having a smear involves removing your undergarments and having a small instrument called a speculum inserted into the vagina in order that the cervix can be visualised. Using a small wooden spatula or brush, a few cells are gently scraped off the cervix and wiped on to a glass slide which is sent to the laboratory. The test takes just a few minutes, and relaxation often helps to minimise the mild discomfort of this procedure (see diagram).

TAKING A CERVICAL SMEAR

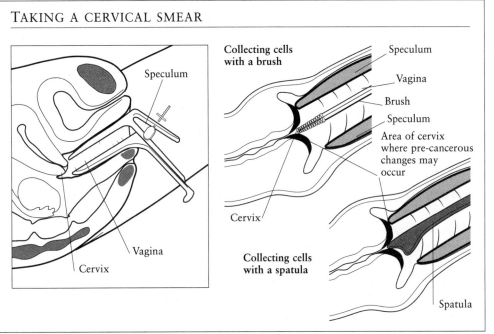

Left: A cervical smear may be taken using a brush or a wooden spatula.

The cells from the cervix are then closely examined under a microscope. The cervical screening laboratory will issue a result to the woman and her GP. This report will indicate when the next cervical smear test should be performed.

Women who have never had sexual intercourse or have had the cervix removed do not need to have cervical smear tests taken. Smear tests can be safely discontinued at sixty years of age if all previous smears have been normal. The GP or nurse may offer a smear below the age of twenty to women who have started having sexual intercourse below this age. Some regions in the UK run a computer recall system to remind women when the next smear is due. For this system to work, it is important that changes of name and address are registered.

PELVIC EXAMINATION

At the time of a cervical smear test, the doctor may offer to do an internal pelvic examination to assess the size of the uterus and the ovaries. For those women who are troubled with pain or swelling in the lower abdomen, or with abnormal periods, this pelvic examination may provide useful information. Depending on the results of this examination, the doctor may advise an ultrasound scan or referral to a gynaecologist. A pelvic examination involves the doctor inserting his/her fingers into the vagina and also pressing on the lower abdomen with the other hand. This usually involves only minimal discomfort for a few seconds.

ABNORMAL CERVICAL SMEARS

Approximately five per cent of all smear tests taken will show some abnormality. The majority of abnormal smears are not due to cancer but are caused by cells that are pre-cancerous. If the smear is abnormal, clear instructions are given on the report on what action is needed.

Frequently, smear tests may need to be repeated in three, six or twelve months' time. Occasionally infections can cause abnormal smears which will need to be treated before the smear is repeated.

If the smear is abnormal, a detailed examination called a **colposcopy** is usually required. Colposcopy involves the assessment and treatment of pre-cancerous abnormalities of the cervix. A specialist doctor inserts a speculum, a device to gently part the walls of the vagina, in order to visualise the cervix in detail with a magnifying lens. In order to highlight any abnormal areas, the doctor may paint some liquids on the cervix with a cotton wool bud. If areas of abnormality are found, these may be biopsied and sent to the laboratory for further analysis. The biopsy may completely remove the abnormal area, or further treatment may be required.

Very occasionally, the cervical smear test detects that a woman actually has cervical cancer. In this situation, she would be seen urgently by her local gynaecology department for further advice and treatment.

LOOP DIATHERMY EXCISION

This is a treatment for women with abnormal smears. It removes the area of the tissue that may be changing and provides a good tissue sample to send to the laboratory. Furthermore, it cuts a piece of cervix out rather than destroying it so a better biopsy is obtained (see diagram below).

THE LOOP AND HOW IT WORKS
A loop is a specially insulated fine stainless steel wire (about one-hundredth of an inch thick). By attaching the loop to a diathermy

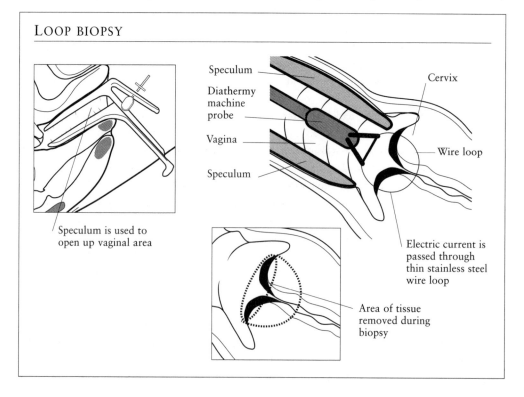

LOOP BIOPSY

Speculum is used to open up vaginal area

Speculum

Diathermy machine probe

Vagina

Speculum

Cervix

Wire loop

Electric current is passed through thin stainless steel wire loop

Area of tissue removed during biopsy

machine (a machine that delivers a specially modulated electric current) and by connecting the patient to another part of the machine the loop, when touching the cervix, completes an electric circuit and generates heat just around the edge of the fine wire. This heat allows the fine wire to cut easily through the tissues and also seal off all of the very small blood vessels. A smooth cut can be obtained easily with virtually no bleeding and removes all of the abnormal tissue in a matter of minutes (two minutes is the average treatment time). Before treatment is started a small amount of local anaesthetic is injected into the cervix. This effectively makes the treatment painless.

In the next six weeks after loop excision, most women will notice a discharge that might be blood stained initially. This is because the area from which the piece of cervix was removed has to heal. During the first six weeks it is advisable to avoid sexual intercourse and not to use tampons or anything else that might cause irritation to the cervix. This is standard advice following all treatment methods.

After six months a smear test will be performed and often a colposcopy as well. In over ninety per cent of cases all has returned to normal at this visit and by twelve months ninety-five per cent of treated women will have a normal smear test. Most patients can be discharged from the clinic after one normal examination although it is important to have regular yearly smears for five years. This can be arranged through the doctor or well woman clinic.

COMPLICATIONS

These are very uncommon. Some women (about three per cent) will have some heavy bleeding following treatment that may necessitate further treatment, although in most cases the bleeding

settles following bed rest and antibiotics (it is probably due to the healing area becoming infected). In an even smaller proportion of cases, the cervix can become very narrow when it heals; this is called cervical stenosis. This does not always cause problems but might make menstruation painful and occasionally requires further treatment. There is no evidence that fertility or childbearing are affected by the treatment.

Once the cervix has been allowed to heal women can enjoy a normal sex life. Treatment of the cervix neither alters enjoyment nor makes sex unsafe in terms of future health. It is important to ensure that adequate contraceptive measures are used unless pregnancy is desired.

If a coil is in place at the time of treatment this will generally be removed. It will therefore be necessary to employ alternative methods of contraception until either a coil has been refitted (about six weeks after treatment) or another method has been chosen. There is no need to stop the oral contraceptive pill.

Women who use a diaphragm or vaginal rings should refrain from inserting these until the cervix has healed. However, as intercourse is unwise until healing is complete then a change in method will not be necessary.

Theoretically a couple could embark upon a pregnancy as soon as the cervix has healed. Some doctors advise that a pregnancy should be delayed until the first check-up at six months. If any further treatment is required (unlikely) this could then be performed. It is not advisable to have treatment in pregnancy but if this occurs it does not appear to harm the pregnancy.

In a very small proportion of women the first treatment will fail to remove all of the abnormal cells. These will be detected at the time of re-examination six months after treatment. In most of these cases a simple repeat treatment is all that is necessary.

SCREENING FOR CANCER OF THE OVARY

Unlike breast and cervical cancer, there is no established screening programme for cancer of the ovary. This is because no test has yet been found which is sufficiently reliable for use in the general population. However, some cases of ovarian cancer run in families. Those women with several close relatives with ovarian cancer may be offered the opportunity to attend a familial ovarian cancer screening clinic. Although an ovarian cancer gene has been identified, widespread testing for this is not yet available. Regular pelvic examinations and ultrasound scans may be of help in those women at increased risk of ovarian cancer. A blood test for ovarian cancer called CA125 may also be offered regularly. A high level does not necessarily mean that there is cancer as it is increased in many other conditions which irritate the lining of the abdomen (peritoneum). However, a very high level in conjunction with an abdominal ultrasound scan is suggestive that ovarian cancer is more likely. Not all regions in the UK have ovarian cancer screening clinics.

ULTRASOUND BY VAGINAL PROBE

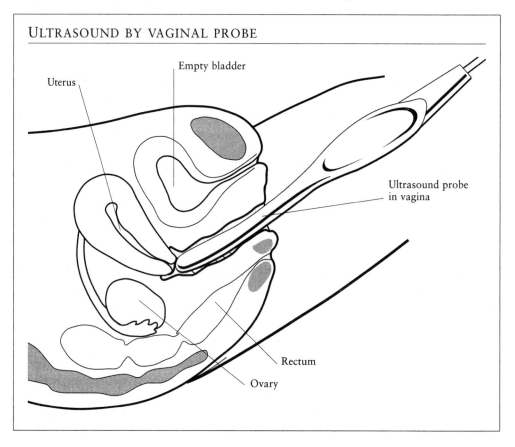

Uterus

Empty bladder

Ultrasound probe in vagina

Rectum

Ovary

OTHER HEALTH CHECKS

BLOOD PRESSURE

Blood pressure checks should be done regularly in those women taking the contraceptive pill or hormone replacement therapy. Your doctor may offer this every six months. High blood pressure does not usually cause symptoms, although occasionally it can cause headaches. Persistent untreated high blood pressure can increase the chance of strokes, so maintaining a normal blood pressure is part of general good health.

RUBELLA SCREENING

Rubella infection (German measles) causes a mild illness like 'flu with a skin rash. Unfortunately, when rubella affects a pregnant woman it can seriously affect the unborn baby. A safe and effective vaccine is available to prevent rubella infection which is now given to all young children. All women of reproductive age, who are not using contraception should ensure that they are already immune to rubella.

WEIGHT

Most people feel better when they are at or around the average weight for their height and build. A number of health problems, such as high blood pressure and diabetes, are more common in the overweight. Similarly, being severely underweight is not healthy and may have serious implications for the risk of conditions such as osteoporosis in later life.

For those who wish to lose weight, a healthy diet combined with a regular exercise programme is usually the best way of keeping the weight off and improving general health and well being. Many GPs can offer referral to a dietician or special clinic for those who wish to lose weight.

CHOLESTEROL AND BLOOD LIPIDS

These blood tests are offered occasionally as a screening test mainly for older women. A high cholesterol level or abnormal lipid levels can mean an increased chance of having a heart attack. Although heart disease is quite rare in women before the menopause, these blood tests may be useful for those who have a strong history of heart disease in their family.

BONE DENSITY

Post-menopausal women are more prone to osteoporosis and fractures of the hip, wrist and spine. Other factors such as family history, as well as diet, exercise, weight and smoking habits, also affect an individual's risk of developing osteoporosis. Women 'at risk' may benefit from knowing their current bone status by having a bone density screen. This is a simple non-invasive X-ray investigation which takes about ten minutes. More about osteoporosis can be found on page 282.

Chapter five

CANCER

There are few words that can strike as much fear as the word 'cancer'. It conjures up thoughts of suffering and pain. Many women who are diagnosed as having cancer immediately consider their future in the short term, with an awful outcome. Yet, advances in medical science and the treatment and prevention of cancer are being made continually and the outcome is not as depressing as it is sometimes perceived. In this chapter, some of the most commonly occurring cancers in women are examined – breast cancer and the gynaecological cancers, i.e. those affecting the pelvic organs, the womb (uterus), ovaries, cervix and vulva.

WHAT IS CANCER?

The human body is made up of tiny building blocks called cells. There are many different types of cells and those that are similar are grouped together to form tissues, such as muscle and skin. Within most tissues, cells eventually die and are replaced by new ones. If, however, the mechanisms that control cell death and replacement break down, more cells are made than are needed. If a large number of excess cells are made, a swelling will occur. This is known as a tumour and it may be either benign or malignant. Benign tumours are generally harmless but they may grow large enough to cause symptoms as they press on adjacent structures.

Cancer is the common term for a malignant tumour in which the cells grow into or invade the surrounding normal areas. They may enter the lymphatic vessels, which are part of the body's defence mechanisms and become deposited in lymph nodes where they may grow to form secondary tumours. Lymph nodes are found in many places; they are also referred to as glands and they may be felt in your neck if you have a throat infection. A malignant tumour may also penetrate arteries and veins from where they may be carried in the blood to other parts of the body.

CHANGES IN GYNAECOLOGICAL CANCER CARE

All regions in the UK now have specific clinics specialising in gynaecological cancers staffed by gynaecologists, oncologists, radiotherapists and specially trained nurses. This results in a more rapid access to the specialist required by the individual cancer patient.

These specialist cancer nurses and counsellors forge greater links with all specialists, in both hospitals and the community, thus providing improved continuity of care. Hospitals are assessed in an ongoing programme to ensure that the necessary structure is in place before they can claim to be a Cancer Centre or Unit. Not only have these recent changes benefited the patient in the holistic care setting, but may also increase survival rates.

SCREENING (SEE PAGE 75)

Screening is a way to detect abnormalities that have the potential to become cancerous, and, through early treatment, the development of a cancer can be prevented. Alternatively, screening can be used to detect a cancer at an early stage, allowing treatment and a greater chance of cure. Such is the case in breast cancer screening. In gynaecological cancers, the main screening programme is in the prevention of cervical cancer, through women having regular cervical smears. There are now more women having smears than ever before and this has resulted in a reduction in deaths from cervical cancer. Studies have commenced in the UK, Europe and the United States to assess methods of screening in ovarian cancer. These studies (clinical trials) will hopefully provide information as to the role of screening in this disease (discussed in the previous chapter).

ADVANCES IN RESEARCH

There is always the inevitable question: why does cancer occur? It is known that certain factors, such as genetic, environmental, social and personal, are all associated with humans developing cancer. Yet, some people do and some don't develop cancer, even though they have been in the same circumstances. There are indeed many unresolved questions, but progress is being made. For example, we can now recognise abnormal genes associated with an increased risk of ovarian cancer. These genes are also associated with breast cancer. This discovery is allowing scientists to further unravel the complexities of cancer and to identify other possible genes that may be involved, although it is important to stress that few women carry these abnormal genes. Applicable, not just to gynaecological cancers, is the greater understanding of how cancers grow, how the body's immune system fails to attack the cancer, and also how the cancer evades such attacks.

ADVANCES IN CLINICAL CARE

Although new ways of treating cancers carry great hope, improvements continue in the use of presently available therapies. For example, not long ago patients who required chemotherapy needed to stay in hospital and some problems associated with this treatment, such as vomiting, were difficult to control. Now many patients can be treated as outpatients, and new drugs practically eliminate the problems of nausea and vomiting.

For people requiring surgery, advances in anaesthetics and pain relief have resulted in many patients being discharged earlier than before. Anybody having treatment now may not recognise these changes yet these are equally important advances, albeit less publicised.

WHAT ARE CLINICAL TRIALS?

Most clinical trials compare different types of treatment. This may be drug treatment or a surgical procedure. A clinical trial is undertaken to resolve the question of whether one treatment is superior to another. It is not uncommon for patients to be concerned about these studies, particularly the feeling that they might be 'guinea pigs'. This is immediately understandable but misplaced. Unless a treatment is always effective and without side effects (which none are) it must be subject to comparison with other treatments. It is by studying the results of these studies that progress can be made. The treatment for many cancers today was at one time recognised as the best from the participation of patients in past clinical trials. Becoming involved in clinical trials is voluntary, and there are strict rules before a trial is even allowed to commence. Rather than viewing trials in a negative manner, patients should enquire about them. As already stated, the concept of a Cancer Team has evolved, but the most important person in that team is, of course, the patient.

PALLIATIVE CARE

Anyone involved in cancer care wants to improve the chances of cure and survival for patients. When this is not possible, the emphasis of care is alleviating symptoms and at all times maintaining the patient's dignity. This involves palliative care (relieving symptoms rather than curing the underlying disease). Unfortunately, the words palliative and terminal care are considered synonymous. Although terminal care is part of palliative care, the brief is much wider. Specialists in this area have a vast knowledge of symptom relief and, in fact, care for many patients who do not have cancer. Palliative care is now an intrinsic part of the Cancer Team. Their involvement is much earlier than previously, and should not be misinterpreted.

QUALITY OF LIFE

Defining quality of life is difficult, and each individual has a different perception as to what is a good or bad quality of life. There is a much greater awareness of the importance of quality of life, and many new treatments are assessed with this in mind. Although endeavours to cure remain the main objective, more attention is paid to using therapies which afford not just the best outcome but also optimum quality of life. Quality of life is not just a side effect of treatment. It is very individualistic, and the patient (not the doctor) determines how this quality is at any

given time. Again, the role of the patient as part of the Cancer Team is evident. With this information, a new dimension will be added to treatment decisions, increasing the possibility of 'best therapy with least harm'.

IS SURVIVAL IMPROVING?

The most basic yardstick to evaluate progress in cancer is the death rate from the disease. It is welcome news to see that there is a continued fall in the annual death rate from cervical cancer. This is, in part, due to more women having regular cervical smears. In ovarian cancer, the survival chances are also greater than before. With endometrial and vulval cancers, we still have to see the impact of new therapies, but there is no reason to consider that the future looks other than hopeful. Today, those women unfortunate enough to develop cancer have a greater chance of cure, and live longer with treatment side effects better controlled. Of course, there is no place for complacency and much work is still needed, but every year improvements and advances continue to be made. The road may seem long but we are heading in the right direction.

CHEMOTHERAPY

At its simplest, cancer can be described as an abnormal growth of cells where the normal mechanisms for its control have broken down. Increases in cell numbers occur in many situations – after all, we all develop from a single cell produced at conception and eventually grow into normal adult size. Similarly, when injury occurs, cells divide and grow in numbers to heal that injury. However, normal growth 'switches off' when the demand for repair or enlargement is no longer required. In the case of cancer, growth continues because the normal control of this process is defective. The control is lost because the genetic code within the cancer cell has been altered from that of a normal cell, sometimes by chance and sometimes by external factors, such as smoking or X-rays.

Patterns of growth and spread vary with the tumour type and site but it is the characteristics of invasion and spread that are the most difficult to tackle and this is why drug treatment (chemotherapy) has been developed to attack the cancer wherever it may be growing.

THERE ARE THREE MAJOR WAYS FOR TREATING THE CANCER:
1 To cut it out by surgery
2 To destroy the tumour by radiotherapy
3 To attack it with drugs.

RADIOTHERAPY

This uses specialised X-ray techniques to destroy the tumour cells. It can be focused on a very small area or used to treat a larger area, depending on the type of tumour. The surgical or radiotherapy approach is directed towards getting rid of the initial or primary tumours but does not address the problem of spread from the site of origin, which may already have taken place.

Cervical cancer may be treated with radiotherapy, which can be given by placing the radiation source in the vagina (see illustration on page 96). If there is distant spread then external beams will be directed towards the pelvis. For breast cancer these beams are aimed at the chest wall and arm pit. The position of these beams and the dosage of radiation are calculated with great care. Radiation kills rapidly dividing cells, including the cancer cells. However, it will also damage other healthy tissues such as the lining of the gut,

which leads to diarrhoea and abdominal pain. These symptoms usually respond well to medication. Pelvic radiotherapy may lead to urinary symptoms and in the long term the tissues become scarred with narrowing of the bladder and vagina. Scarring may also occur in the chest and lungs after treatment of this area.

There have been huge advances in the use of radiotherapy and complications are very much less than in years gone by.

GYNAECOLOGICAL CANCERS NEEDING CHEMOTHERAPY

Not all cancers need to be treated by drugs. Sometimes surgery with or without radiotherapy may be sufficient and in some cases chemotherapy has not proved very useful as yet and cannot be recommended. However, the subject is developing very rapidly and new drugs are coming on the market all the time, so that chemotherapy may, in the near future, be recommended for many more tumours than it is today. They decrease the rate at which cells divide. Since cancer cells tend to divide more rapidly than normal cells, they are affected to a greater extent.

GYNAECOLOGICAL TUMOURS
WHERE CHEMOTHERAPY IS USEFUL
■ Ovary
■ Uterus and cervix
■ Carcinoma
■ Trophoblastic disease
■ Germ cell tumours
■ Late stage carcinoma
■ Sarcoma in young people
The above list shows the kinds of gynaecological cancers for which chemotherapy is usually recommended but choice of treatment

COMMON CHEMOTHERAPY AGENTS	
Cytotoxics	**Biologicals**
Cisplatin/carboplatin	Interferon
Cyclophosphamide	Colony stimulating factors
Adriamycin	Tumour necrosis factors
Chlorambucil	Antibody therapy
Ifosfamide	
Vincristine	

in any particular case will be based on several factors. The doctor will need to know the extent of the tumour when it is first diagnosed – often called the stage of the disease. He/she will need to weigh the benefits to be expected against the unpleasantness or harm that may occur as a result of treatment. The doctor must also take into consideration other factors, such as the frailty of the patient or any other diseases that may complicate or undermine therapeutic benefits. Last, but not least, the doctor and the patient will need to discuss together the best way to go forward in the management of her illness. It is particularly important in all cancer treatment that she not only knows the diagnosis but also understands the treatment and investigation programmes that are being recommended and collaborates with the cancer team to get the best possible outcome.

WHAT DOES CHEMOTHERAPY INVOLVE?

The table above lists the common drugs (cytotoxics) used today for gynaecological cancer.

Biological therapies are becoming increasingly useful but as yet their place in overall treatment is still being assessed.

Treatment with cytotoxic drugs is usually given via injections into the arm vein (intravenously), either singly or, more commonly, as a combined chemotherapy, e.g. cisplatin plus cyclophosphamide. Intravenous treatment is necessary to get the right dose into the blood stream and therefore to the cancer.

Drugs are usually given over one to five days and this may mean you need to be admitted to hospital during the treatment. However, courses of treatment are normally given every three to four weeks and it is possible to be at home in between. The total length of treatment usually lasts about six months and it is important that during this time progress is monitored. A few cytotoxics are best given by mouth (e.g. chlorambucil) and the tablets are generally prescribed for five to fourteen days once monthly. Monitoring of the tumour on treatment tells the doctor whether a good response is occurring. If this is not happening, treatment will need to be changed or stopped altogether.

MONITORING THE STATE OF THE DISEASE

In gynaecological cancer this takes the form of general examination, including vaginal and rectal examination, blood tests, X-rays and specialised scans (including ultrasound) which may give better visualisation of remaining areas affected by cancer. The scans show whether the known areas of tumour are shrinking on treatment and the blood tests may reflect any shrinkage by a reduction in the level of what are called blood tumour markers. These are substances in the blood that tend to increase when a tumour is enlarging and decrease when it is shrinking.

SIDE EFFECTS OF CYTOTOXICS

Most drugs produce some unwanted results and cytotoxics are powerful agents which therefore produce other effects which can be very unpleasant and sometimes damaging. Thus it is very important that the treatment is given by experts in the use of these agents who know how best to overcome or avoid their worst aspects.

The most common side effects are nausea, vomiting and loss of head hair (alopecia). Nausea and vomiting have now been very much reduced or eliminated by the use of modern anti-vomiting agents, and sometimes hair loss can be prevented by the use of a scalp tourniquet. It should be remembered that the hair regrows normally as soon as treatment stops and sometimes earlier than that. In the meantime, a wig can be worn, or some patients prefer a headscarf.

While chemotherapy is being given, blood tests will need to be done to make sure that the drugs are not damaging the production of blood cells or kidney function. These tests are usually performed at the time when the next treatment is planned in order to avoid extra hospital appointments.

During treatment questions may arise that hadn't been thought of earlier and should be discussed with a doctor or nurse at the earliest opportunity. It is often useful to write down these questions as they come to mind and to take a list to the clinic as a reminder.

Other effects of chemotherapy that might occur with some drugs are tingling in the fingers or toes, noises in the ears or blood in the urine. If these do occur, the doctor or nurse specialist should be told so that the treatment can be modified if necessary.

Biological therapies are now being introduced into treatment of gynaecological cancers and many of them have very different effects from those of cytotoxics. Some are given into the abdominal cavity via a needle and with accompanying local anaesthetic. Others are given under the skin (subcutaneously) or by vein. If any of these agents are to be given then a full discussion of their use should occur so that you understand what is involved.

BENEFITS OF CHEMOTHERAPY

In association with surgery, and sometimes radiotherapy too, the purpose of chemotherapy is to reduce the number of cancer cells to zero. When the number of tumour cells is greatly reduced, the problems arising from the presence of the tumour will begin to disappear and when treatment stops you will begin to return to normal health. Full recovery may take up to twelve weeks. But one of the advantages of chemotherapy is that, in most cases, despite its immediate unpleasantness, recovery from the side effects is complete. The regrowth of hair is normal, nausea, vomiting and tiredness stop, and the blood production that may have been reduced will return to normal. Thus most tests can now be stopped and the doctor can simply keep an eye on your general health from time to time as an outpatient.

IMPORTANT AREAS OF CONCERN

SEXUAL FUNCTION AND FERTILITY

Whilst feeling unwell, either due to the illness or the treatment, sex may be unattractive to you but when you return to good health it may become important again. Sexual problems can occur because of the surgery you may have had, such as the removal of the uterus or ovaries. If the surgery has resulted in your periods stopping earlier than normal, it is important to discuss with your doctor the possibility of having hormone replacement treatment (HRT). This will prevent the problems that can arise from an early menopause.

In the case where you have still got at least one ovary and a womb, then the chemotherapy that is given in gynaecological cancer usually does not affect fertility. The younger you are when you have chemotherapy, the less likely that drugs will reduce fertility. This should be discussed with your doctor before starting treatment. When you feel well again and if you want a pregnancy this should also be discussed. It is important that during chemotherapy, however, you do avoid a pregnancy since the drugs might damage the baby, particularly in the first three months of a pregnancy when the baby's cells are growing rapidly.

PSYCHOLOGICAL AND OTHER SUPPORT

The diagnosis of any cancer can be a shocking experience and the consequent treatment is hard. Thus no one should be surprised if you need help from a variety of sources in the more difficult periods. Most cancer centres can help with psychological support, and there are many patient support groups. Ask your local hospital staff or your doctor for information about these groups.

It is important that you talk with your family too and that they have the knowledge to help you in the best possible way. Hiding the facts from your family is rarely helpful and often leads to misunderstandings and lack of trust, which can make a difficult situation much worse.

ALTERNATIVE TREATMENTS

Not all cancers can be cured, even today, and some patients may look for cure and greater hope outside conventional medicine.

Most doctors understand this need and will readily agree if you want to go to one of the clinics that are operating to support and treat cancer patients by other means. It is important, however, that you ask at those clinics the same questions you would ask your own doctors. The benefits and drawbacks of modern medicine have been tested and are known because of scientific enquiry and testing, whereas in some alternative areas there is more belief and very much less testing.

BREAST CANCER

There are 25,000 new cases of breast cancer in the UK annually and approximately 13,000 deaths. This is a very important fact, which affected women should be told because what it means is that overall about half of the patients who develop breast cancer are cured. Many women obviously think the worst when the diagnosis is made. They are full of morbid thoughts, and that basic fact about incidence and death incidence gets the whole illness/disease into context.

SCREENING

The basic premise underlying screening for breast cancer is that if it can be detected before it becomes palpable, then there is a higher chance of cure. (Screening has been discussed in depth in Chapter Four.) In other words, the single most important fact that governs survival in breast cancer is whether or not the cancer has spread outside the breast. The smaller the tumour, the less the chance of spread. So the smaller the breast cancer at the time of diagnosis, the more likely it is that the woman can be treated by breast conservation and without removing the breast (mastectomy).

TREATMENT OPTIONS

Overall, probably about eighty per cent of women with breast cancer can be treated by removing the lump (which is called breast conservation) probably with some breast tissue, whereas the remaining twenty per cent will need to have to have mastectomies. Having said that, there are some surgeons who are much more enthusiastic about breast conservation, and other surgeons who tend to favour mastectomy, so that there is some variation in the breast conservation/mastectomy ratio of individual surgeons. But overall, about eighty per cent of women diagnosed with breast cancer are suitable for treatment by breast conservation.

Who then is suitable for breast conservation and who is more suitable for mastectomy? Well, the women who are more suitable for breast conservation have smaller tumours, and particularly the tumours that occur towards the outside of the breast. The women who perhaps are better suited for treatment by mastectomy are those with central breast cancers and, of course, those with the larger breast cancers.

The next thing to stress is the importance of tumour spread. Tumour cells (or metastases) break off and start growing elsewhere

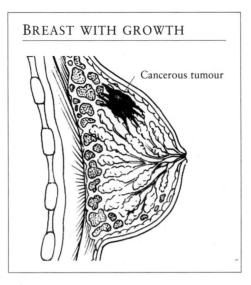

BREAST WITH GROWTH

Cancerous tumour

in the body. Initially, spread is often to lymph nodes which are glands normally involved in defending the body against infection. All tissues have lymph nodes and those principally associated with the breast are found under the arm (in the axilla). Involvement of these lymph nodes alters the type of treatment required. For example, if the nodes under the arm (axillary nodes) contain no tumour, then there is a seventy to eighty per cent cure rate. If the axillary nodes contain tumour, then the cure rate overall is forty to fifty per cent. Apart from giving information about the future, the status of the axillary nodes also determines what additional therapy should be advised, and that is particularly true in pre- and peri-menopausal women.

There have been two major advances in the treatment of breast cancer over the past ten years which have contributed to the beginnings of a reduction in mortality. The first is the screening programme to detect early breast cancers, and the second is the use of additional chemotherapy for pre- and peri-menopausal women who have tumour cells in the axillary nodes.

The other important additional treatment is tamoxifen. This is a drug that blocks the effect of oestrogen in the breast and this is particularly useful in post-menopausal women. Tamoxifen is a non-toxic agent and will give a small survival advantage. The problem with tamoxifen is that it can produce miserable side-effects, in terms of precipitating or worsening menopausal symptoms. Women taking tamoxifen may complain of flushing, which in many cases can be intolerable.

The other initial treatment used for breast cancer is radiotherapy. Virtually all women who are treated by breast conservation have to have radiotherapy to the breast. Women who have had a mastectomy do not need post-operative radiotherapy, but if a woman has been treated by breast conservation then she will be advised to have radiotherapy. This is usually given five working days per week and the treatment lasts for four to six weeks, depending on the amount of radiotherapy given per day.

TREATING ADVANCED BREAST CANCER

This involves treating women whose breast cancer has spread (or metastasised) from the breast and axilla to distant sites, and the commonest sites of metatastic disease in breast cancer are the bones, lungs and liver. If a patient has developed metastatic disease, e.g. bone, then they will experience bone pain, or possibly a fracture. If it has gone to the liver, the woman may present with jaundice. If it goes to the lung, then women get shortness of breath.

When it comes to treating metastatic disease, chemotherapy really is the most effective treatment, although it may be associated with unpleasant side effects. Drugs are used in this situation to prolong life.

There are lots of hormones that are used to help the symptoms of metastatic disease, particularly in the treatment of bone pain. For example, Tamoxifen, which has been described above, and drugs similar to progesterone can only be given in high doses.

CERVICAL CANCER

The impact of screening programmes on an organised basis is dramatically reducing the incidence of invasive cancer of the cervix. Cervical cancer is the third commonest gynaecological cancer in the UK. It appears to be occurring in the younger age groups, with approximately a third of cases occurring in women under the age of thirty-five. There is also an increase in the type of cervical cancer known as adenocarcinoma, which in the past has been relatively rare, accounting for only fifteen per cent of cases. There has also been a real and apparent increase in the incidence of pre-invasive (pre-cancerous) disease of the cervix over the last few decades. This is more than can be accounted for merely by a greater number of women taking advantage of the screening programmes.

We should be winning in this disease because we have quite a number of factors in our favour. There is a defined high-risk population, the cervix is reasonably accessible and there is a good screening test in the form of the smear. The disease process persists in a pre-invasive state for a number of years and, even if there is a failure to diagnose it at this time and the woman gets invasive cervical cancer, it generally shows itself at an early stage in its evolution by inappropriate bleeding, when cure rates are in excess of ninety per cent. The bad news, however, is that still 14,000–16,000 women die, perhaps unnecessarily, in England and Wales each year.

RISK FACTORS FOR CERVICAL CANCER

The traditional list of causes includes:
- Low socio-economic status
- Early age of first intercourse
- A large number of sexual partners
- Smoking
- Certain strains of human papilloma (wart) virus
- The unidentified male factor.

The list is, however, only helpful to a certain extent in providing a general profile of the woman most at risk, but many of the above factors are inter-linked, and in many instances women with cervical cancer do not fall into these risk groups. However, the combination of smoking, together with exposure to human papilloma virus, appears to be significant. This means that women who have this virus may reduce their risk of precancer or perhaps of cervical cancer by stopping smoking.

TREATING PRE-INVASIVE CERVICAL CANCER

The most commonly employed practice in the UK these days for pre-invasive cancer is loop diathermy excision of the lesion. The cervix is assessed under magnification, a process known as colposcopy (see page 82), and once the area of abnormality is diagnosed, it is excised using this technique which employs an electric current passed through a wire loop, and the superficial layer of skin on the cervix is removed and sent for analysis. This process is also aimed at removing all the abnormal area. It has a primary cure rate of approximately ninety-five per cent, but follow-up smears are recommended six months after treatment, to ensure that the patient is not in the five per cent who require re-treatment for persistence or recurrence. Thereafter, annual smears for three years are recommended.

TREATING INVASIVE CERVICAL CANCER

Unfortunately, however, some women develop invasive cancer of the cervix. This is more common in women who have not been having regular cervical smears. The symptoms associated with cervical cancers are irregular bleeding; between periods or after sexual intercourse, and vaginal discharge. In older women, post-menopausal bleeding may occur. The diagnosis of invasive cervical cancer may be suspected visually, but confirmed following biopsy. Following diagnostic confirmation, the woman is admitted to hospital for assessment of the disease under an anaesthetic. Usually, disease that is confined to the cervix is managed surgically. More advanced disease is treated by radiotherapy.

In its earliest form cervical cancer is classed as micro-invasive. This means the tumour is superficial with no spread. In these cases, if the woman is young and wishes to have children, removing part of the cervix (known as cone biopsy) is sufficient to provide adequate treatment. If her family is complete, however, a simple hysterectomy is the treatment of choice. Disease that is deeper but still confined to the cervix or just reaching the vagina is traditionally treated by a more extensive hysterectomy.

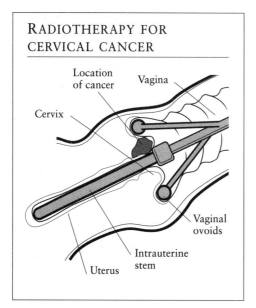

RADIOTHERAPY FOR CERVICAL CANCER

Location of cancer

Vagina

Cervix

Vaginal ovoids

Intrauterine stem

Uterus

If there is no spread, no further treatment is required and there is a ninety-two per cent chance of living five years. If there is spread, then the rate is reduced to forty-five to fifty per cent over five years. Traditionally, radiotherapy is given in these cases in addition to surgery. More advanced disease may not be suitable for surgery and radiotherapy alone is the best treatment. Long-term survival is lower when the patient presents with advanced disease.

Recurrent disease is treated with radiotherapy, if this has not previously been used. If the cancer recurs in the middle of the pelvis, surgery may be an option in some women. The extent of operation may be modified in some women very keen to have a pregnancy.

ENDOMETRIAL CANCER

The endometrium is the specialised lining of the womb, which in normally menstruating women is shed on a regular basis. Under the influence of the hormones manufactured by the ovary, a new layer of tissue develops which is very responsive to hormones. Oestrogen causes it to grow, whereas progesterone (made by the ovary after ovulation has occurred) causes it to organise and stabilise. Withdrawal of these hormones causes the endometrium to break down and bleed.

WHAT CAUSES ENDOMETRIAL CANCER?

Cancer of the endometrium is not common and is very uncommon before the menopause. Only ten per cent of all cases occur before the menopause and many of these are associated with conditions where there is excess oestrogen in relation to progesterone. The relationship between oestrogen and endometrial cancer is further shown by the increased risk of endometrial cancer in women who use hormone replacement therapy that does not contain progesterone. This is why, in women who have not had their womb removed, oestrogen and progesterone should always be given together as part of HRT.

Endometrial cancer is also more common in women who have not had children and/or who have a delayed menopause.

There is also an association between endometrial cancer and obesity which may be due to altered production and breakdown of oestrogen in obese women. There also appears to be an association between diabetes and endometrial cancer; again, obesity may be a common factor.

SYMPTOMS

The disease initially starts in the lining of the uterus and may cause bleeding at an early stage. This is why bleeding after the menopause should always be investigated thoroughly. Most women who bleed after the menopause will not have endometrial cancer but a minority will, and if diagnosed and properly treated at this point, they will have an excellent outlook (more than eighty per cent should survive beyond five years).

As the tumour enlarges, it erodes into the muscular walls of the womb and can spread to local lymph nodes or via the blood stream to more distant organs, such as the lungs. Before any treatment is planned for this disease, it is important to try and exclude the possibility that it may have spread beyond the womb.

TREATMENT

For early cancers, the treatment is removal of the womb and ovaries and, in some circumstances, the local lymph nodes will also be removed. Once the tumour has spread deeply into the wall of the womb, or, if on analysis it appears to be an aggressive type of tumour,

radiotherapy is given to the area after surgery to reduce the chance of the cancer recurring in this area. Radiotherapy is described on page 89.

Radiotherapy, alone or with hormone treatment, can be used in more advanced disease to help prevent symptoms such as bleeding but in these situations the outlook is not good.

Because there is some evidence that oestrogen can make the cancer grow, all but the most early cases should avoid the use of oestrogen after treatment.

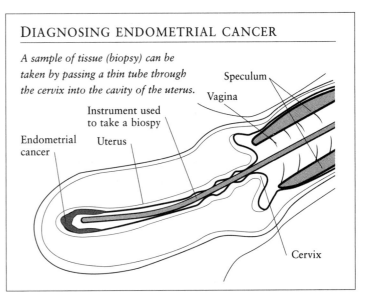

DIAGNOSING ENDOMETRIAL CANCER

A sample of tissue (biopsy) can be taken by passing a thin tube through the cervix into the cavity of the uterus.

Speculum
Vagina
Instrument used to take a biospy
Endometrial cancer
Uterus
Cervix

OVARIAN CANCER

Ovarian cancer afflicts a significant number of women each year and it is a disease that is often not well understood. There is a lack of symptoms in the early stages and up to two-thirds of patients will present with advanced disease. Consequently, due to this late diagnosis, it has a higher mortality than cancers of the cervix and uterus combined.

RISK FACTORS

Ovarian cancer occurs more commonly in the post-menopausal woman, and the peak incidence is in women in their sixties. There is a slightly increased risk in women who have not had children, and use of the contraceptive pill over a long period of time appears to confer some protective effect. Lifestyle habits, such as diet, exercise, smoking and alcohol, do not have an effect on the incidence.

SYMPTOMS

Patients with ovarian cancer can be asymptomatic (without specific symptoms), especially in the initial period. They often present to doctors in other specialties because of the non-specific nature of their complaints. The more common symptoms include an increasing abdominal girth, and the woman might have felt a lump in the abdomen. If she is pre-menopausal there may be irregular periods or bleeding, though post-menopausal bleeding is not a usual complaint. When the tumour becomes large enough to compress the bladder and rectum, there may be urinary or bowel symptoms. Other complaints are feeling generally unwell, loss of appetite and other symptoms that are really not specific to ovarian cancer.

WHEN TO CONSULT A DOCTOR
If you have any of the symptoms described, you should see your local doctor first. These symptoms do not mean that you have ovarian cancer, and only your doctor can make the diagnosis. An examination will be carried out, when a lump may be felt.

HOW DOES OVARIAN CANCER SPREAD?
A common route of spread is transplantation of cancer cells in the abdomen and pelvis. Spread can occur by means of blood and other fluids which circulate around the body.

ASSESSING THE CANCER

A staging system allows doctors to determine the extent of cancer in a particular woman. Staging in ovarian cancer is done at operation when a thorough assessment will be made of the abdomen and pelvis. Accurate staging is essential as any subsequent treatment will be based on this.

TREATMENT OF OVARIAN CANCER

The treatment in ovarian cancer is primarily surgical. Surgery allows the location and extent of disease to be determined, and the correct stage to be assigned. It usually involves the removal of the involved ovary as well as the other ovary, the uterus and both tubes. The fatty membranes, coverings over the intestines, called the omentum, are also removed as they are a common site of spread.

Occasionally removal of part of the bowel is necessary if it helps to remove as much of the tumour as possible. Rarely, a colostomy may be necessary if the two ends of bowel cannot be joined. These issues will be fully discussed with the patient prior to surgery, but the decision to carry out these procedures can only be made at the time of surgery.

The main aim at the end of surgery is to leave as little disease behind as possible, as this will influence the subsequent response to treatment and the prognosis.

In young women who want to have children in the future **conservative surgery** is indicated, but only in a select group of patients. Conservative surgery is only appropriate when the disease is confined to one ovary without evidence of involvement anywhere else, and it is imperative that the patient attends for close follow-up.

■ **Conservative surgery** may consist of removing just the tumour mass, leaving behind the ovarian remnant, the other ovary, both tubes and the uterus. Alternatively, the whole affected ovary is removed with preservation of the other reproductive structures.

In younger women, **ovarian germ cell tumours** are more common. Conservative surgery is usually carried out for these tumours as they tend to occur in the younger patient, and they respond well to various chemotherapy regimes. They are also associated with certain tumour markers which makes monitoring easier.

POST-OPERATIVE TREATMENT

This is indicated when there is advanced disease or disease that is not confined to the ovaries. Either single or combination chemotherapy can be given, the regime consisting of several courses over a few months.

TESTING FOR OVARIAN CANCER

Tests may be carried out if they are felt to be warranted on the basis of a woman's history or abnormal clinical signs which are found.

■ **Blood tests**: These include having blood taken for estimation of tumour markers. These markers are either substances released by the tumour into the blood or they are part of the body's response to the presence of a tumour. They only give an indication that a tumour may be present, and the levels may be raised in other non-cancerous conditions. In short, raised levels are not confirmatory evidence of cancer and they are useful mainly for monitoring purposes only.

■ **Ultrasound scan**: This useful test can detect a mass (lump) in the pelvis that cannot other-wise be felt. It can provide some information on the nature of the mass, especially when colour Doppler flow studies are carried out, but again they do not confirm or refute the presence of cancer.

Other tests are more specialised and include contrast studies to outline the urinary tract and computerised tomography (CT scans) which looks at the characteristics of tumour masses and the status of lymph glands in the body. They will guide your doctor in deciding whether surgery is necessary.

Your doctor will take a Papanicolaou smear from the cervix for screening. Cervical smears by themselves do not have any value in the diagnosis of ovarian cancer.

WHEN IS DIAGNOSIS CERTAIN?
Women, especially when they are premenopausal, may have enlarged ovaries due to the presence of totally benign cysts. These cysts result from cyclical hormonal changes and are functional; they do not in any way indicate the presence of cancer.

Other conditions that must be differentiated from ovarian cancer include benign tumours, endometriomas, pelvic inflammatory disease and pedunculated fibroids. In ovarian cancer, the diagnosis often can only be made at surgery, and confirmation by laboratory tests on the removed tissue is necessary.

FOLLOW-UP AFTER TREATMENT

The patient will be seen at more frequent intervals during the first two years after treatment as recurrence is more common during this period. At each visit, a thorough clinical examination will be carried out, followed by measurements of tumour markers at periodic intervals and computerised tomography (CT scans). The follow up will be for life.

Further surgery may be necessary for assessment and when recurrent disease is detected. Laparoscopy involves a telescope being introduced through a small cut below the umbilicus to look around the abdominal cavity; a more formal open operation may be necessary if a more thorough assessment is required. The main objectives of these further surgical procedures are to assess the response to treatment, and to remove more tumour if this contributes to an improved quality of life.

THE OUTCOME OF OVARIAN CANCER

The outcome in ovarian cancer is mainly dependent on the stage of disease. Eighty to ninety per cent of patients with early disease will survive five years or more and the proportion decreases to five per cent for advanced disease. But altogether over thirty five per cent will survive five years and this figure has hardly changed over the last thirty years.

DEVELOPMENT OF TREATMENT FOR OVARIAN CANCER

In specialised units, trials are constantly being conducted with different surgical approaches and using different combinations of drugs to improve the outcome in ovarian cancer. These trials do not in any way compromise the likely outcome in any individual patient, and may point the way towards an eventual cure for ovarian cancer.

IN THE FUTURE

As new drugs become available, the role and timing of surgery and chemotherapy may change in an attempt to select more effective treatment methods for individual patients. Multi-disciplinary specialised units are being developed to treat patients with gynaecological cancer in order to ensure that all aspects of patient care are taken care of. Advice is then freely available to the family and community as well as the patient herself.

VULVAL CANCER

Cancer of the vulva is not a common disease and it is unlikely that you and perhaps even your doctor will know anyone who has suffered from this condition. The vulva is the area of skin around the opening of the vagina. There are many different types of vulval cancer but the most common is a cancer of the skin, which is usually treated by means of an operation to remove the vulval skin and the lymph nodes in the groin. The chances of cure are excellent.

THE VULVA

In medical terms, the vulva is a diamond-shaped area of skin and subcutaneous tissue around the entrance to the vagina. At the front is the mons pubis and the anus is at the back. It is an area of skin, which on the larger outer lips, or labia majora, is hairy, whilst on the smaller inner lips or labia minora, which start at the front near the clitoris, it is hairless and smooth. Beneath the skin there is fat, even in very thin people: connective tissue, which supports the skin and glands which lubricate the area.

Special glands are located around the external opening of the urethra, which is the tube through which urine is passed from the bladder. Others are found at the back of the vagina, and these are called Bartholin's glands. These glands occasionally become infected and this may lead to an abscess being formed. Muscle is found in the deeper layers of the vulva beneath the skin and fat. This is arranged as a ring around the entrance of the vagina.

THE SKIN

The skin is a complex tissue which protects the body from damage. It contains a number of different cell types, the most numerous of which are the squamous cells. These give the skin its strength because they are arranged in many layers. Beneath these cells are nerves, blood vessels, both arteries and veins, pigment cells or melanoctyes and the cells of adjacent glands.

THE CANCERS

There is not only one specific type of cancer related to the vulva, but malignant changes may occur in any of the tissues although it is usually the skin that is affected.

■ **Squamous cell cancer** of the vulva accounts for nearly ninety per cent of all cases.

■ The swelling may also develop into a **warty cauliflower-like growth**. Spread occurs by direct extension and also to the lymph nodes in the groins and the pelvis.

■ **Verrucous** and **basal cell cancers**, which are also cancers of the squamous cells, rarely spread to the Lymph nodes.

■ The **melanocytes** or pigment cells may develop into a malignant melanoma, which usually arises as a painless black swelling, although it can occasionally be flesh coloured. It is very rapidly growing and spreads quickly to the lymph nodes. Because it can invade blood vessels it can also easily spread to other parts of the body.

■ Cancers may occasionally develop within the glands and these are called **adenocarcinomas**. The majority arise in one of the Bartholin's glands and start as a swelling just beside the back of the vagina. Bartholin's gland cancers may also be of the squamous type.

■ Very rarely cells of the fat, muscle, nerves or blood vessels may develop into a cancer called a **sarcoma**. In some cases, these are slow growing whilst in others they develop rapidly.

OTHER CANCERS

If there has previously been a cancer elsewhere, it is possible that spread to the vulva might occur. Spread from cancers of the cervix, the womb, the ovary and the bowel have all been reported. These are known as secondary cancers or metastases.

WHO GETS VULVAL CANCER?

Cancer of the vulva is usually seen in women who are over sixty. Only fifteen per cent of women with vulval cancer are under the age of forty, although those with a sarcoma are generally in a younger age group.

There is no known cause, although vulval cancer may develop from other areas of abnormality. These areas have a variety of appearances. They may be white, red or have a brown discoloration. The areas may be flat or raised but they may also resemble a wart. Any such areas should be shown to your doctor for evaluation.

WHAT ARE THE SYMPTOMS?

It usually starts as a small painless lump which grows to become an ulcer which may eventually become infected and painful. Despite the variety of cancers that may occur on the vulva, the symptoms are fairly constant. Very occasionally, bleeding may occur and, under rare circumstances, a vaginal discharge or an offensive smell may be noticed, particularly if an infection is present.

Often, in very elderly patients, the symptoms may be ignored. This is when the infection is more likely and leads to the symptoms described above. The lump can also get quite large. It is very important therefore that if any of the above symptoms are noticed they are immediately reported to a doctor for their advice.

THE SPREAD OF VULVAL CANCER

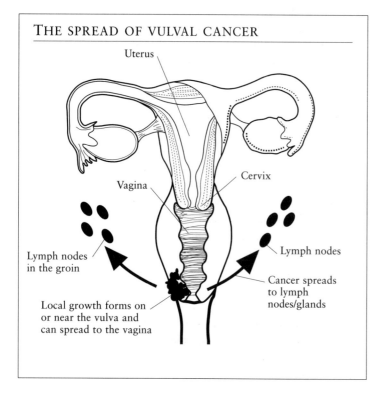

Uterus

Vagina

Cervix

Lymph nodes in the groin

Lymph nodes

Cancer spreads to lymph nodes/glands

Local growth forms on or near the vulva and can spread to the vagina

WHAT IS THE TREATMENT?

The treatment of cancer of the vulva depends on the type and its location. The usual treatment is radical vulvectomy and bilateral inguinal lymphadenectomy. This means that the skin and underlying tissue of the vulva are removed in addition to the lymph nodes in the groins. The nodes are removed because tumour cells may have spread there.

■ During a **radical vulvectomy**, the vulva, including the labia minora, the labia majora and the clitoris, is removed together with the underlying subcutaneous tissue. The vagina remains as a simple opening.

There are a number of ways of performing the operation. One method involves removing the skin and Lymph nodes of the groin and the vulva as one piece. In another procedure, the inguinal Lymph nodes are removed through separate incisions on both sides. The vulval skin is removed separately.

Following the operation a catheter is usually placed temporarily in the bladder and if the lymph nodes have been removed, there may be plastic drains beneath the skin of the groins. These help to release the excess lymphatic fluid which may become infected if it accumulates.

■ If the cancer is small, a simpler operation to remove just the cancer may be all that is required, with no need for further treatment.

■ If the cancer was not completely removed at the first operation or if the lymph nodes were found to contain tumour, **further surgery** or **radiotherapy** might be necessary.

Some types of cancer, the verrucous and basal cell cancers, very rarely spread to the lymph nodes and thus the treatment of these will not usually involve lymph node removal.

■ For cancers such as **malignant melanoma** and **sarcoma**, the lymph nodes are removed, only under special circumstances. If the cancer is diagnosed very early and lymph node spread is unlikely, they will not be removed. If the cancer is very advanced and there would be no advantage in removing the nodes, they may be left untouched. Under these circumstances chemotherapy might be suggested.

■ In rare circumstances, the cancer may spread widely around the vulva but will not spread to any other part of the body. In these cases, a large operation may be performed called a pelvic exenteration. This involves the removal of the vulva and all other internal pelvic organs, including the bladder and the rectum. This will mean that a colostomy and an ileostomy will be necessary to collect faeces and urine respectively.

ARE THERE ANY COMPLICATIONS?

In general, the operations for vulval cancer require prolonged surgery. If a radical vulvectomy and bilateral inguinal lymphadenectomy is performed the surgery may last between two and three hours and a hospital stay of several weeks will be necessary.

Because of this the women who undergo these operations are more prone to develop post-operative complications. The formation of a blood clot in the veins of the leg or deep venous thrombosis is not uncommon. Occasionally part of the clot may become dislodged and it may settle on the lung but special precautions are taken to prevent this. Heparin, a drug which is given by regular injections, helps to prevent both deep venous thrombosis and pulmonary embolism. Special stockings to compress the veins in the legs may also be worn for the same purpose. Sex after a radical vulvectomy may be more difficult. The vaginal opening may be narrower and if the clitoris is removed, sensation will be diminished.

WHAT ARE THE CHANCES OF BEING CURED?

The chances of being cured of vulval cancer are excellent. Because it is a skin cancer, it is usually detected at a time when surgical treatment is possible and no further therapy is required. Over ninety per cent of early squamous cancers of the vulva are cured. A successful outcome is less likely if the lymph nodes are involved or if there is an aggressive type of cancer present. Melanomas or sarcomas which have spread beyond the vulva are, unfortunately, rarely cured.

CAN IT BE PREVENTED?

Because we are unaware of any factors that may predispose to the development of cancer of the vulva, there is no easy answer to its prevention. Early recognition and prompt treatment are more likely to lead to a successful outcome. In this respect the treatment of precancerous areas may prevent the cancer developing.

If a swelling in either the vulva or the groin, vulval irritation or pain, bleeding or discharge develop, particularly in a woman in her sixties or older, she must visit her doctor or gynaecologist as a matter of urgency.

SUMMARY

Cancer of the vulva is uncommon but if it is detected early it has a high chance of being successfully treated. If there is any abnormality in the skin of the vulva medical advice should be sought as soon as possible.

Chapter six

SEXUAL INTERCOURSE

Human sexual expression is more than procreational, it is also recreational. Usually sex takes place in a non-exploitative environment of trust and affection and is part of confirming the bond that exists in the relationship between partners. However, sexual expression can have a darker side and be used or withheld to demonstrate domination or humiliation.

A normal physiological response to sexual arousal takes place when the physical and psychological components are healthy. Within this environment, a couple can choose and enjoy a full range of mutually agreed sexual behaviours. However, when there is a physical or psychological sexual problem this cannot

happen and failure can be devastating for the individual and the relationship.

Studies suggest that at least half the population will experience a sexual difficulty sometime during their lifetime. Women are more likely to seek help than men.

The biological function of sexual intercourse is to ensure that the man's sperm are released into the woman's vagina so that the sperm can fertilise an egg. In Western societies the most common position used to achieve this is with the man on top of the woman who lies on her back with her knees flexed and legs apart. The man positions himself between her thighs, supporting himself on his hands and knees. This enables the man's penis to enter the woman's vagina. In this position, the man can control his movements more than the woman but he can tire more easily. The female superior position gives the woman more control. Many couples enjoy a variety of positions – the Karma Sutra lists sixty-four elements in love play and forty-one positions in copulation! Side to side, and rear entry are other common positions enjoyed by both men and women.

Slang words used to describe sexual intercourse usually depict the act as being male active and female passive. However, both partners can enjoy being active or passive and may change roles during the same sexual encounter. It is not just that the penis enters the vagina, the vagina can also actively draw the penis inside.

Right: The male and female genitalia during intercourse.

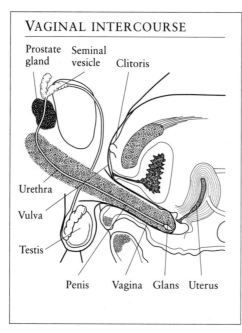

VAGINAL INTERCOURSE

Prostate gland
Seminal vesicle
Clitoris
Urethra
Vulva
Testis
Penis
Vagina
Glans
Uterus

ALTERNATIVES TO SEXUAL INTERCOURSE

Vaginal penetration is just one form of sexual expression although the method if pregnancy is desired. Couples may enjoy giving or receiving oral sex, anal intercourse or non-penetrative mutual masturbation. It is not uncommon for couples to change their pattern of lovemaking as they get older. Time taken in sensual non-penetrative love-making tends to increase, confirming the couple's affection. This places less pressure on the need to achieve prolonged intercourse which may become more difficult if the man has problems achieving an erection as he gets older and the woman has problems with vaginal dryness. Physical illness is also likely to affect sexual performance, either because of the disease process itself or because of side effects of medication. This is more likely to be a problem for the older couple. The ability to talk through any sexual difficulties and arrive at a mutually acceptable compromise, given the realities of any physical problem, will be essential to maintain the role that intimacy has in the relationship.

STAGES OF HUMAN SEXUAL RESPONSE

All humans possess a biological sex drive to maintain the species. The stages of the human sexual response cycle arise from this drive, beginning with desire progressing through arousal to orgasm.

Imagine that progressing from desire to orgasm is progressing up a staircase.

■ **Ground level** is non-sexual.

■ **Step 1** is desire without any physical change.

■ **Step 2** is when arousal begins and the man's penis begins to get firm but not firm enough for penetration, and the woman begins to lubricate.

■ **Step 3** is the stage when arousal progresses to give the man a firm erection that could penetrate, and in a woman more lubrication

---

STAIRCASE TO HEAVEN AND BACK

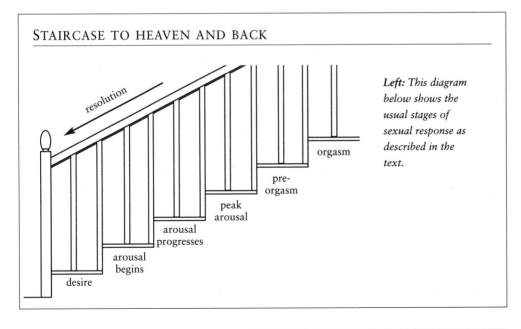

Left: This diagram below shows the usual stages of sexual response as described in the text.

resolution

orgasm

pre-orgasm

peak arousal

arousal progresses

arousal begins

desire

occurs, the inner part of the vagina opens and widens (balloons) and the lower third becomes engaged.

■ **Step 4** is like step 3 but excitement is more intense.

■ **Step 5** is when orgasm is recognised as being imminent.

■ **Step 6** is orgasm itself.

■ **Sliding down the banisters** is the process of returning to the ground.

With this analogy you can understand that you can climb on to the banister from any step on the staircase. As you slide, you take with you all the thoughts and feelings surrounding that particular sexual encounter. It is normal for both men and women to spend time going up and down some of the steps and not to go directly to step 6 in one dash up the stairs.

Men and women often progress up the stairs at different rates. Physiologically a man on step 3 can penetrate a woman who could still be on step one or even on the ground. The reverse is impossible. A common problem occurs when a man reaches step 3 and his partner is still on step 1. He wants penetration but she has little or no arousal response and experiences penetration as painful which blocks her from going further. He pushes on up to step 6 and slides down the banister passing her feeling frustrated, still on step 1 or 2. This scenario frequently precedes a woman losing interest in sex.

The important concept for both partners to understand is that each is responsible for their own progression up the staircase. The man is responsible for his orgasm and the woman for hers. Communication is therefore essential. There is no need to aim for synchronicity or even to make orgasm the goal. What is important is that each individual is comfortable with their own progress and that the thoughts and feelings that are around when returning down the banister are of fulfilment and contentment, not anger and resentment or a sense of failure.

SPECIFIC SEXUAL PROBLEMS

LACK OR LOSS OF DESIRE

This can affect men and women and means that the individual has reduced or no interest in sex. The situation may have always existed or may develop after a period of normal sexual interest. It is possible for low libido to exist in isolation but commonly it is secondary to some other sexual problem so that repeated unsatisfactory sexual experiences lead to a loss of interest. Deep seated personal problems or relationship difficulties often present with loss of desire. Chronic physical illness frequently leaves low desire because of fatigue, loss of self esteem, altered body image, or as a side effect of medication.

LOSS OF DESIRE FOLLOWING CHILDBIRTH

The transition to parenthood itself can be very challenging to the new mother and the new father as well as to their relationship. Depending on the individual's past role models it may be hard for either the man or the woman to accept that the mother can also be a sexual person. Sheer exhaustion is another common factor in loss of libido in new parents. An altered body image due to weight gain, stretch marks, altered breast size and shape or scars can also have an effect. Women who are breast-feeding may occasionally experience a temporary loss of sexual interest which is related to the changed hormone pattern necessary for breast feeding. They will have a high level of the hormone prolactin which is known to reduce interest in sex, and because they are unlikely to be ovulating they will have low oestrogen levels and may notice that they have reduced natural lubrication so that when sex does take place more added lubrication is needed.

A traumatic pregnancy or birth experience, post-natal depression or a sense of failure in the role of parent may all lead to a fear of future pregnancy and mistrust of contraception being adequate. This could present as reduced frequency of love-making which is really a demonstration of sexual avoidance rather than true loss of desire which may still be present.

LOSS OF DESIRE AFTER THE MENOPAUSE

This may arise because of hormonal changes. Loss of oestrogen itself does not seem to be linked to loss of interest in sex, more specifically to a problem with lubrication. However, if sex is perceived as painful then this is quite likely to lead on to sexual avoidance and therefore apparent loss of interest. There does seem to be a link for some women with low testosterone levels after the menopause. Testosterone is particularly thought of as the male hormone but it is also known to be relevant to the female sexual libido. It is produced in part by the ovaries and therefore for some women not only do they lose the female hormones oestrogen and progestogen at the

menopause but they may also significantly lose testosterone. This seems to be a particular problem for women who undergo a premature surgical menopause if they have their ovaries removed often at the time of hysterectomy.

LOSS OF DESIRE FOLLOWING HYSTERECTOMY OR STERILISATION

Loss of desire following hysterectomy is likely to be psychological unless the ovaries have also been removed. For some women their uterus is identified with their femininity and creative role. The loss of this important part of their body can be traumatic and it then becomes difficult to switch into a role of becoming sexual active for fun without the possibility of procreation. Occasionally sterilisation can have a similar effect. Usually those who have problems post-hysterectomy have had problems pre-hysterectomy.

LOSS OF DESIRE DUE TO HYPERPROLACTINAEMIA

Prolactin is a hormone produced by a small gland at the base of the brain known as the pituitary gland. It is the hormone that is released to stimulate milk production when breast feeding. Occasionally the pituitary gland can over-produce this hormone at times when the woman is not breast feeding. When prolactin levels are high, most women stop ovulating and would therefore also notice that their periods are absent or infrequent. The high prolactin levels may also stimulate milk production and so some leakage of milk from the breasts known as galactorrhoea may occur. High prolactin levels are also associated as a side effect of some medication – for example, drugs used in the treatment of severe depression or schizophrenia.

LOSS OF DESIRE SECONDARY TO MEDICATION

People are very individual in the way they respond to different medication. Certain treatments for high blood pressure and depression are particularly known to affect interest in sex. Some women find that the contraceptive method with hormones related to progesterone may reduce their sexual interest. If loss of interest in sex occurs with the onset of any form of medication, it is worthwhile considering this as a possible side effect and discussing this with a doctor to see if an alternative can be found. It may be that coming off the medication briefly will help to prove whether or not this particular medication is responsible or whether the problem has come about because of the illness itself or other problems.

TREATMENT OPTIONS FOR LOSS OF DESIRE

The treatment options for loss of desire are usually as follows:

1 Appropriate treatment of any underlying chronic physical illness may be beneficial
2 Individual or couple therapy
3 Drug options, including bromocryptine for hyper prolactinaemia; testosterone for post-menopausal women; and anti-depressants if clinically depressed.

SEXUAL AVOIDANCE, AVERSION & LACK OF SEXUAL ENJOYMENT

Sexual avoidance, aversion and phobias may stem from traumatic sexual experiences in childhood or adult life, or they may arise from receiving strong negative messages about sex so that sex leads to feelings of guilt shame or fear. Fear of pain may also be a trigger for sexual avoidance. It can be hard to differentiate between sexual avoidance and low desire because both will present as reduced frequency of lovemaking. However, it is important to differentiate between the two because the management approach will be different.

Sexual aversion and phobias can be total and therefore all sexual activity is avoided, or situational when only specific sexual activities trigger the aversion or phobia response. For example, a woman may be phobic about the male penis, semen, breast stimulation or oral sex. Sometimes the sense of possible loss of control during mounting sexual arousal can trigger a panic response so that low levels of arousal are tolerated but high levels of arousal are avoided. Sexual pleasure can also trigger a panic response if childhood conditioning has led to the belief that sexual pleasure is wrong.

TREATMENT OPTIONS

■ Gradual reintroduction of previously painful activities to regain confidence that sex is no longer painful. Vaginal trainers may help.
■ Gradual desensitisation to the sexual activity that is being avoided.

■ Deeper individual therapy may also be required where past trauma or past conditioning are responsible for the aversion or phobia.
■ Treatment with medication, e.g. serotonin re-uptake inhibitors or beta blockers if there is a strong physical component to the phobic.

PROBLEMS WITH ORGASM

This problem is related to either inadequate stimulation or to difficulty in letting go and losing control. Around ten per cent of women never experience orgasm. There should be a biological component to this and it has been speculated that because the woman does not need to be orgasmic to become pregnant there is less of a biological urgency to achieve orgasm and therefore women who cannot reach an orgasm would not be biologically selected out. There is a link between orgasmic problems and women who have chronic constipation, or are late starting their periods when teenagers. Therefore possibly there is a hormonal or nervous system component.

Another myth around female orgasm is that it is only a proper orgasm when it occurs during full sexual intercourse. Studies suggest that fifty per cent of women find it difficult or impossible to achieve orgasm during penetra-tive sex, but are readily orgasmic when their clitoris is stimulated either when they masturbate themselves or when their partner participates in their masturbation. Orgasmic problems can be helped by either individual or couple therapy. Group work with women has also proved a successful treatment approach. Two important concepts are needed for success with moving on to becoming orgasmic. One is the ability to lose control, and the second is the ability to take responsibility for one's own sexual arousal and stop feeling that the partner is responsible and stop the anxiety of feeling responsible for the partner.

TREATMENT OPTIONS FOR ORGASMIC PROBLEMS
■ Sex therapy: individual, couple or woman's group
■ Self help: to experiment with self pleasuring (masturbation)
■ Nipple stimulation at the height of sexual arousal: this has been found to help some women, possibly through the release of a hormone oxytocin thought to be involved in the orgasmic response
■ Use of sexually erotic material or sexual fantasy
■ Use of vibrators.

PAINFUL INTERCOURSE

Many women suffer painful intercourse (dyspareunia) on one or two occasions but most of them are unaccustomed to talking about this aspect of their life and find it difficult and embarrassing. Consequently individuals may not come forward with their complaint and may simply stop having sexual intercourse.

Delay in seeking help has, in the past, led to avoidable breakdown in family relationships.

Hence, the problem of painful intercourse requires a sensitive and understanding approach by professionals. An accurate diagnosis, with a detailed explanation, and prompt treatment will allay fears, prevent marital disharmony and increase the quality of life for both partners.

CAUSES OF PAINFUL INTERCOURSE

The causes of can be divided into two groups:
■ Those that result in pain on penetration (insertion of the penis)
■ Those giving rise to pain during, and sometimes continuing after, intercourse.

Those conditions responsible for deeper pain during intercourse often result in apprehension about sex and a reflex spasm of the sphincter-like muscle in the wall of the vagina, accompanied by lack of secretion, making penetration impossible. Consequently, the two groups overlap considerably.

PAIN ON PENETRATION
Causes under this heading are usually easily diagnosed following discussion of the symptoms and past events and a simple examination, seldom requiring any further tests. Both the woman and her sexual partner will experience pain on intercourse in most of these situations. The causes are:
■ Lack of vaginal secretions
■ Infections in the vulva and vagina
■ Spasm in the vagina muscle (vaginismus)
■ Pain from the scars of childbirth or vaginal surgery.

LACK OF VAGINAL SECRETIONS
The excitement phase of the female sexual response is accompanied by release of fluid by the vaginal skin. Prolongation of this 'fore-play' is rewarded by an increase in secretions. However, in the same way as fear leads to a dry mouth, the vaginal fluid is not released unless the woman is relaxed and confident in her love-making.

The vaginal fluid has a role in preventing the ascent of infection through the vagina, and its effectiveness depends on harmless bacteria which promote a mildly acidic environment. These conditions prevent growth of most other microbes. Cervical mucus changes through the normal cycle, being more copious and characteristically 'stringy' at the time when eggs are released at midcycle. Some women learn to use this sign to control their fertility, but it makes little contribution to lubrication.

The amount of vaginal fluid produced varies from person to person, according to the degree of stimulation and to women's habits with respect to vaginal hygiene. A fastidious approach to hygiene may paradoxically lead to reduction of anti-microbial protection and loss of natural lubrication. For a few days after using vaginal tampons secretions are often reduced.

Women approaching, or after, the menopause often suffer from vaginal dryness. The vaginal skin is thinned and produces a reduced amount of fluid and intercourse may be painful.

In all situations of reduced vaginal secretion the problem is remedied by use of lubricating agents. Water-based agents (such as K-Y Jelly) are rapidly absorbed and give transient relief from painful intercourse. More effective is a cream that binds to the skin of the vagina, holding water between its molecules and at the same time increasing anti-bacterial vaginal acidity. It can also be purchased without a prescription from most retail pharmacies under the name of Replens (or Senselle).

A long-term answer in menopausal women is the use of hormone replacement in the form of implants, tablets, patches, vaginal creams or pessaries.

INFECTIONS IN THE VULVA AND VAGINA

■ **Candida** and **Trichomonas**: Infection with Candida (thrush) will cause discharge (typically resembling cottage cheese), inflammation and pain on intercourse. Treatment is with anti-fungal cream or pessaries and, if recurrent, the sexual partner, who may not have symptoms, should be treated. Similarly, Trichomonas infection causes inflammation and superficial pain on intercourse. The vaginal discharge is usually light green in colour and frothy.

■ **Herpes virus**: Herpes infection is manifest as small, extremely painful blisters on the vulva and sometimes around the bladder outlet. Affected individuals should not have sexual contact until the ensuing scabbed-over areas have completely healed, as the infection will be passed on. Attacks last for between one and two weeks, and both sexual partners should be seen in the local genito-urinary medicine (GUM) clinic. Saline baths may ease the pain the drug, Acyclovir, may reduce the length of attacks. The disease is often recurrent and the same drug administered to the skin early in an attack can prevent its return.

■ **Bartholin's cysts**, abscesses and infected sebaceous cysts. Bartholin's glands produce mucus, and the ducts are present in the fold of skin at the back of the vulva. The ducts may become blocked with the appearance of a mucus-filled cyst which is usually painless unless infection occurs when an abscess forms. An infected cyst causes severe pain and requires surgical treatment. Unfortunately, recurrence can occur. Other infected cysts in the area are likely to be sebaceous cysts or boils.

MUSCLE SPASM IN THE PELVIC FLOOR

The vagina is supported by muscles which are usually relaxed prior to penetration. If contracted when penetration is attempted, severe pain will prevent insertion of the penis.

In extreme cases, the inner thigh muscles will not relax. Fears of becoming pregnant, despite contraception, sexual abuse or fear of recurrence of pain experienced during previous sexual intercourse may be responsible. The advice of a specialist in psychosexual medicine is essential; therapy will be directed at the couple together and includes exploring the causes of anxiety, counselling and understanding of the normal human sexual response.

PAIN FROM THE SCARS OF CHILDBIRTH OR VAGINAL SURGERY

■ **Childbirth**

There is no evidence of an increased tendency to painful intercourse when **episiotomy** is done compared to following natural tearing, when assessed at three months after childbirth. Either can heal with a painful scar, a web of tissue posteriorly or an area of **granulation tissue** (see below). Occasionally a cyst may form as a result of trapping surface cells underneath the skin and this is termed an **inclusion cyst** or an **epidermoid cyst**.

Ordinarily resumption of sexual intercourse is possible within six weeks of vaginal delivery. Breastfeeding mothers have reduced levels of vaginal fluid and may notice the vagina is drier and less compliant while this method of feeding continues. If pain occurs artificial lubrication is often helpful and careful perseverance is recommended as many problems will respond to the dilating effect of intercourse itself. Should pain persist, this should be reported at the six-week check and the area examined.

If scar tissue is the problem, special smooth glass dilators will be helpful. These are passed into the vagina several times each morning and evening. They are available in different sizes and dilation starts with the largest tolerable and continues with small increases in size until intercourse is again painless. A further check-up will be organised.

A small web of skin can form at the back of the entrance to the vagina. As a result of scarring this can be painful but will usually respond to regular massaging with a well-lubricated finger, pushing backwards.

A raised area, sometimes frond-like, which is red and bleeds easily is **granulation tissue**. If present at six weeks, it can be removed by cautery to the surface. The cause is overgrowth of the healing process, either in response to low-grade infection or irritation by suture material. A few sessions of treatment may be required to remove it.

■ **Painful intercourse after vaginal operations**
Intercourse is usually not recommended until six weeks after vaginal operations to allow healing and often the surgeon will want to do a check-up at this time. The success of operations performed for prolapse of the vaginal walls or womb depends on tightening the muscles and tissues around the vagina. An inevitable consequence of an effective operation is a narrowing of the vagina. In younger women, and older women who wish to remain capable of intercourse, a compromise can be reached. The desire to retain this function is discussed before the operation, but sometimes slight narrowing is unavoidable but should not ultimately have any adverse effect on the comfort of intercourse.

■ **Incomplete formation of the vagina**
This problem is extremely rare and varies from the vagina being represented by a shallow pit to the presence of two vaginas.

Treatment is highly specialised and

requires referral to a consultant gynaecologist. Modern therapy involves giving support to the couple and often no more than regular perseverance with sexual intercourse will improve or produce a functional vaginal tube. Plastic surgery operations can fashion a new vagina which functions well.

PAIN DEEPER IN THE PELVIS

Pain is caused during and after intercourse when there is pressure on ovaries, fallopian tubes or other organs of the pelvis, which may or may not be affected by a disease process. Only the woman will feel this pain and partners sometimes have difficulty understanding the problem. The causes are:
■ Pelvic inflammatory disease (see page 56)
■ Endometriosis (see page 58)
■ Ovarian entrapment with uterine retroversion
■ Pain only at mid-cycle
■ Inflammation of the bladder or bowel.

1 PELVIC INFLAMMATORY DISEASE
This is discussed in detail in Chapter Three (see page 54).

2 ENDOMETRIOSIS
This is discussed in detail in Chapter Three (see page 58).

3 RETROVERSION OF THE UTERUS
One fifth of women have a backward tilt to the uterus and most are unaware of this as it produces no symptoms. Some gynaecologists believe that painful intercourse can result because the ovaries intermittently come to lie behind the top of the vagina and between it and the back of the pelvis. The ovaries may then be caught during intercourse. This is

most likely with the woman in the dorsal position (lying on her back) and an alteration to the left side is recommended. An operation may be required to bring the uterus and ovaries forward and is successfully performed through the laparoscope .

4 PAINFUL INTERCOURSE AT MID-CYCLE

A small amount of blood may ooze from the surface of the ovary at ovulation. The result may be some local inflammation of the lining of the abdomen which is irritated by intercourse. The contraceptive pill will stop ovulation and help this problem.

5 INFLAMMATION OF THE BLADDER AND BOWELS

Infection in the bladder causes cystitis and during attacks intercourse is painful. Similarly, bowel inflammation from Crohn's disease, ulcerative colitis or irritable bowel syndrome will cause pain. If the urinary tract is at fault the pain will be reproduced by pressure forwards on vaginal examination, and if the bowel is affected then pressure posteriorly will elicit the pain. Disorders in these areas are usually short-lived and easily identifiable and treatable.

Chapter seven

CONTRACEPTION

Safe and effective contraception is now available free to couples in the United Kingdom from a number of different centres. In addition to general practitioners, Family Planning Clinics, the Brook Advisory Centre and most genitourinary medicine clinics all offer contraceptive services. Emergency contraception may be available from Accident and Emergency departments in general hospitals.

The Brook Advisory Centre is targeted at young people under twenty-four years of age. Many Family Planning clinics also offer services aimed at teenagers and young people. These clinics have a policy of confidentiality, although

---

EFFICACY OF CONTRACEPTIVE METHODS

% per 100 women per year

*Methods that have no 'user' failure

Injectable contraception	over 99% effective
Implant	over 99% effective in first year (over 98% per year over five years)
Intrauterine system (IUS)	over 99% effective
Intrauterine device (IUD)	98 to over 99% effective (depending on IUD type)
Female sterilisation (tubal occlusion)	over 99% effective
Male sterilisation (vasectomy)	over 99% effective

*Methods that have 'user' failure

Combined pill	over 99% effective
Progestogen-only pill	up to 99% effective
Male condom	up to 98% effective
Female condom	up to 95% effective
Diaphragm or cap + spermicide	up to 96% effective
Natural family planning	up to 98% effective

Note: The success of the first six methods in the table is not dependent on following any instructions on a daily basis or at the time of intercourse - there can be no 'user' failure.

The efficacy of the second six methods depends on how they are used - they are subject to 'user' failure. The efficacy rates given in the table for the second six methods reflect correct and consistent use. Where these methods are used less well, lower efficacy will be seen.

Table adapted from FPA Contraceptive Handbook by Toni Belfield, FPA 1997, with permission.

---

clients younger than sixteen will be encouraged to include their parents or guardians in making important decisions about contraception. However, unless in exceptional circumstances, neither the general practitioner nor the client's parents will be contacted without the express

permission of the client who attends the clinic.

In many centres, couples can seek additional advice about other aspects of sexual health. Contraception is offered free of charge when obtained on the National Health Service.

CHOICE OF CONTRACEPTIVE

There are many factors that may play a part in an individual woman's decision about which contraceptive to use. Some of these factors are discussed below.

EFFECTIVENESS

Contraceptive methods vary in their reliability. However, some women are prepared to accept a less reliable method according to their personal circumstances, A method of contraception that may not be sufficiently reliable for a young woman may be quite acceptable for an older woman who is less fertile.

AVAILABILITY

Women (and men) may be put off by having to talk to the pharmacist, nurse or doctor about contraception. However, condoms are available by mail order, in slot machines and from garages and shops.

COST

Although contraceptives are free under the NHS, local NHS Trust budgets do not always allow ordering of sufficient supplies to meet demand. This means that not all methods are available in all areas, depending on demand, but choice may be greater in larger clinics. In each

centre, the available options will be discussed by a specially trained health professional.

ACCEPTABILITY

Contraception can be viewed as a nuisance which interferes with the pleasure of sex. Also, perceived health risks may be a worry, although health professionals can make sure that the method chosen is not unsafe for the individual concerned. Some methods are not associated with intercourse and so do not reduce spontaneity (pills, implants, injectables, IUS and the IUD). Others may reduce sensitivity (male condoms) or be felt to be messy (diaphragms or caps with spermicide).

INFLUENCE OF PARTNER, FRIENDS AND THE MEDIA

A partner will obviously have their own views on preferred methods. Friends may have had particular experiences of contraception. Lastly, the media sometimes exaggerate papers published in medical journals into a scare story which puts undue emphasis on the disadvantages of a method. If there is concern about health risks or side effects, it is helpful to get more information to give a balanced view of the available methods which results in an informed decision.

PERSONAL, RELIGIOUS AND CULTURAL VIEWS

Ideas about contraception may well have been influenced by sex education received and attitudes to marriage, having children and abortion. Some religions are opposed to contraception of any type as interfering with a divine process.

LIFESTYLE AND RISK OF SEXUALLY TRANSMITTED INFECTION

Some methods are highly protective against sexually transmitted infections (male and female condoms) while other methods give no protection (natural method, oral contraception (the pill)).

HORMONAL METHODS

COMBINED PILL

This is so called because it combines two hormones: oestrogen and progestogen. It works mainly by suppressing egg development within the ovary (ovulation). One pill a day is taken for twenty-one days and then there is a seven-day break. During the break a 'Withdrawal bleed' takes place which is generally lighter than a period. The pill is taken every day, with seven placebo (without an active ingredient) tablets taken during the withdrawal bleed time. Many women are reassured by a regular monthly bleed.

By the time seven pills have been taken, the ovaries become inactive. However, egg development will start during the 'pill-free' week and if the pill is not taken for more than seven days, even with a break of eight or nine days, there is a risk that ovulation may occur and thus pregnancy. It is therefore essential that a woman does not forget to restart her pill on time. Luckily a packet of pills is always started on the same day of the week which helps with the routine. Pills should be taken at the same time of day and no longer than twelve hours late. Some manufacturers incor-

porate seven inactive pills in the pack (ED; every day). This can be useful for women who prefer to take a pill every day.

ADVANTAGES OF THE COMBINED PILL

■ Very reliable when taken according to the instructions
■ Usually makes periods shorter and lighter
■ Often relieves painful periods
■ Often relieves premenstrual symptoms
■ Reduces the risk of cyst formation in the breast
■ Reduces the risk of fibroids and ovarian cysts
■ Significant protection against cancer of the ovary and the lining of the womb (endometrium)
■ Decreases the chance of developing anaemia.

DISADVANTAGES OF THE COMBINED PILL

■ Potential for forgetting pills and misunderstanding instructions
■ Minor side effects in some women when first starting the pill, such as headaches,

■ Weight gain, bleeding during the pill-taking days

■ Some women develop high blood pressure

■ There is a very small risk of serious circulatory disorders: heart attack, stroke or a clot in a vein (venous thrombosis). For this reason the pill is not suitable for smokers over the age of thirty five

■ Some drugs may reduce the effectiveness of the pill, particularly those taken for epilepsy, and occasionally antibiotics. Pregnancy is then more likely. The effectiveness of the pill may also be reduced by severe diarrhoea and vomiting

■ No protection against sexually transmitted infections

■ A very small extra risk of having breast cancer diagnosed during pill use and for ten years afterwards

■ A possible small extra risk of cancer of the entrance to the womb (cervix).

Note: If a woman is properly assessed by a doctor or nurse before taking the pill, any factors that would make it too risky to take the pill can be ruled out or, if present, alternative methods can be recommended.

PROGESTOGEN-ONLY PILLS

These pills, which used to be known as 'mini-pills', contain no oestrogen. They act mainly on the mucus in the cervix, making it impenetrable to sperm. The method is slightly less effective than the combined pill, but reliability is good, particularly for older women who have lower fertility.

DISADVANTAGES

■ There is less margin for error in pill-taking than with the combined pill, this pill needs to be taken no longer than three hours late

■ Periods can be different: either erratic or absent

■ Possible side effects include acne, depression, headaches, fluid retention and loss of sex drive

■ When a pregnancy does occur, there is a very slightly higher chance that it may be ectopic (outside the uterus)

■ A small chance of developing ovarian cysts which can cause pain but usually disappear without treatment.

ADVANTAGES

■ It is suitable for older women (particularly those who smoke or who have 'risk factors' for heart disease or for stroke)

■ It can be taken while breastfeeding

■ It can be used by women who have other reasons for not being able to take the combined pill, e.g. repeated bad migraines.

CONTRACEPTIVE IMPLANTS

The currently available implant consists of a small rod which is inserted into the upper arm. This rod releases a continuous low dose of contraceptive hormone. A local anaesthetic is used to numb the arm during insertion and when the rod is removed, which takes just a few minutes.

ADVANTAGES OF CONTRACEPTIVE IMPLANTS

■ Long-acting

■ Very effective

■ Instant return of fertility on removal.

DISADVANTAGES OF CONTRACEPTIVE IMPLANTS

■ Fitting is by a minor surgical procedure and must be performed by trained personnel since removal can be more difficult if the fitting has been carried out incorrectly

■ A few women will develop ovarian cysts.

INJECTABLE CONTRACEPTION

There are two injectable contraceptives:
■ A twelve-week injection (Depo-Provera®)
■ An eight-week injection (Noristerat®).
The injection is given into the buttock or upper arm. The hormone injected is released very slowly into the body. These preparations are highly effective as they work in several ways, including suppressing ovulation. Side effects include weight gain in a few susceptible individuals (particularly with Depo-Provera®) and others as for all progestogen-only methods (acne, depression, headaches, fluid retention and loss of sex drive). Particularly with Depo-Provera®, most women's periods will eventually stop, since the endometrium (lining of the uterus) becomes extremely thin and inactive. This is not harmful.

ADVANTAGES OF INJECTABLE CONTRACEPTIVES
■ Very effective
■ Can be used while breastfeeding
■ Stops symptoms related to menstrual cycle e.g. premenstrual syndrome
■ Associated with most of the benefits of the combined pill

DISADVANTAGES OF INJECTABLE CONTRACEPTIVES
■ Possible delay in the return of normal fertility
■ Cannot be removed once given
■ Requires regular attendance at a medical centre.

INTRAUTERINE SYSTEM (IUS)

This is like a combination of an IUD and a progestogen-only method. Instead of copper wound round the plastic frame, there is a chamber containing progestogen, which is released slowly for up to five years. The device is inserted into the uterus in the same way as an IUD (see right). The only such device available so far is called Mirena®, which currently has a licence for five years. The hormone released into the cavity of the uterus makes the endometrium very thin but most women ovulate most of the time. Irregular bleeding often occurs and may persist although eventually many women experience virtually no bleeding. The hormone does get into the blood stream at a level similar to the progestogen-only pill and so similar side effects are possible (acne, depression, headaches, fluid retention and loss of sex drive). Mirena® costs much more than an IUD and is not available in some parts of the United Kingdom.

ADVANTAGES OF IUS
■ Highly effective
■ Immediate return of fertility after removal
■ Menstrual loss is reduced (in fact, the IUS is being extensively used for the treatment of heavy periods, particularly for women in their forties. It is more effective than tablet treatments, and may lead to avoidance of hysterectomy)
■ Reduces painful periods
■ Reduces the chance of an ectopic pregnancy
■ Reduces the chance of pelvic inflammatory disease.

DISADVANTAGES OF IUS
■ Has to be fitted by a doctor, and rarely perforation of the uterus may occur at fitting
■ May be expelled by the uterus
■ A few women develop ovarian cysts.

The depot preparations (Depo-Provera® and Noristerat®), contraceptive implants and the Mirena intrauterine system are more effective than female sterilisation.

NON-HORMONAL METHODS

INTRAUTERINE DEVICES (IUDS)

These are flexible devices providing a plastic frame or thread round which copper wire or tiny copper sleeves are fixed. The device is inserted into the uterus by a trained doctor or nurse. An internal examination is necessary to check the size and position of the uterus. A speculum is inserted into the vagina in the same way as when a cervical smear is taken. A special device is used to measure the length inside the uterus and then the IUD is carefully inserted through the cervix into the uterus. Some cramping, like a period pain, takes place but is usually over within a few minutes of the procedure being finished. The threads hang a little way down into the top of the vagina and can easily be checked by self-examination.

INTRAUTERINE DEVICE

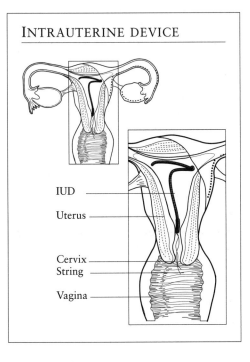

IUD
Uterus

Cervix
String

Vagina

IUDs work mainly by stopping fertilisation; they do not cause abortion. The newest IUDs are very reliable and are effective for up to ten years. Women who have not had children can have an IUD fitted, but it may be more difficult to fit than in women who have had children.

ADVANTAGES OF IUDS
■ Long-term reversible contraceptive
■ Hormone-free
■ Very effective.

DISADVANTAGES OF IUDS
■ Has to be fitted by a doctor or nurse; rarely, uterine perforation may occur
■ Periods may be heavier, longer and more painful, particularly at first
■ Expulsion can occur
■ Pelvic infection can occur – usually immediately after fitting (the chance is low in those women not at risk of sexually transmitted infection).

DIAPHRAGMS AND CAPS

These female barrier methods are made of latex rubber or plastic, are inserted into the vagina, and cover the cervix. Diaphragms and caps are different. They come in different sizes and must be fitted initially by a doctor or nurse to make sure that they cover the cervix adequately; the doctor or nurse will teach the woman exactly how to use the method. They are used with spermicides (see page 121). There is no limit to the number of times they can be used. Devices which are currently available must not be worn for longer than thirty hours at a time because of the possible

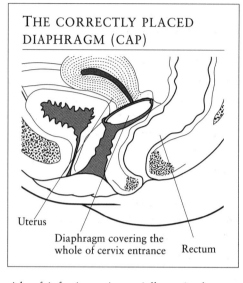

THE CORRECTLY PLACED
DIAPHRAGM (CAP)

Uterus

Diaphragm covering the
whole of cervix entrance

Rectum

Right: The diaphragm in position, covering the cervix.

■ May protect against cancer of the cervix, some sexually transmitted infections (but not HIV) and against pelvic inflammatory disease
■ No health risks
■ Under the direct control of the woman.

DISADVANTAGES OF DIAPHRAGMS AND CAPS

■ It can take time to learn how to put a cap in easily and correctly
■ Needs forethought so that it is in place prior to intercourse
■ Must be positioned carefully
■ Women have an increased chance of having cystitis (a smaller cap may be needed)
■ Latex types must not be used with oil-based products, such as bath oils and certain vaginal creams and pessaries
■ Local irritation can occur from the rubber or the spermicide.

risk of infections. A specially trained nurse or doctor should check the diaphragm or cap annually to ensure that it does not need changing. Occasionally they become damaged or a different size may be required. Weight gain (or loss of 7 kg/15 lb) abortion, pregnancy or miscarriage will mean that the size needs to be checked.

ADVANTAGES OF DIAPHRAGMS AND CAPS

■ Can be put in at any convenient time before intercourse and so need not interfere with spontaneity

FEMALE CONDOM

This is made of polyurethane, is larger than most male condoms, and has two flexible rings. Like a male condom it is used once only and comes in a single size. The method is available from pharmacies and from certain family planning clinics. The condom is inserted into the vagina using the inner ring as a guide. The outer ring lies flat against the body, covering the vulva.

ADVANTAGES OF FEMALE CONDOM

■ No known side effects
■ Protects against sexually transmitted infections (including HIV) and may protect against cancer of the cervix and pelvic inflammatory disease
■ Under the direct control of the woman
■ Can be inserted at any time before intercourse takes place

Right: The cap in position over the cervix.

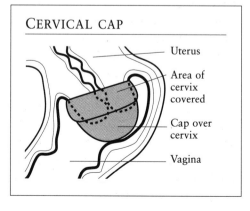

CERVICAL CAP

Uterus

Area of
cervix
covered

Cap over
cervix

Vagina

FEMALE CONDOM

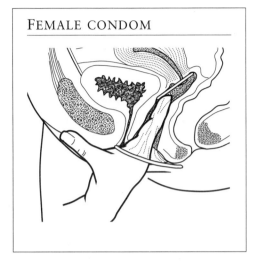

- Does not need male erection before use
- No hurry for man to withdraw after ejaculation
- Does not need spermicide
- Can be used with oil-based products
- Odourless.

DISADVANTAGES OF FEMALE CONDOM
- Requires careful placement
- Off-putting size and appearance
- Less sensitivity for the woman
- Can get pushed into the vagina by the penis during intercourse reducing its effectiveness.

MALE CONDOMS

These are made from latex rubber, many now of the hypoallergenic type which is less likely to cause irritation, or they can be made from polyurethane. Recommended condoms to use are those that carry the BSI Kitemark and a BS EN mark. Condoms come in a variety of types: unlubricated, lubricated with silicone or spermicide, coloured, ribbed, teat-ended, plain-ended, shaped and flavoured.

Like all other barrier methods, condoms must be used before there is any genital contact. The closed or teat end of the condom is squeezed to expel any air and leaves about a centimetre to receive the ejaculated semen. It is then rolled down over the full length of the erect penis. After ejaculation, and before erection is completely lost, the condom should be carefully removed, holding it firmly at the rim as the penis is withdrawn.

ADVANTAGES OF MALE CONDOMS
- No side effects
- Easy to obtain and use
- The man takes responsibility for birth control
- Can protect either partner against some sexually transmitted infections, including HIV
- Can protect the woman against cancer of the cervix and pelvic inflammatory disease
- Needs no medical supervision.

DISADVANTAGES OF MALE CONDOMS
- **Requires forward planning**
- **Loss of sensitivity during intercourse (not with polyurethane condoms)**
- **May interrupt intercourse (but putting on the condom can be enjoyed as part of foreplay)**
- **Can split or come off**
- **Latex condoms cannot be used with oil-based products (water-based lubricants such as KY Jelly® are OK) but polyurethane varieties can be used with any products.**

SPERMICIDES

These chemicals kill off sperm. They are inserted into the vagina before intercourse. They come in the form of creams, jellies, aerosol foams or pessaries. They are not effective enough to be used alone for contraception, except for women going through their

Left: Fitting the female condom into position in the vagina.

menopause. They are useful for use together with barrier methods as described above.

ADVANTAGES OF SPERMICIDES
- No serious side effects
- Easily available and simple to use
- Provide lubrication.

DISADVANTAGES OF SPERMICIDES
- Can cause irritation or sensitivity
- Regarded as 'messy' by some.

NATURAL FAMILY PLANNING

Natural family planning or 'fertility awareness' is a method based on recognising ovulation by bodily symptoms and signs and thus working out whether the woman is in her fertile or infertile phase. Usually, a combination of daily temperature recordings, observing the mucus from the cervix, checking for characteristic changes in the cervix itself and certain other symptoms is used. Very few general practices or family planning clinics are trained to teach natural family planning. Personal instruction from a specially trained teacher is essential.

A fertility device, Persona®, is a way of using technology instead of symptoms and signs. The system consists of a hand-held monitor and disposable urine test sticks. The system detects hormone changes in the urine. A woman performs eight tests a month at key times in her cycle and these are interpreted by the device. A red light shows for fertile days and a green light for non-fertile days. Despite the 'high-tech', the method is not very effective, with a six per cent failure rate.

THE FERTILE PERIOD

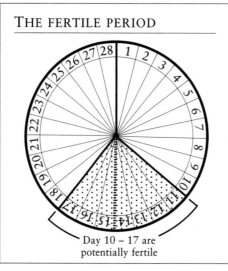

Day 10 – 17 are potentially fertile

Right: In a 28-day cycle, days 10-17 are those on which conception is most likely to occur.

STERILISATION

As sterilisation is a permanent non-reversible method, it is important to be aware of the choices now available before such a final decision is made. Today there are very effective, acceptable, long-acting, reversible methods that may not be considered carefully enough before a decision is made to opt for sterilisation.

Couples thinking about sterilisation should seek information and counselling from a doctor or nurse. This helps to minimise subsequent regret. Regret is unavoidable for some individuals with around one in three of all marriages breaking down.

Having made a decision to undergo sterilisation, couples will reap the benefits of a lifetime of protection against pregnancy by a single action and no need for subsequent medical care under normal circumstances.

FEMALE STERILISATION

Female sterilisation is achieved by blocking or cutting the fallopian tubes (tubal occlusion). It is usually carried out under general anaesthetic, although in some centres local anaesthetic may be an option. The usual method is by laparoscopy. A doctor makes two tiny cuts, one just below the navel and the other just above the bikini line, to reach the fallopian tubes. A laparoscope is then inserted into the abdomen – this is a thin, telescope-like instrument. It has magnifying lenses which allow the doctor to clearly see the reproductive organs. The doctor seals or blocks the Fallopian tubes, usually with clips or rings. A woman will need forty-eight hours of rest away from heavy work after the operation.

It is important to know that tubal occlusion is not 100 per cent effective. There is a failure rate of one in every 200 women.

Pregnancy resulting from failure of the method does not necessarily occur immediately after the operation, but may occur some years later. Pregnancies resulting from failure of sterilisation are more likely to be ectopic than usual.

ADVANTAGES OF FEMALE STERILISATION

■ Effective immediately

■ No further contraception is required, but other means of contraception must still be used for the initial period after sterilisation.

DISADVANTAGES OF FEMALE STERILISATION

■ Means having an operation in hospital with an anaesthetic

■ Reversal is very expensive (not readably available on the NHS in all areas) and may not be successful.

FEMALE STERILISATION BY LAPAROSCOPY

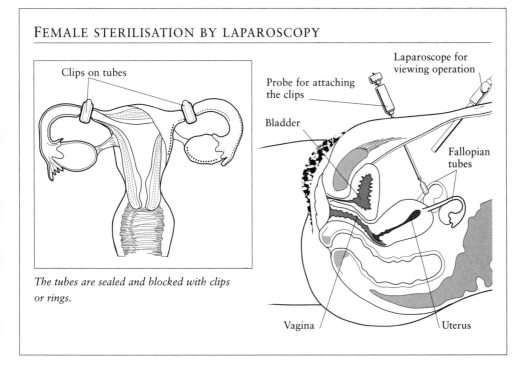

Clips on tubes

The tubes are sealed and blocked with clips or rings.

Laparoscope for viewing operation

Probe for attaching the clips

Bladder

Fallopian tubes

Vagina

Uterus

VASECTOMY

Male sterilisation involves cutting the vas (the tube that carries the sperm from the testis to the penis) each side so that sperm cannot be ejaculated. It is almost always carried out under local anaesthetic and does not need to be performed in an operating theatre. After freezing the skin, a tiny incision is made to locate the vas, the vas each side is brought out onto the surface and a section removed. The ends are treated in such a way that they are not likely to grow back together.

After the operation a man may have some bruising and swelling in the scrotum; he should wear tight underpants day and night for a week and avoid heavy lifting, vigorous sport, intercourse and masturbation until the swelling is settled.

There is no effect on male sexual function; sex drive is unaffected as testosterone is still produced in the testis and the semen appears the same in quantity although there are no sperm in it.

Research shows that there are no serious long-term health risks from vasectomy. A small minority of men develop chronic testicular pain.

ADVANTAGES OF VASECTOMY
- The operation is a minor one
- Very reliable (more effective than female sterilisation)
- No further action will be needed about contraception.

DISADVANTAGES OF VASECTOMY
- Not effective immediately (two semen samples must be produced and checked for absence of sperm before stopping contraception)
- Reversal is very expensive (not available on the NHS in all areas) and may not be successful (less reversible than female sterilisation, especially if it is a long time since the vasectomy was performed).

EMERGENCY CONTRACEPTION

Emergency or postcoital contraception can be used in the event of unprotected intercourse. This is contraception which works after fertilisation but before a fertilised egg implants in the lining of the uterus; it is not abortion. The episode(s) of unprotected intercourse may be the result of no contraception being used, failure of a method being used regularly, forgotten pills or accidents with a method. It is best to seek medical advice even if unprotected intercourse took place during a non-fertile part of the cycle. Treatment is extremely safe.

THE HORMONAL METHOD

Hormonal emergency contraception aims to prevent the fertilised egg from implanting, thus preventing pregnancy. These methods comprise either oestrogen plus progestogen in combination, or progestogen-only tablets. Having taken emergency contraception after one episode of unprotected sex, another reliable contraceptive method must be started immediately. If the next period is delayed by more than fourteen days, then a pregnancy test should be performed.

Emergency contraception is available from family planning clinics, general practitioners and Accident and Emergency departments and should be taken within 72 hours of intercourse.

FITTING AN IUD

The other form of emergency contraception is to fit an IUD. This method is used less often but it is more effective than the hormonal method and works even if there has been more than one episode of unprotected intercourse. The IUD can be inserted up to five days after unprotected intercourse or known ovulation, so there is more leeway.

The IUD can either be taken out after the next period or left in as an ongoing method.

ABORTION

Abortion is not a method of contraception. However, it has been legal in Great Britain for the last thirty years in certain specific circumstances and is an important back-up if pregnancy occurs when not wanted, either due to failure of contraceptives or because contraception was not used for whatever reason. It may be that emergency contraception will reduce the need for abortion, but accidents do happen and there will always be unintended pregnancies (see page 138).

Chapter eight

SEXUALLY TRANSMITTED INFECTIONS AND VAGINAL DISCHARGE

The majority of women will have a troublesome vaginal discharge at some point in their lives, and many women will have contact with sexually transmitted infections.

In order that infections are recognised and correctly managed, it is essential that sexually active couples have an understanding of these conditions. The great majority of infections can be easily managed, and confidential help is available regarding the avoidance, recognition and treatment of sexually transmitted infections and vaginal discharge.

Genital infections may cause a variety of symptoms, or may be completely asymptomatic. Sexually active men or women may be infected by a partner who is a long-term carrier of infection yet is completely unaware of this. Some of the long-term risk of certain sexually transmitted infections are infertility, due to Fallopian tube damage and pelvic pain. Both of these conditions can be difficult to treat.

For these reasons it is vital that sexually active women have an understanding of sexually transmitted infections, know where to seek information and advice and how to act to protect their future fertility. Because there is no single ideal contraceptive method which effectively protects against pregnancy and provides protection against sexually transmitted infections, couples are often advised to consider using barrier contraception to prevent infection in addition to other (e.g. hormonal) methods in order to protect against unwanted pregnancy.

TYPES OF INFECTION

Infections are classed as sexually transmitted because they are only passed between the moist and fragile skin surfaces of the genitals, mouth and, occasionally, the eye by intimate contact via vaginal secretions, seminal fluid, blood and, very rarely, saliva. Some of these infections can be transmitted from mother to baby during, or sometimes before, delivery. The organisms do not generally survive or remain infectious when cooled or dried, and so are not passed from towels or toilet seats. The most important groups of infection are:

■ **Bacteria**: Chlamydia, gonorrhoea, syphilis, which are curable with antibiotics

■ **Viruses**: Warts, herpes, hepatitis, HIV, which can usually be treated to improve symptoms.

Since chlamydia, warts and herpes are common, they will be discussed in some detail. The rarer conditions will be discussed briefly before concluding with a consideration of the main causes of abnormal vaginal discharge – candida and bacterial vaginosis – which are not sexually transmitted infections.

The hidden nature of most sexually transmitted infections means that it is not possible to rely on any simple check-list of symptoms before deciding to get tested. It is much more important to think about individual risk, and the type of protection against sexually transmitted infections used. The younger the individual, the less well developed are defences against infection, and the more serious the consequences. The older the couple, the greater the opportunities there may have been to acquire infections in the past.

WHEN TO CONSIDER A CHECK-UP

■ As part of a general health check when initiating a new relationship
■ When not using condoms
■ When trying to conceive.

WHEN TO SEEK HELP

■ Following unprotected sex
■ If either partner suspects infection

■ If either partner has sex with others
■ Following sexual assault
■ When symptoms are present.

SYMPTOMS WHICH MAY SUGGEST A SEXUALLY TRANSMITTED INFECTION

■ Lower abdominal pain
■ Pain during or after sex
■ Bleeding after sex
■ Irregular spotting/bleeding between periods
■ Suddenly heavier periods after starting a new relationship
■ Pain or difficulty when passing urine
■ Increased or smelly vaginal discharge
■ Rash, spots, lumps, ulcers or itching over the genitals.

The most obvious need for thorough infection testing comes from a combination of recent symptom and recent risk. Having a cervical smear will not, by itself, identify a sexually transmitted infection. If the possibility of infection is present, then it is advisable to ask a health professional for the appropriate tests.

COMMON INFECTIONS

CHLAMYDIA AND PELVIC INFECTION

Chlamydia (*Chlamydia trachomatis*) is the most serious and the most common curable sexually transmitted infection. It is the main cause of infection of the uterus and fallopian tubes (pelvic inflammatory disease or PID) and the main preventable cause of pain with

intercourse (dyspareunia), infertility and ectopic pregnancy. As seventy-five per cent of both women and men with chlamydia will have little or no sign of the infection, neither they nor their partner may suspect that anything is wrong.

WHO DOES IT AFFECT?
Nobody knows exactly how common chlamy-

dia is, because only a few of those infected seek screening, and even women with symptoms were not offered tests in the past. The infection is found most commonly among women in their late teens and men in their early twenties, with studies in women in general practice showing between five and fifteen per cent of women infected at the age of twenty. The highest recorded infection rates – of around twenty-five per cent – occur in women under twenty seeking abortion, which is why it is essential to be checked and treated for chlamydia before termination of pregnancy to prevent the infection spreading.

Nine out of ten chlamydial infections are acquired before the age of twenty-five, as are most other sexually transmitted infections. However, some sources estimate that, for people currently aged thirty-five to forty-five, one-quarter to one-third may have been infected at some time.

SCREENING TESTS AND SYMPTOMS

Screening tests for chlamydia are done by cervical swab, and the accuracy is improved by taking a urethral sample. Since some routine tests are not 100 per cent effective at picking up chlamydia infection, antibiotic treatment may be advised before the results of tests are available. Long-term problems, such as infertility and pelvic pain, may be avoided by immediate treatment.

When symptoms of infection occur in women, they tend to be subtle and non-specific, which means they are common to other conditions. Some of the more severe symptoms are lower abdominal pain, which may be similar in nature to period pain but unrelated to menstruation and, most important, pain with sex on deep penetration (deep dyspareunia). These symptoms may indicate spread of infection into the pelvis (PID), but can

also be caused by other conditions such as endometriosis, ovarian cysts, gut pain or bladder infection, and, in emergencies, by ectopic pregnancy or appendicitis.

Chlamydia can occasionally infect the throat and the eyes and can be transmitted at birth; it is one cause of 'sticky eye' (opthalmia neonatorum) in babies, and causes infant pneumonia at around six to eight months of age. It is easily treatable.

The chlamydia organism usually lodges in the urethra and cervix, where it may remain undetected. However, in about half of all cases it spreads into the uterus and fallopian tubes. This spread may be triggered by menstruation, the insertion of an intrauterine device, or by abortion, and may be months or even years after the initial infection. Repeated infection (continuing intercourse with an infected partner) increases the chance of damage.

Chlamydia inflames the lining of the uterus and destroys the hairs that waft the egg down the fallopian tubes. This damage – salpingitis – which occurs in a minority of women is usually silent. It is the most common cause of tubal factor infertility and is strongly linked with ectopic pregnancy.

PELVIC INFLAMMATORY DISEASE (PID) (SEE ALSO PAGE 54)

The consequences of one episode of painful PID can be serious, and are multiplied by repeated infection.

Damage after one episode of PID

■ Fifteen per cent chance of tubal infertility (doubles per recurrence)

■ Twenty per cent chance of chronic pelvic pain

■ Seven- to ten-fold increased risk of ectopic pregnancy

■ Eight-fold increased risk of hysterectomy

Treatment of PID

The sooner it is treated, the better. The outcome is much improved by starting treatment within two days of the onset of pain using appropriate antibiotics (doxycycline or azithromycin) and making sure that the partner is also treated. In research studies, very many partners of women with PID are found to be infected unknowingly. If sexual partners are not treated it is very likely that the woman may become reinfected and may have further episodes of PID. In Scandinavia, PID has almost disappeared due to widespread chlamydia screening of women and education targeted equally at men.

If there has been pain with intercourse, seeing the couple together provides an important opportunity to advise on the need for care when intercourse is resumed after treatment, to avoid triggering any further pain. This might be due to residual physical damage, inadequate treatment, or a wrong diagnosis, in which case other investigations will be required. Alternatively, a cycle may develop where anticipation of pain may cause a failure to relax, which will cause further deep pain. This produces stress in the relationship, making it very difficult to unravel the physical and psychological factors.

PARTNER TREATMENT

It is important to abstain from intercourse during treatment of a sexually transmitted infection until the partner has also been checked and treated, to protect from reinfection. Broaching the subject with a partner or contact can be daunting and stressful for many people. Advice is available from the nurses or doctors in gynaecology wards or outpatients, and practical advice will be offered by the health advisor if seen in a sexual health clinic. They can help by talking through how a conversation might be started. Explanatory leaflets are available for both partners, and the health advisors can make the initial contact.

What a partner needs to be told depends on whether there is pelvic pain – possibly due to infection – or whether tests for infection have proven positive. As the advice is similar, the following points should be of assistance in de-stressing and de-stigmatising the situation to achieve the desired result of the partner attending for a check-up, with minimum recrimination:

■ Infection may be without symptoms
■ Infection may have been present for some time and may precede the relationship
■ Treatment should be finished before recommencing intercourse in order to prevent reinfection
■ Infection is one of the many causes of pelvic pain
■ All attendance and discussion at sexual health clinics are confidential.

In the case of sexually transmitted infections due to viruses – which are not cured by antibiotics – the above principles still apply, but the advice given to women and their partners on the chronic nature of the infections must be put into sensible and pragmatic perspective.

WARTS

Most sexually active people – possibly around ninety per cent – will have been exposed to the wart virus (human papillomavirus or HPV), but relatively few ever develop visible genital warts, which appear as small growths around the vaginal opening and labia. Physically, they are not a serious disease (as they do not spread to other parts of the body and rarely bleed or cause discomfort), but are more of an unsightly cosmetic nuisance, often having a profound effect on body image and sexual self-esteem.

It takes a minimum of two to three months for warts to grow after exposure, but the interval varies widely. A reasonable analogy is the sowing of poor quality seed into soil – most of it never grows but, occasionally, a shoot will appear. New growth is probably triggered by healing of small cuts in the skin after the friction of sex. Thus it is often impossible to say how long ago an individual was infected. In pregnancy, warts grow more easily, often appearing for the first time – this does not mean they were 'caught' recently. They cannot harm the baby during the pregnancy, and very rarely cause difficulty with delivery. Although briefly exposed during birth, their transmission and growth in the baby is exceptionally rare.

TREATMENT OF WARTS

In most cases, genital warts eventually heal by themselves. This takes longer in smokers and recurrences are more likely, because smoking damages the immune defence cells in the skin, hindering the natural elimination process. The wide variety of available treatments are designed to remove the visible wart by simple destruction – freezing, cutting or burning – or applying a chemical cream or fluid to reduce the growth. They can do nothing about hidden wart particles in the nearby skin.

It is now known that visible genital warts are mostly of HPV types 6 and 11, which are not the wart virus types associated with cancer of the cervix (most commonly HPV 16, which infects the skin without producing growths). Thus, contrary to advice given in the 1980s, women with visible warts do not require more frequent (annual) smears.

HERPES

Genital herpes is caused by the herpes simplex viruses (HSV types 1 and 2) which infect the skin of the mouth and genitals, travelling along the nerves that supply touch and pain sensation, to lodge in the nerve roots in the spine. Although the nerves are not damaged the virus reproduces in the spine and travels back to the skin, causing blisters which itch and then burst to form painful ulcers which often cause pain on urination, and should heal within one to two weeks.

The herpes virus is present throughout the population. By their mid-twenties, some sixty per cent of people carry it – mostly as cold sores acquired at some point during their childhood or adolescence. Most genital herpes in the under-twenty-fives is nowadays HSV type 1, transmitted in monogamous relationships, usually from a partner who is unaware that they have had cold sores or genital infection. This is almost certainly due to oral sex being a regular part of the sexual repertoire of the majority.

SYMPTOMS OF HERPES

First exposure to herpes is usually preceded by 'flu-like symptoms and sometimes headache for around a week before the appearance of blisters, and accompanied by tingling or numbness over a wider area of skin (mostly the buttocks and backs of the thighs) and occasionally complicated by constipation and inability to pass urine if the rectum or urethra are infected, although those infected may have all or none of these symptoms.

Most people suffer very little from the virus, and the symptoms are often confused with candida or bladder infections. Many women assume they have thrush or cystitis, as the symptoms recover in a few days without treatment, or regardless of incorrect self-treatment.

For ninety-five per cent of those infected, recurrences happen infrequently, and are very rarely as severe as the first attack. Episodes are usually preceded by numbness or tingling – the prodrome – which acts as a warning. Many are triggered by other acute illnesses, stress during major life events, or in the pre-menstrual period.

MISUNDERSTANDINGS ABOUT HERPES

Three important misunderstandings about herpes require clarification:

■ Contrary to what was thought up to the late 1970s, it is now clear that herpes is not the cause of cervical cancer, so women do not require annual smears.

■ Mother-to-baby transmission of herpes is exceptionally rare in Britain. Some eighteen babies will be severely affected by herpes each year, only three born to women with a known past history of genital herpes (out of 700,000 deliveries annually). There is no value in routine swabs for herpes before delivery, and caesarean section is now reserved for cases where ulceration occurs during labour. If you have genital herpes, discuss with your obstetrician what plans are in place if your herpes is present during labour.

■ Genuine first-attack herpes in mid-pregnancy is rare, but can be successfully and safely treated with intravenous anti-herpes drugs. When a woman experiences genital herpes for the first time during a pregnancy, it is almost always her first visible episode, rather than newly acquired infection.

The biggest problem with herpes is not the physical symptoms, which can be suppressed or prevented with one of the three specific anti-herpes drugs (aciclovir, valaciclovir or famciclovir) in the five per cent or so of people who experience them frequently or severely, but what, when and how to tell the next partner. Treatment, and detailed, sympathetic advice and assistance with these issues is available from sexual health clinics.

OTHER INFECTIONS

GONORRHOEA

Gonorrhoea causes the same spectrum of disease as chlamydia: genital symptoms are more obvious, pelvic pain is greater, yet long-term complications tend to be less severe. Discharge and bleeding or painful urination more often appear sooner after infection, with perhaps two-thirds of men and one-third of women noticing a problem. Medical care is the same, with swab testing, antibiotics and urgent partner treatment.

Gonorrhoea is now rare in Britain outside large inner city populations or business travellers and holidaymakers returning from abroad. This means that tests for gonorrhoea are rarely offered outside sexual health clinics.

SYPHILIS

Syphilis and gonorrhoea were the original 'venereal diseases', infecting about one-tenth of the UK population at the beginning of the twentieth century. With careful tracing of contacts, the arrival of penicillin in the 1940s, routine screening in pregnancy since the 1950s and HIV prevention in the 1980s, syphilis had almost disappeared in Britain, with fewer cases per year in women than the number of STI specialists in the country.

The recent epidemic in Eastern Europe and parts of Asia has reintroduced the infection to Britain. As it is transmitted during pregnancy, causing severe crippling disease to babies, and is completely curable with antibiotics, antenatal screening will remain an essential part of both personal and national prevention.

HUMAN IMMUNODEFICIENCY VIRUS (HIV)

HETEROSEXUAL RISK

For most women, concerns about HIV will be greatest around the beginning of a new relationship, when planning a pregnancy or, most acutely, after sexual assault. While a full consideration of how HIV affects women's lives and health, and advice on protection is well covered elsewhere, a few important facts may help clarify women's realistic risk of infection and help with decisions regarding testing.

Although HIV, like all other sexually transmitted infections, is more easily transmitted from man to woman, some female partners in long-term relationships with HIV-positive men remain uninfected, regardless of how long they had practised unprotected sex before their partner's diagnosis was discovered. HIV may be most highly infectious for a short time (from two to three weeks to two to three months) at the start of the infection.

HIV can be transmitted at any time and it is sensible in a new monogamous relationship to use condoms until you and your partner

have been tested for HIV if there are concerns that either partner might have been exposed in the past. Following unprotected sex in a short-term or casual relationship, it is important to remember that there is a three month interval before tests can be certain to be negative (they can become positive within one to two weeks at the earliest). This does not mean that there should be a delay in getting a full sexual health check-up for other infections, but it is advisable to be re-tested at three months.

Because it is possible that very early treatment with anti-HIV drugs (within a few hours) can reduce transmission from a known positive source in blood injection accidents, all hospitals have policies and facilities for treating staff and patients who may have been exposed to HIV.

TESTING AND PREGNANCY

HIV can be transmitted by an infected mother to her baby. This may occur during pregnancy perhaps most frequently during delivery and also via breast feeding. The risk of transmission in women who carry HIV and breast feed can be as high as thirty per cent. This risk of transmission can be very substantially reduced to around eight per cent in women who know they are HIV positive. It is recommended that HIV positive women have their pregnancy managed by an obstetrician with approved experience. The same factors as above – including trauma during delivery – determine the chances of mother-to-baby transmission during pregnancy and at birth. Depending on local maternity unit policy, at the booking visit, the midwife may strongly suggest that an HIV test is done as part of the routine screening, or the opportunity to have an HIV test should be available to those who wish it.

The main benefits of testing are: if negative, reassurance; if positive, the ability to markedly reduce risks of transmission to the baby by anti-HIV drug treatments, better medical treatments for HIV to maintain the mother's health during and after the pregnancy, or the option of considering termination. This latter course is uncommonly chosen by women, or recommended by doctors, except when the woman is found to be unwell with late-stage HIV disease – as these have the greatest transmission risk.

Although there is no ideal time to be found to be HIV positive, the blow will be greater halfway into a pregnancy. In England, less than one-fifth of the HIV infected mothers identified by anonymous screening are known to their antenatal team. This means that some women will only discover that they are infected when, for instance, their newborn child becomes unwell. It is sensible for woman to seek HIV testing before pregnancy, as a normal part of good preconceptual preparation.

■ Think about being tested before pregnancy, at the start of a new relationship, or three months after a 'risky' contact.

■ A negative test says nothing about the current partner.

■ A negative test in the partner says nothing about personal risk.

■ A negative HIV test as part of pregnancy screening will not affect insurance.

■ Results of tests performed at a sexual health clinic will not be revealed to anyone without consent. This includes insurance companies.

HEPATITIS B AND C

Hepatitis B is the only sexually transmitted infection that can be prevented by vaccination. While in some parts of the world, such as South-east Asia, twenty per cent of the population are infected, in Britain less than one in a thousand heterosexual men and women are positive. The proportion of infected intravenous drug users is falling, thanks to widespread use of vaccination.

Individuals with Hepatitis B are much more highly infectious than HIV, and, unlike HIV, it is relatively easily acquired from blood splashes or minor skin abrasions as well as sharing razors and toothbrushes. Following infection, some ninety per cent of people develop protective antibodies to the virus and pose no further sexual risk to others. A small group do remain infectious – so-called chronic carriers – who are more likely to suffer long-term liver damage, and these individuals may reinfect their sexual partners.

Sexual transmission of Hepatitis C is probably low. The infection is found in some seventy to eighty per cent of current or former intravenous drug users in Britain, and a small proportion of those who received blood transfusions prior to screening tests being developed in 1990 – but very few of their partners. Mother-to-baby transmission is likewise rare, probably confined to those who acquired the virus during pregnancy.

VAGINAL DISCHARGE

A change or increase in discharge is one of the commonest symptoms assumed to be associated with STI, yet this may be difficult to tell apart from normal healthy fluid loss which varies with the menstrual cycle and is increased by sexual arousal. Both gonorrhoea and chlamydia cause increased discharge of pus from the cervix, but this may not be sufficient to cause a noticeable change in loss from the vagina. Three main infections cause increased vaginal inflammation:

■ *Trichomonas vaginalis* (TV)
■ Bacterial vaginosis (BV)
■ Candida, commonly known as 'thrush'.

Of these, only TV is entirely sexually transmitted. Like gonorrhoea, it is nowadays rare outside large inner city areas. It usually starts within a week of the sexual contact, causing copious yellow or yellow/green discharge, swelling of the labia and intense genital itching with widespread red rash. It is usually easily treated with metronidazole. This organism does not seem to survive long in men so it is less commonly diagnosed. Sexual partners must obviously be checked and treated at the same time. Candida and bacterial vaginosis occur naturally, so are not considered to be sexually transmitted infections, and do not usually require the partner to be checked as an essential part of prevention.

BACTERIAL VAGINOSIS

BV is the commonest cause of increased vaginal discharge, affecting around one-third of women. At its most obvious, the discharge is off-white, creamy or watery and has a characteristic fishy smell. Although it is increased by sex, and, in some cases, may be linked with acquisition of chlamydia, it often occurs in women who are not sexually active.

It is caused by a change in the normal balance of bacteria in the vagina – the healthy acid-producing lactobacilli are replaced by an overgrowth of mixed organisms which are naturally present in small quantities. One of these, called Gardnerella, was previously, and wrongly, thought to be the cause of the infection. It is not known whether menstrual cycle variation or chemical irritants trigger these changes, or why some women are more severely affected than others – most will not notice symptoms and it often gets better by itself.

The condition is important in pregnancy, as it may be associated with early rupture of the membranes (breaking of the waters), early onset of labour and premature delivery. However, it is not yet proven whether routine antenatal testing for bacterial vaginosis is useful in preventing preterm labour.

Treatment is straightforward, with metronidazole tablets or newer vaginal creams. A few women are frequently troubled by recurrences, and should seek specialist assessment. Even in these cases, treatment of the partner does not seem to change the situation.

CANDIDA (THRUSH)

The yeast infection *Candida albicans* causes 'thrush' with symptoms of vulval itching, soreness and curdy white vaginal discharge. Seventy-five per cent of women will get it at some time in their lives, because the organism is naturally present in small numbers in the skin, bowel and vagina in everyone. Changes in this natural balance cause the yeast to overgrow. This damages the skin resulting first in irritation, then a visible rash with pain. Rarely, ulceration occurs, which can be confused with herpes.

CAUSES OF THRUSH
■ Antibiotic treatment
■ Pregnancy
■ Diabetes
■ Poor general health
■ Immunosuppressive drugs
■ HIV
■ Predisposition to skin allergy

■ Tight clothing
■ Poor genital hygiene (wiping from back to front)
■ Excessive genital washing (soap scrubbing)
■ Bubble baths and other chemical irritants.

TREATMENT OF THRUSH

Thrush usually occurs after an obvious triggering event, and simple treatment with vaginal creams and pessaries, or the newer single tablet preparation, is most effective. Thrush is one of the many causes of external (rather than deep) pain with sex – if this does not improve after simple treatment, specialist advice should be sought. Men are unlikely to be affected except when infection is severe. A man may get a slight rash over the head of the penis (glans), which will be more obvious if he is uncircumcised or diabetic, and treatment is by simple cream application.

PREVENTING THRUSH

Candida grows best in hot, sweaty conditions. Careful attention to general health, hygiene, appropriate clothing and avoiding chemical irritants should prevent frequent problems. Despite this, a minority of women suffer recurrent and sometimes severe symptoms, often in the week or two prior to menstruation. This is because the hormone progesterone promotes the growth of candida, increasing the quantity in the vagina. This natural cyclical variation is not noticed by most women. Specialist advice should be sought to exclude other conditions and plan treatment, which can involve regular administration of carefully timed preventive anti-fungal drugs to start earlier in the cycle.

GETTING A CHECK-UP

Some infections may be successfully screened and treated in general practice, contraception clinics or gynaecology services. Facilities for men and women are provided by sexual health clinics, which are the only services offering routine check-ups for the full range of infections.

SEXUAL HEALTH/GENITOURINARY MEDICINE CLINICS

These confidential clinics – variously called Department of Genitourinary Medicine, Centre for Sexual Health or simply a number or person's name – give advice, screening and free treatment for sexually transmitted infections, providing condoms, pregnancy testing and emergency contraception as a minimum. Most have a range of other services – family planning, colposcopy, psychosexual advice, rape care, abortion advice. Facilities vary depending on local resources; some clinics aspire to provide a complete women's sexual health service under one roof.

■ All visits are completely confidential regardless of the client's age.
■ No doctor's letter is required.
■ All treatment is free – there are no prescription charges.
■ See the local telephone directory or Health Education Authority website for local clinic addresses. An appointment may not be needed at many clinics.

Chapter nine

UNPLANNED PREGNANCY

Unplanned pregnancies are common. About one-third of all births are not planned pregnancies. There are many reasons why pregnancies are unplanned. All contraceptive methods have some failures. Sometimes women have not used contraception at all, because they had difficulty getting access to the right advice and supplies, or difficulty using the method they chose, or they thought they were not fertile at that time. Some women will have planned a pregnancy, but a change of circumstances makes having a baby problematic. Every woman's situation is unique. Making decisions can be difficult. This chapter is about what choices are available, and how to find out more about them.

FINDING OUT FOR SURE

For most women, the first suggestion that they might be pregnant is a late period. Some may also be aware of changes in their body, such as tender, swollen breasts, nausea or vomiting, or an inability to tolerate certain foods, smells or cigarette smoke. It is important to find out for sure as soon as possible, so you can begin to plan for the future. The first thing is to have a pregnancy test.

These detect a rise in a pregnancy hormone which is known as hCG (human chorionic gonadotrophin). The levels of this hormone go up almost immediately after the embryo has attached to the wall of the uterus and may be positive before a missed period.

HOME PREGNANCY TESTS
- Are easy to follow and only take a few minutes to do.
- Work on a urine sample (the first one of the day is best).
- May be useful if you want the first result quickly and in private.
- Cost about £10.
- Are available from most pharmacies and some larger supermarkets.

PREGNANCY TESTING IS ALSO AVAILABLE AT:
- Some GPs (free)
- Some local family planning clinics (free)
- Brook Advisory Clinics if you are under twenty-four years old (free)
- British Pregnancy Advisory Services (fee payable)
- Marie Stopes clinics in London, Leeds and Manchester (fee payable)
- Some pharmacists will do a test for you (fee payable).

THE TEST IS POSITIVE
Depending on personal circumstances, it may be useful to discuss your feelings with your partner. Sometimes it is useful to talk to a person outside your relationship first, such as a close friend, a health professional or counsellor.

THE TEST IS NEGATIVE
If this comes as a relief, it could suggest that you may not be using the appropriate contraception for your situation.

CONSIDERING MOTHERHOOD

Many women find that a pregnancy, however unplanned, forces them to think differently about their priorities. You may be delighted that you are fertile, or may simply know that having a child is one of the things you want. Although many births in Britain were unplanned, by the time the child is born most of them are very much wanted. Some of the things you need to consider can be broken down into some practical questions:

■ If you are working, what maternity leave arrangements are available?

■ Can you go back to work part-time if you want to?

■ What local childcare is available? How much will it cost?

■ If you do not go back to work, what options are available?

■ If you are not working, can you afford to live on your available income or benefits?

■ Can you continue to live where you are now once the baby is born?

■ What about the people you share the house with? How will they cope with a baby about the house?

YOUR EDUCATION

If you are still at school or at college, you may need to interrupt or modify your studies to accommodate the changes in your life. The services available will vary from area to area. The local Educational Welfare Services Department should be able to help you.

WHAT ABOUT YOUR PARTNER?

■ How do they feel about being a parent?

■ What is the likely future of your current relationship?

■ If there is no possibility of an ongoing relationship, how will you manage being a single parent?

■ What financial contribution can you realistically expect him to make?

■ What about family and friends?

■ Who can you trust to talk to about your situation?

■ Will they provide support? If so how much help can you count on?

■ Will you be isolated by your choices?

■ What resources in yourself can you count on if that happens?

■ Who will baby-sit when you want a night off?

■ Who will be there for you at three in the morning if there is a problem?

■ How will people respond to you? How will you cope with that?

This may be particularly important to you in certain circumstances, for example if you are very young or if your partner is married.

WHAT ABOUT ADOPTION?

Adoption provides the child with new legal parents. This is a difficult choice, and is becoming far less common as society changes. However, some women who feel unable to bring up a child consider it a positive alternative to abortion, and there is a long waiting list of couples who wish to adopt a baby. It is usual for them to be of the same ethnic group as the child, and the mother may specify other types of family that she wishes the child to go to – for example, a particular religion.

Those considering this alternative need to contact their local Social Services Department. The midwife or health visitor and the British Agencies for Adoption and Fostering can provide further support (see Useful Addresses).

Counselling before adoption will include discussion of how you will feel about handing over your baby once it is finally born; how you will explain to interested people where your baby is or how he/she is doing; and perhaps wondering about that yourself. Some women experience deep sadness and regret about this choice; others may wonder how it might have been but feel sure the right decision has been made.

You may wish to write a letter to your child and maybe include a photograph. This can be kept by the adoption agency. If you wish to remain anonymous you may do so – ask the social services or adoption agency staff about that.

If you are considering adoption, it is best to arrange as much as possible while you are still pregnant, and to tell the staff at the hospital where you will deliver. They should be able to accommodate your wishes about such things as how much contact you want with your child once he or she is born.

You can also mentally prepare yourself for how you will cope with practical things, like engorged breasts, and how soon you will want to go home and what support you will need. Once the baby is born, and you have left hospital, usually when the baby is about five days old, your child will go to its adoptive parents or a temporary foster mother. After the baby is about six weeks old, you will be visited by a reporting officer who will ask for your consent to the adoption agreement. You can still change your mind until this is done. Unless your child were to be at risk in your

care, the social services must comply with your wishes. Once the adoption agreement is signed it becomes much more difficult to regain care of your child if you change your mind. If there is any doubt, you should consider fostering your child until you decide.

WHAT IS FOSTERING?

Fostering is a temporary arrangement. Your child is cared for in someone else's family, until your circumstances permit you to provide a settled home for your child. You may visit your child regularly during this time. If you think you will need this sort of help contact the Social Services, tell them the sort of problems that make it difficult to look after your baby at home yourself, and they will make the arrangements to help you, for example with accommodation difficulties, or counselling to help you decide about adoption.

The foster mother with whom your child is placed can sometimes be a good source of support and can help you gain confidence in looking after your baby. You should keep up contact with the foster family and your child so that your baby is used to your company when he or she comes home.

Sometimes the difficulties that led to you placing your child in foster care are not easily resolved, and it may take longer than you planned to have your child back in your care. Your social worker will usually be the most helpful person in this situation.

CONSIDERING ABORTION

Those who feel that they cannot continue with their pregnancy may seek advice about termination of pregnancy. It is prudent to book an appointment to discuss this early, and cancel it if you change your mind and decide you can continue your pregnancy.

Since 1967 abortion has been legal in Great Britain (not in Northern Ireland) under the following circumstances:

■ The continuance of the pregnancy would involve risk to the life of the pregnant woman greater than if the pregnancy were terminated

■ The termination is necessary to prevent grave permanent injury to the physical or mental health of the pregnant woman

■ The pregnancy has NOT exceeded its twenty-fourth week and that the continuance of the pregnancy would involve risk, greater than if the pregnancy were terminated, of injury to the physical or mental health of the pregnant woman

■ The pregnancy has NOT exceeded its twenty-fourth week and that the continuance of the pregnancy would involve risk, greater than if the pregnancy were terminated, of injury to the physical or mental health of the existing child(ren) of the family of the pregnant woman

■ There is a substantial risk that if the child were born it would suffer from such physical or mental abnormalities as to be seriously handicapped.

Two doctors will need to certify that in their opinion this request for termination meets the requirements of the law. Abortion is available in the NHS system, but provisions vary throughout the UK, and for various reasons almost half of the women having abortions are seen outside the NHS.

WHO DO YOU ASK ABOUT ABORTION?

■ **The GP,** who has a legal duty to provide advice and referral. If your GP is likely to be sympathetic and you feel able to talk to him or her, make an appointment as soon as possible to discuss your options, and arrange a referral if that is what you want. Some women would rather not involve their GPs for reasons of privacy (although your GP is duty bound to respect your confidentiality). If your GP is unable or unwilling to help, ask them to refer you to someone who can.

■ **The Family Planning Clinic** You can phone your local family planning clinic for information and advice, and make an appointment for counselling about the pregnancy. They may also confirm your pregnancy and check your dates with you, discuss your options, offer to screen you for important infections, and if you know abortion is your choice, refer you to an appropriate clinic.

■ **Brook Advisory Centres** If you are under twenty-four, check if there is a Brook Advisory Centre near you, which will offer pregnancy diagnosis, counselling, and Charitable clinics. These, such as British Pregnancy Advisory Service and Marie Stopes Clinics, are charitable organisations which have branches across the country. They charge fees to cover costs, but if you are in financial difficulties, let them know and they may be able to help (see Useful Addresses).

■ **Private gynaecologists** These specialists, at private hospitals or clinics, may see you more quickly than in the NHS. Their fees are higher than the charity clinics, so it is worthwhile checking what other help is available.

WHAT HAPPENS NOW?

■ The pregnancy will be confirmed by a urine test even if you have done that already. Your pregnancy dates will be worked out from the first day on which bleeding started in your last period.

■ You should be offered counselling to help

you with your decision, if you have not already talked to someone. It is not necessary to have counselling; you may be sure in your mind already, but sometimes it is very useful, as it is vital that you are 100% sure of your decision. The availability and types of help available vary from region to region. The first doctor you see will:

■ Ask you about your medical history including any pregnancies or gynaecological problems in the past

■ Ask you about your reasons for wanting to terminate this pregnancy

■ Ask you what alternatives to abortion you have considered

■ Perform an abdominal and internal vaginal examination

■ May perform an ultrasound

■ Take a blood sample to decide your blood group.

If this first doctor agrees that termination is right for you, they will sign the appropriate legal document (HSA1) and refer you to another doctor for a second opinion.

The second doctor will usually be a gynaecologist at the outpatient clinic of your local hospital, the charity clinic or private sector. They will have the referral letter from the first doctor, but may still want to ask some of the same questions again to help them decide for themselves that you are making an informed choice about abortion. Some or all of the examination may need to be repeated – if you are not sure why in your case, ask the gynaecologist to explain.

If the second doctor agrees with the first doctor that termination is appropriate, they will sign form HSA1 and offer you an appointment for termination of pregnancy as soon as possible. If the second doctor does not agree, arrange to see the first doctor again as soon as possible or they may arrange an immediate second opinion.

WHAT TYPE OF ABORTION?

There are two different types of abortion: medical termination and surgical termination.

MEDICAL TERMINATION

If you are early in pregnancy (less than nine weeks pregnant) you may be offered medical termination, although this is not available everywhere. This usually avoids the need for an operation but involves the use of special drugs. If you choose medical termination, you will make three visits to the hospital or clinic.

1 You take a mifepristone tablet (a hormone that blocks the production of progesterone, which is produced by your body to maintain the early pregnancy). A small number of women will have bleeding and pain after this; you should have the hospital's number to phone if this is more than you would expect with a period or if you are worried.

2 Two days later you will return to the hospital, and a doctor or nurse will insert a vaginal tablet (pessary), which is like a tiny waxy tampon. This contains prostaglandin, which will bring on uterine cramps. The lining of the womb breaks down and the pregnancy is expelled with the bleeding, which can be heavy. Some women have headaches, sickness and diarrhoea. Over the next few hours you will probably expel the pregnancy completely. Afterwards you will be examined, and discharged home.

For a small number of women this will not be successful and they may need to go to the operating theatre to have their uterus emptied by surgery under anaesthetic.

3 You may continue to bleed for up to ten days. Many clinics offer a follow-up visit at

about two weeks to check that there are no complications. Other clinics suggest you see your own doctor or family planning clinic. It is important that if there are any things that concern you, you know who to contact sooner.

SURGICAL TERMINATION

Up to nine weeks, you may be offered the choice of surgical or medical termination. Up to and including fourteen weeks, you will be offered a surgical termination of pregnancy.

This procedure is done in an operating theatre in a hospital or special clinic. It is usually done under a light general anaesthetic, so you will be asleep. If you wish, some clinics will perform this procedure under local anaesthetic.

Often the doctor will insert a prostaglandin pessary an hour or more before the operation. This helps to soften and open your cervix. Sometimes you will be given an injection to make you relax, just before the operation.

Once in the theatre, you will be anaesthetised and your legs supported in stirrups. The surgeon will then clean the vaginal area, insert a speculum to hold the vagina open and let him or her see your cervix, hold the cervix steady with a pair of forceps (tenaculum) and open the cervix a little way with rods called dilators. He or she will then insert a thin plastic tube into the uterus. This is attached to a suction machine or hand-held syringe, which gently removes the contents of the uterus. A check will be made that the uterus is empty with an instrument called a curette. This whole procedure usually takes ten to fifteen minutes, and the anaesthetist will then wake you up.

You may feel quite drowsy and sick for a few hours, but if you live close by, you will usually be well enough to go home in four or five hours. You should expect some period-like cramps and bleeding for a few days.

ABORTION AFTER TWELVE OR THIRTEEN WEEKS

The procedure for termination of pregnancies later than twelve to thirteen weeks is more complex. The techniques offered will vary depending on the stage of pregnancy and across the country. Surgical methods are rarely used to terminate pregnancies over twelve weeks. Alternative methods which lead to uterine contractions (similar to labour) are more usually advised. Adequate pain relief will always be available.

At the end of this time, you will expel the pregnancy, assisted by a nurse. You do not need to see the fetus if you do not wish to. Sometimes after this sort of abortion you will need to go to the operating theatre to have the uterus emptied under anaesthetic.

COMPLICATIONS OF ABORTION

In general, the earlier in pregnancy that an abortion is performed, the safer it is. In Britain, the rate of minor complications is low, less than five for every hundred women; serious complications are extremely rare.

The most common complication is infection, which can cause pain, abnormal discharge and prolonged bleeding after the abortion. This is more common if you have an untreated infection already, which is why some doctors screen women for infection before abortion, and others will give antibiotics at the time of the procedure. Infection is usually easily treated with antibiotics.

Other problems are incomplete abortion and, far less commonly, tears to the cervix or perforation of the uterus. Long-term complications, such as ongoing infection and damage to the fallopian tubes which can lead to difficulty in conceiving, are very uncommon in Britain. If you have any concerns afterwards about complications, see your doctor for information and advice.

SEX AND CONTRACEPTION

The right time to restart a sexual relationship is when you are ready. You may have all sorts of emotions you wish to sort out before you think about resuming that part of your life again. Every woman is different.

Couples are advised to avoid penetration until the bleeding has settled, and some gynaecologists would recommend waiting until six weeks after your abortion. This should lessen the chances of any infection.

The best time to think about and plan future contraception may be in the time leading up to abortion. Pregnancy can occur almost immediately afterwards, and some of the methods of family planning are best started at the time of the abortion if they are to be effective by the time intercourse is resumed.

A new method of contraception may need to be started if the previous method failed or was unsatisfactory. Your GP or family planning doctor or nurse should give you the information you need to help choose the right method.

HOW WILL YOU FEEL AFTERWARDS?

For most women the decision to have an abortion is difficult. However, following termination, most women feel that they made the right decision. Despite this, many benefit from the opportunity to talk to a counsellor about their feelings and concerns. This can be organised by the centre where the termination was arranged.

Chapter ten

PREGNANCY

Pregnancy produces many changes in the body to cope with the demands of carrying the baby inside the uterus until it is able to survive outside. These changes are often noticed by the mother and some may cause differing emotions, from excitement to discomfort and worry. These changes will be described with an explanation of why they occur and when symptoms noticed by a pregnant woman should be a cause to seek advice.

This chapter also describes what happens at the antenatal visits to the doctor/midwife.

It also aims to discuss some conditions that are rare but about which little information may be available elsewhere. This information will be irrelevant to most women.

CHANGES IN THE BODY DURING PREGNANCY

The placenta produces large amounts of hormones that are designed to maintain the pregnancy and lead to changes in the mother's body which will help her adjust to the pregnancy and nourish the body when it is born.

One of the earliest signs of pregnancy is the missed period. This occurs since the period involves the shedding of the lining of the uterus which would lead to the loss of an early pregnancy. Some women may not miss a period, but will have significantly less bleeding, giving a period that is shorter and lighter than usual. Any period which is significantly different to a normal period where there has been unprotected intercourse in the previous month should be checked out.

Other early signs are 'early morning sickness' and also tender enlarged breasts. The nausea and vomiting occurs due to the high levels of oestrogen in the blood but it is not inevitable. Some women will even notice it in some pregnancies and not in others. The changes in the breasts occur in preparation for milk production. They may even leak fluid. Make sure that you wear a supportive bra that fits well, as this will minimise any discomfort (you may need to go up a few sizes over the course of the pregnancy).

EARLY CHANGES IN PREGNANCY

The huge increase in female hormones produces changes from very early in pregnancy. Some women feel wonderfully well and healthy, but are still likely to experience some of the following signs of pregnancy:

■ Enlarged and tender breasts
■ Fluid retention
■ Sickness and nausea (especially in the morning)
■ Tiredness

- Constipation
- Emotional upsets
- A tendency to faint
- Going off certain foods, e.g. coffee, alcohol.

CHANGES LATER IN PREGNANCY

High hormone levels continue to produce the symptoms listed above throughout pregnancy, although fortunately the sickness usually settles after twelve to fourteen weeks. Later in pregnancy, as the baby and the womb grow, pressure effects are added to the above. These include:

- Heartburn
- Passing urine frequently (also a common early pregnancy sign)
- Backache.

CHANGES IN THE HEART AND BLOOD VESSELS

Changes in the heart and blood vessels are also an early feature. The heart beats approximately twenty per cent faster during pregnancy; this starts in the first three months. In addition, the heart pumps out more blood with each beat. These changes result in up to forty per cent more blood circulating each minute. Blood pressure falls in early pregnancy when blood vessels increase in size to allow more blood flow. This low blood pressure can give symptoms of dizziness and even fainting.

The volume of blood in the body increases by almost fifty per cent. It is slightly thinner in pregnancy as the increase in plasma (fluid) is larger than the increase in blood cells. The effect of this dilution is to reduce the work done by the heart in pumping this extra blood, and to increase the amount reaching the tissues. Thinner blood, however, also results in more fluid escaping from the circulation, which sometimes leads to swelling, especially of the hands and feet.

In later pregnancy, the womb and its contents are large and heavy and in certain positions can press on the main blood vessels that run to and from the heart at the back of the abdomen. This reduces blood returning to the heart and brain and may even cause dizziness and fainting. To avoid this, slightly tilt your body forwards while sitting, lie on your side rather than flat on your back, and get up slowly from sitting or lying down. If you do feel faint at any time, then lie down on your side until it passes.

FLUID RETENTION

This is apparent as an increase in weight during the first few weeks, and increases notably in the last weeks before delivery. It can also cause swelling of the fingers and ankles. This usually occurs gradually and sudden or dramatic swelling is best checked by your doctor as it can occasionally be a sign of high blood pressure

Finger swelling is usually mild, but can be severe enough for you to have to remove your rings. It is better to anticipate this happening

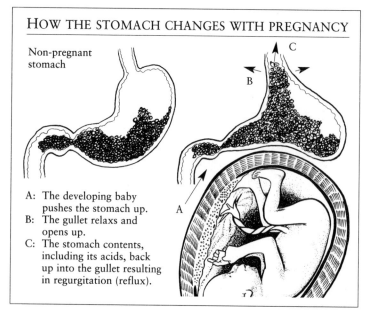

HOW THE STOMACH CHANGES WITH PREGNANCY

Non-pregnant stomach

A: The developing baby pushes the stomach up.
B: The gullet relaxes and opens up.
C: The stomach contents, including its acids, back up into the gullet resulting in regurgitation (reflux).

and remove the rings yourself when they become tight.

The extra accumulation of fluid in the body during pregnancy can cause swelling in the wrists. In this situation, very limited space is available and the pressure within the wrist begins to rise and can squash the nerve that supplies the hand. Tingling of the thumb, index and middle fingers can occur (often worst at night) and this is called carpal tunnel syndrome.

It may be advisable to see your doctor for these symptoms. Treatment includes sleeping with the hand outside the covers to keep it cool and lifting it up. In more severe cases, specially designed wrist splints can help. The condition usually resolves after pregnancy.

Ankle swelling can be relieved by gentle exercise and sitting with your feet up. Occasionally, support tights can be useful to limit the amount of swelling if prolonged periods of standing are anticipated.

VARICOSE VEINS

These are most likely to develop or get worse in pregnancy, due to the increase in size of blood vessels, the increase in blood volume, the weakening of the valves of the veins, and the pressure effect of the pregnant womb reducing blood returning from the legs up to the heart. Varicose veins occur most commonly in the legs, but can also occur in the vulva. Treatment with support tights or stockings, gentle exercise and elevation of the legs when sitting improves symptoms of itching, aching or throbbing.

THE DIGESTIVE SYSTEM

The best way to minimise the sickness associated with early pregnancy is to eat a little and often and to maintain an adequate intake of fluids.

The high levels of the hormones are responsible for the digestive problems of pregnancy. These hormones relax the smooth muscle surrounding the gut, resulting in reflux of acid from the stomach into the gullet causing heartburn. It also results in reduced activity of the large gut, causing constipation.

YOUR TEETH

The growing baby needs lots of calcium and it is therefore important to eat foods containing calcium to keep bones strong and teeth healthy. The diet should include:

- Dairy products – milk, hard (pasteurised) cheeses (but not soft cheeses, which may be a source of listeria), yogurt
- Citrus fruits
- Dark green leafy vegetables – cabbage and spinach
- Broccoli.

General dental hygiene and gum care are encouraged as are regular dental check-ups, which are available free to pregnant women.

HEARTBURN

Although many women do not experience heartburn while pregnant, those who do often find that it gets worse as the pregnancy progresses due to increased pressure from the baby.

To reduce it, try sitting up straight while eating, and eat small meals often.

You can also try lying more upright in bed; this can be achieved by simple measures such as using an extra pillow at night or raising the head end of the bed with books or bricks.

To minimise the irritation, drink milky drinks or take an antacid from your doctor to reduce the acidity of the stomach contents. This also helps coat, and therefore protect, the gullet from the burning effect of acid. Antacids can be safely taken as directed by the manufacturer.

CONSTIPATION

This is best avoided by eating a diet with a high fibre content (bran, fresh fruit and vegetables) accompanied by plenty of fluid. If additional help is needed, lactulose, bran or ispaghula husk can all be taken safely in pregnancy. Iron tablets can make things worse, but there are different preparations of iron and a change may solve the problems (iron tablets make the motions black).

PILES (HAEMORRHOIDS)

These are distended veins in the anus which occur commonly in pregnancy as part of the general dilatation of the veins. They are made worse by constipation and straining. They can cause itching and bleeding and occasionally 'prolapse' out of the anus to feel like small lumps. These can usually be avoided by a diet which helps prevent constipation. If necessary a gentle laxative can be taken. If they become sore, special creams and/or suppositories are a great help.

CHANGES IN THE BLADDER

In pregnancy there is a desire to pass urine more frequently than normal. This may be due to the high levels of pregnancy hormones in early pregnancy, and due to a pressure effect of the womb and baby in later pregnancy.

The hormone progesterone relaxes all smooth muscles, and the bladder and ureters (which join the kidney to the bladder) become rather floppy and work less well. This is why pregnant women are more likely to get urinary tract infections, such as cystitis. It is very important that these are treated quickly with one of the many antibiotics that are safe to take during pregnancy.

Urine may leak with sudden movements later in pregnancy due to the pressure effect of the baby on the bladder and the softening of the ligaments and supports in the pelvis. It usually corrects itself after the birth but pelvic exercises may reduce the leakage during pregnancy, and hasten recovery after your baby is born. For further information on exercises, see page 198.

VAGINAL DISCHARGE

Due to hormone changes, you may notice an increase in the vaginal secretions and this is usually completely normal.

The vaginal secretions in pregnancy are less acidic than in the non-pregnant state which increase the likelihood of candida infection (thrush). This infection causes an itchy white discharge, which can be treated safely with vaginal pessaries or cream. However, it is sometimes more difficult to eradicate the infection completely. Live yoghurt may also help if put around or inside the vagina as it restores the natural balance of germs, reducing the risk of an overgrowth of thrush.

Vaginal bleeding, however, is not normal and if this occurs you must consult your doctor immediately (see page 167).

THE BONES AND JOINTS

Pregnancy puts many stresses on the skeleton, ligaments (which support the bones) and muscles. These are caused by the enlarging uterus in the abdomen, the softening of ligaments and the extra weight being carried.

THE ENLARGING WOMB

Stretch marks are caused by changes in the hormones in pregnancy. They are not affected by the size of the baby, and cannot be avoided by creams or tablets. Some women are just more prone to stretch marks than others.

They are reddish-purple lines which can be itchy, but after pregnancy the colour fades and they finish as pale smooth lines on the skin. they can form in other areas as well as the abdomen, such as the thighs and breasts.

In the last few weeks of the pregnancy the pressure of the womb can cause the lower rib cage to splay out. This can be a painful condition and may require simple painkillers.

SOFTENED LIGAMENTS AND EXTRA WEIGHT

The joints become loose as the ligaments soften and stretch in response to the pregnancy hormones. The excessive movement of some joints can cause anything from discomfort to fairly severe pain. This is most common in women who have had several children but usually resolves after the pregnancy is over. Pain is usually felt in the lower back but can also occur in the pubic bone.

A woman's centre of gravity moves forward as her abdomen swells outwards in advancing pregnancy. This, together with the softened ligaments, adds strain on the back. Well-toned abdominal muscles can help the back by limiting the forward shift of the centre of gravity. If you do have a bad back, then physiotherapy may also help. If there is any possibility of disc problems or sciatica (where pain goes into the buttock or down the leg), you should see your doctor. You should also take care when lifting heavy objects, carrying shopping or bending over.

The softening of the ligaments results in backache for many women, although it rarely causes a significant problem. The backache can be lessened by paying great attention to posture and by avoiding standing for long periods. Very occasionally, those who get problems as described above may require some sort of support and this will be provided by the physiotherapist or doctor (see also page 191).

MUSCLE CRAMPS

These occur most commonly in the calves and feet at night. if they occur, just stretch and gently massage the affected muscle.

SLEEP DISTURBANCES

Insomnia occurs very commonly, especially in advanced pregnancy, due to difficulties in getting comfortable. Try sleeping lying on your side, using pillows to help support you. It is advisable to cat-nap in the afternoon in later pregnancy to catch up on some of the sleep missed at night.

YOUR EYES

During pregnancy there is a reduction in tear formation and the size and shape of the eyeball can alter slightly. For both these reasons, contact lenses can become uncomfortable. Wear them for shorter periods of time, although if problems persist, seek advice from your optician.

FEELING SHORT OF BREATH

During pregnancy there is an increased need for oxygen which is achieved by deeper rather than more rapid breathing. Most activities are more tiring than normal as any exercise is harder work due to the increased demands of pregnancy on the body. Shortness of breath occurs throughout and is especially common in later pregnancy. It is due to the increased need for oxygen and the increased weight of the pregnant uterus. It can be made worse by anaemia.

Anybody who normally suffers from

asthma may continue to do so in pregnancy. For more information, turn to page 174.

TIREDNESS

All women feel tiredness during pregnancy. It means that over-exertion is less likely to occur and also that it will be important to rest as much as possible, so you may find it necessary to curtail some of the activities you would pursue outside of pregnancy. Tiredness is rarely caused by anaemia, although it may be worsened by it. There is no cure apart from rest.

HEADACHES AND MIGRAINES

Often these are improved by pregnancy although some migraine-sufferers have more attacks in pregnancy, particularly during the early months. Simple painkillers, such as paracetamol, are safe to take. In later pregnancy, headaches may be due to high blood pressure and this should be checked if headaches persist. Preparations specifically designed to treat migraine should not be taken without asking your doctor first.

THE WATERS

The waters are the fluid that surrounds the baby as it grows and develops in the womb. In medical terms, this is called amniotic fluid or 'liquor'. The waters are maintained within a sealed bag, known as the membranes or amnion. Within this fluid-filled bag the baby is nourished while it grows by way of the

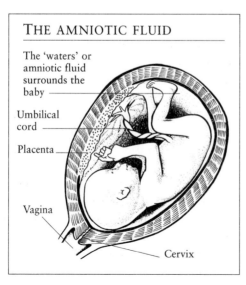

THE AMNIOTIC FLUID

The 'waters' or amniotic fluid surrounds the baby

Umbilical cord

Placenta

Vagina

Cervix

placenta or afterbirth via the umbilical cord.

The waters are produced by both the mother and baby. In early pregnancy, the mother contributes more, but as the baby grows and develops, its contribution increases and eventually outstrips that of the mother. From the moment the fertilised egg enters the womb fluid is being produced. The amount of fluid increases steadily from 30 ml at ten weeks to almost 900 ml by thirty-six weeks. The volume of fluid around the baby is not static and is constantly being filtered, very much like the water in a swimming pool. This continuous filtering process ensures that the waters are maintained at ideal conditions for the growth and development of the baby. This continuous filtering of liquor occurs every twenty-four hours. By the time the baby reaches thirty-eight weeks the liquor is at its maximum volume. From then on the volume reduces very slightly so that by forty-two completed weeks the amount of liquor may have been reduced by half.

AMNIOTIC FLUID

Amniotic fluid is like blood without the red blood cells, giving it a clear opalescent colour. It contains proteins, fats, minerals, hormones and cells shed by the baby. The composition of liquor changes throughout pregnancy as the baby matures. Occasionally it is useful to take a sample of liquor and test the maturation of the baby's lungs. This test measures fatty substances produced by the baby's lungs at about thirty-two weeks of pregnancy which are important in helping the lungs to work when the baby is breathing air.

Occasionally, this clear fluid may change as the baby passes some of its bowel contents into amniotic fluid. This is known as 'meconium'. Depending on the quantity of meconium passed relative to the volume of amniotic fluid, the waters may be lightly contaminated or heavily stained. If a woman should go into labour before thirty-six weeks gestation it is unusual to find meconium in the amniotic fluid. Its presence may indicate that the baby is becoming stressed and lacks oxygen. This distress generally results from insufficient oxygen or nutrients passing to the baby through the placenta, and passing meconium may be a response to this. After forty weeks gestation, however, babies often pass meconium, so that by forty-two weeks almost fifteen per cent of babies will be surrounded by meconium-stained fluid. In this situation it may not represent fetal distress but instead be a normal finding in a healthy mature baby.

MONITORING VOLUME AND COMPOSITION

A doctor or midwife examining the abdomen of a pregnant woman is attempting to estimate the stage of pregnancy and size of the baby as determined by the height of the womb. What he or she feels is the womb and its contents: namely the baby and also the surrounding fluid. By this examination it is therefore possible to estimate roughly the amount of fluid present. A more accurate method of assessing the volume of the amniotic fluid is by means of an ultrasound scan. Every time a woman has an ultrasound scan to monitor the baby the volume of amniotic fluid is also assessed.

The production of the fluid relies on the baby's kidneys, bladder and placenta working normally. If the volume of waters is reduced below that expected it can mean that either some is leaking out vaginally or that not enough is being produced. If a woman reports leaking of fluid a speculum examination will be performed by the doctor or midwife in order to look directly at the neck of the womb and discover if there is any fluid leaking from it. He or she may also notice fluid pooling in the vagina and sometimes it is helpful to test this fluid, using what is known as an amnicator (a cotton wool ball tipped swab impregnated with a special chemical). If the waters are leaking it means there is a hole in the bag of membranes. The significance of this finding depends very much on how mature the baby is. Pregnant women who suspect that their waters have broken should contact their midwife or the labour ward for advice. If the waters have not broken, too little fluid around the baby may indicate that the placenta is not working adequately and act as a warning sign that the baby may need delivery sooner rather than later. It is a common reason for starting (inducing) labour early (see below).

Although breaking of the waters is usually followed by labour, this is not always the case, particularly when early in the pregnancy.

DIAGNOSIS OF PREGNANCY

PREGNANCY TESTS

Urinary pregnancy tests which can be obtained at most pharmacies and many supermarkets are very accurate, and may be able to diagnose pregnancy around the time of a missed period. The test detects the hormone human chorionic gonadotrophin in urine. This is made by the outer layers of the implanting embryo, part of which will eventually become the placenta. As early as nine or ten days after fertilisation (i.e. twenty-four days after the last menstrual period or four days before the next expected period), sufficient concentrations of this hormone are in the urine to turn the standard pregnancy test positive.

Occasionally, a test may be falsely negative if it is carried out too soon or with very diluted urine for then there will not be a high enough concentration of the hormone. Hence, an early morning specimen collected around the time of the expected period should give a correct result.

Ultrasound is used sometimes to confirm the gestation (length) of the pregnancy, and sometimes to diagnose twins or to exclude an ectopic pregnancy (one that has implanted outside the uterus). By about five weeks since the first day of the last menstrual period, the sac in which the embryo is developing can be seen. By six weeks, parts of the embryo can be detected and in the seventh week the fetal heart can be demonstrated. Ultrasound using a probe in the vagina (transvaginal) may be able to see the fetal heart even earlier than this. For more on ultrasound, see page 153. X-rays are not used to diagnose pregnancy for they may have damaging effects on the growing embryo.

MONITORING THE CHANGES: ANTENATAL CARE

The fetus lives and grows inside the uterus. It is therefore well protected against the outside world but this can make checking fetal health difficult. Antenatal care aims to monitor the health of the fetus and mother during pregnancy, and to identify any problems at an early stage where intervention is more likely to be effective. Antenatal care may take place with a doctor or midwife, and the doctor may be a specialist or a GP. Many women will see their GP or specialist on some occasions and their midwife on others. Others will be taken care of completely by their doctor or a midwife. At each antenatal visit the standard tests of blood pressure, testing a urine sample and measurement of the growing uterus will be performed. Blood tests and now HIV testing are also to be offered (see page 132). Antenatal visits are also a good opportunity to discuss any concerns or plans for pregnancy and delivery. In a normal healthy pregnancy very few visits may be needed.

ANTENATAL VISITS

The great number of pregnancies proceed uneventfully to the uncomplicated delivery of a healthy baby to a healthy mother. The aim of antenatal care is to promote the delivery of a healthy baby born to a healthy mother in the most natural and safe way with the minimum of intervention. This is achieved by means of a series of regular check-ups during which both the mother's health and that of her baby are monitored.

Uncomplicated pregnancy and delivery is the remit of the midwife. Problems should be dealt with by the whole team, including the GP, obstetrician and midwife. However, the care of uncomplicated, healthy pregnancy still remains an area of debate. Some obstetricians wish to be involved in the care of 'normal' women. Also, since all women have a nominated consultant obstetrician under whose care they are 'booked', most women wish to meet this person on at least one occasion (and vice versa).

THE BOOKING VISIT

The initial visit to the GP, midwife or specialist is usually referred to as the 'booking visit'. This time is spent gathering information about the health of the pregnant woman, about previous pregnancies and about home and work conditions, all of which may impact on the pregnancy. Specific details such as the date of the last period, the length and nature of the menstrual cycle and methods of contraception used prior to conception will be requested.

A general examination will be carried out, including measurement of blood pressure and testing of a urine specimen for blood and protein.

Screening tests in pregnancy aim to identify those women who may be at risk of developing complications in their pregnancy. The screening tests offered may vary from one hospital to another, and will also depend on the obstetric and medical history of the pregnant woman, and of course her own wishes to be tested or not. An outline of the common screening tests offered, and the reasons for performing them is given below.

HAEMOGLOBIN

This is a blood test to check for anaemia. The growing fetus needs a lot of iron, so this test is usually repeated three or four times during pregnancy. Anaemia is usually treated with iron tablets.

BLOOD GROUP

This test is usually done only once, partly for the records in case a transfusion is required, and also to find out whether the blood group is rhesus positive or negative. This is important because all rhesus negative mothers are offered an injection of 'anti-D' either during the pregnancy or after the birth of the baby in order to protect their next baby from developing severe anaemia. This occurs if blood cells from the rhesus-positive baby pass into the circulation of the rhesus-negative mother. These cells will stimulate the formation of antibodies which 'defend' the mother's body against the baby's cells and destroys them. Pregnant women who experience bleeding or miscarriage are also advised to have anti-D injections, for the same reason.

ANTIBODY LEVELS

Very occasionally, pregnant women develop antibodies to other factors in their baby's blood. Tests for antibodies can detect any antibodies that the women might be developing and which might suggest an incompatibility with their baby's blood cells.

RUBELLA ANTIBODIES

This test is usually only done at the beginning of the pregnancy. It will confirm that there is immunity to rubella (German measles). For those women who are not immune, exposure to rubella in pregnancy can have serious consequences for the baby. All women who are considering pregnancy are strongly advised to ensure that they are immune to this common infection.

SYPHILIS

This test is also done only once, to detect and allow treatment of the few women who have this sexually transmitted infection.

ALPHAFETOPROTEIN (AFP)

This substance is present in small amounts in all pregnancies but can be raised in certain conditions such as when the baby is affected by spina bifida. For some reason not yet fully understood, it is also lower than normal when the baby has Down syndrome.

HAEMOGLOBIN ELECTROPHORESIS

This test allows the mother's blood to be screened for variations in the structure of blood cells, including sickle cell disease and thalassaemia. Sickle cell disease is a condition which can affect people of African and Asian origin. Pregnant women with sickle cell disease are at risk of developing a number of complications in their pregnancy. Thalassaemia generally affects people of Mediterranean origin, but is less likely to lead to pregnancy problems. (see page 185).

TOXOPLASMOSIS

This disease is caused by an organism that is commonly found in household pets, usually cats, and can also be transmitted through handling raw meat or gardening. It can be harmful to unborn babies and since the disease can be treated the test may be worth doing in some circumstances. If you feel that you are at risk because of household pets, discuss this test with your doctor.

CERVICAL SMEARS

The purpose of these is to detect early changes in the cervix which could later lead to cancer. It is quite safe to do a cervical smear in pregnancy, and if it is abnormal it can be investigated further by colposcopy without harm to the baby.

HIV

The number of pregnant women who are HIV positive has increased over the last decade, particularly in the major cities. However, it is still an uncommon condition in pregnancy. Testing for HIV is encouraged in many hospitals since the knowledge that a pregnant woman is HIV positive allows effective antiviral treatment to be given which can greatly reduce the chances of the virus being transmitted to the baby. It is likely that all pregnant women will be offered HIV screening because of the improved care that can be offered to HIV-positive mothers (see page 132).

SCREENING FOR CHROMOSOMAL ABNORMALITIES

The risks of common chromosomal abnormalities, such as Down syndrome, increase with the age of the mother. However, a baby with Down syndrome may be born to a woman of any age, and some pregnant women chose to have screening tests which provide information about the chances of their unborn child having Down syndrome, or a number of other, less common chromosomal abnormalities.

DOWN SYNDROME

Mother's age	Approximate risk of having a Down sydrome baby
25	one in 1,500
30	one in 800
35	one in 350
36	one in 300
37	one in 200
38	one in 170
39	one in 140
40	one in 100
45	one in 30

A blood test (sometimes called the 'double' or triple' test, because it measures a number of factors in the blood) can be performed at 15-19 weeks of pregnancy. The results of this test may take up to two weeks to become available. By combining the blood test results and the age of the pregnant woman, an estimate can be given of the likelihood that this baby has a chromosomal anomaly. If the results show that the chances of chromosomal anomaly are greater than 1:150, most hospitals will offer a diagnostic test, such as amniocentesis (see below). Some women, particularly those who are at higher risk of carrying a child with a chromosomal anomaly, decide to have amniocentesis without having the screening blood test.

One component of this screening test is alphafetoprotein. Raised levels of this protein can suggest spina bifida and can sometimes predict babies at risk of poor growth later in pregnancy.

ULTRASOUND SCANS

Ultrasound scanning uses high intensity sound waves to build up a picture of the baby which can then be shown on a television screen or a photograph. It is a painless and, as far as we are aware, harmless procedure.

Most hospitals encourage pregnant women to have at least one ultrasound scan in pregnancy. Many units perform an ultrasound scan either at the booking visit (often twelve to fourteen weeks) or at about eighteen to twenty weeks. This allows accurate dating of the pregnancy, it can detect twins and can detect a number of abnormalities, such as major defects in the heart, brain, spine and kidneys.

Other scans may be performed at later stages, depending on the need. For example, the position of the baby may be uncertain or its growth more or less than average. If there is any vaginal bleeding, a scan may be advised to try and locate the source of the bleeding.

AMNIOCENTESIS

This test involves taking a sample of amniotic fluid from around the baby, and is usually performed in order to look for chromosomal abnormalities such as Down syndrome. This test is generally performed in centralised units with great expertise. Unlike the screening blood test, amniocentesis involves a small but significant risk to the baby.

Women may be offered amniocentesis if they are thought to be at increased risk of having a chromosome anomaly, particularly Down syndrome. This includes older women, usually those who are over thirty-five to thirty-seven years, depending on local policy; those who have previously delivered a baby affected by a chromosome anomaly and women who have had a positive result from a blood screening test for Down syndrome. Those couples with a family history of inherited disease may also be offered amniocentesis.

The risks of having a Down syndrome

baby based on the mother's age are shown in the table below.

Amniocentesis is usually offered from fifteen weeks onwards. Most commonly, it is performed between fifteen and seventeen weeks from the last menstrual period. The test is performed on an outpatient basis. You should arrange a day off work and arrange transport home afterwards. The doctor will explain the procedure and will also check your blood group. The procedure is normally performed under ultrasound scan guidance. This also allows the doctor to check the size of the baby and to identify the position of the placenta.

Sterile paper towels or drapes may be placed around the area. Local anaesthetic may be used to numb a small area of skin but it is often not necessary. A fine needle is passed through the skin and the wall of the uterus and into the amniotic fluid. Most doctors watch this on the ultrasound scan at the same time to help them guide the needle into the fluid. A syringe is attached to the end of the needle, and 15–20 ml (three to four teaspoonfuls) of fluid is removed and the needle is withdrawn. This is only a small fraction of the fluid and most of it is left inside. Moreover, the fluid that has been removed is rapidly replaced.

Another ultrasound scan is performed immediately afterwards which would allow the mother to see that the fetus is unharmed. A day of rest is usually advised after amniocentesis.

Those with a rhesus negative blood group will need an injection of Anti-D. This is to prevent the formation of antibodies against the rhesus positive blood group, should the fetus be rhesus positive.

Some women experience a little soreness around the needle site afterwards, or even some mild cramping pains. If bleeding or clear fluid is lost vaginally you should contact your family doctor or the hospital.

Amniocentesis carries a risk of miscarriage of one in 100 to 200. There is also a slight risk of infection around the baby, and that the waters will break following the procedure. Much less commonly, there are links between amniocentesis and breathing difficulties in a few newborn babies, particularly if the babies are born early. The effect appears to be temporary and can be treated without long-term problems. Amniocentesis does not cause premature labour.

A lot of women are concerned that the needle will injure the fetus in some way, but the chances of this happening are very small. The use of ultrasound scanning in planning the procedure, guiding the needle and withdrawing the fluid now makes this more unlikely.

Before the cells in the fluid can be examined, they have to be cultured (grown) in the laboratory. This takes from two to four

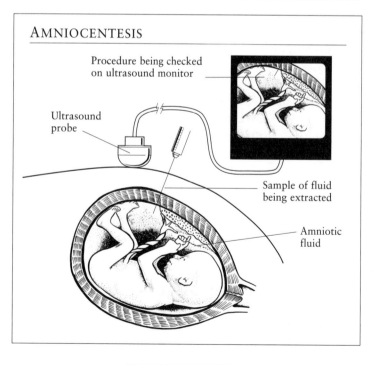

AMNIOCENTESIS

Procedure being checked on ultrasound monitor

Ultrasound probe

Sample of fluid being extracted

Amniotic fluid

weeks. Very occasionally the cells fail to grow and the test may have to be repeated. The test results are extremely accurate and can be relied upon. However, a normal test result cannot guarantee a normal baby although it does exclude chromosome anomalies.

If the results are abnormal, your hospital midwife or obstetrician will contact you and arrange to discuss with you and your partner the implications of the anomaly which has been discovered. In some cases, it may also be appropriate for you to talk with a paediatrician (children's specialist), geneticist or other specialist. Sometimes it is difficult to say with absolute certainty how badly a baby might be affected. Other investigations, such as a detailed ultrasound scan of the fetal heart, may be useful.

If it is found that the baby would be likely to suffer from a significant degree of mental or physical disability, you may wish to consider a termination of pregnancy. By the time these results are available this means the induction of labour and the vaginal delivery of the fetus.

This can be similar to a labour. Some women find that having decided to have the test, and having discovered that the fetus has an anomaly, that they do not want the pregnancy terminated. It is neither essential nor compulsory to terminate a pregnancy if the fetus is significantly affected. However, those women who feel that they would certainly not terminate their pregnancy, even if their child were affected by a chromosomal anomaly, should think very carefully before choosing to have any of the screening or diagnostic tests for these conditions. Sometimes it is useful to know in advance of any anomaly in order to prepare for this and to get the best advice about how to cope in the future.

ALTERNATIVES TO AMNIOCENTESIS

The same chromosome tests can be performed from ten weeks of pregnancy by the technique of chorionic villus sampling (CVS). The results may then be available at a time when a much more straightforward termination of pregnancy can be arranged should the results be abnormal. Unfortunately, the risks of miscarriage and possibly damage to the baby seem to be higher with this test.

A blood sample can also be taken directly from the umbilical cord; 'cordocentesis'. This gives rapid and accurate information, but is associated with significant risks for the baby.

NUCHAL TRANSLUCENCY

Understandably, there has been a great deal of effort made to develop a test which reliably identifies chromosomal anomalies such as Down syndrome early in pregnancy, when a termination is more straightforward, and which does not have a risk of miscarriage.

Some studies have suggested that the measurement of the skin fold at the nape of the baby's neck can be a useful indicator of chromosomal anomaly. This can be done by ultrasound in early pregnancy. However, it is not a diagnostic test, and will only provide an estimate of the risk that the developing fetus has a chromosomal anomaly.

SUBSEQUENT ANTENATAL VISITS

In many centres in the UK, pregnant women carry their own medical notes and bring them to each antenatal visit. In other centres, a 'co-op' card has a similar purpose, and contains all the important information about the pregnancy. During the pregnancy the information is this booklet will be updated and women are asked to keep this information with them at all times.

At each visit the blood pressure and urine will be checked. A rise in blood pressure may indicate 'pregnancy induced hypertension' or pre-eclampsia' (see page 168). A urine specimen will also be checked. The presence of protein or blood in the urine may be an indicator of urinary infection, or may indicate pre-eclampsia when protein is found in conjunction with raised blood pressure.

The size of the growing baby is measured at each visit. This may be done by measurement of the uterus by the doctor, midwife or by ultrasound. In later pregnancy the lie of the baby (whether down or across the uterus), whether the head (cephalic) or bottom (breech) points towards the pelvis and how much the head or breech are engaged will also be assessed. The part of the baby that is closest to the cervix is called the 'presenting part'. The distance of the presenting part from the pelvic brim is usually measured in 'fifths palpable' and recorded on the co-op card. The volume of amniotic fluid (the cushioning material for the baby) is also checked, and should not be increased nor diminished in volume. It is important to remember that about ninety-six per cent of babies are normal and well.

The baby's heart can also be heard using a hand-held instrument.

Antenatal care is also about maximising general health, answering questions about pregnancy and preparing the woman and her partner for labour and parenthood. Advice may also be given about avoidable risk factors, such as smoking, excessive alcohol and drug abuse, and help offered where appropriate.

TYPES OF ANTENATAL CARE

There are several types of antenatal care, depending on local circumstances and your individual needs. Broadly speaking, they fall into the following categories:

FULL HOSPITAL CARE

This is for those women who have specific problems that need specialist attention throughout their pregnancy; for example, women with diabetes or very high blood pressure. In addition, full care will usually be available for women who would not have any other recourse to antenatal care; for example, if they are not registered with a GP who offers antenatal care.

SHARED CARE

The vast majority of pregnant women have this type of care, where visits are shared between the hospital staff, their family doctor's team and the hospital and community midwifery teams.

MIDWIFE-LED CARE

This was the norm many years ago and it is offered to many healthy women who are having uncomplicated pregnancies. If problems arise, the midwife can ask for specialist medical help from the family doctor or hospital team.

BABY GROWTH

An average baby weighs about 450 g (1 lb) at around twenty weeks. This is about halfway through pregnancy and when the mother may feel the baby move for the first time. Six weeks later, it weighs 900 g (2 lb); four weeks later at thirty weeks it weighs 1.3 kg (3 lb), and by thirty-six weeks it will weigh about 3 kg (6 lb).

Although the average baby weighs 3.3 kg (7½ lb) at birth, it does not mean to say that because a baby is 3 kg (6 lb) that it is underweight or because it is 4 kg (9 lb) that it is overweight. Some babies are meant to be big whereas others are meant to be smaller.

A fetus who seems to be much larger than normal, or who is growing at a very rapid rate may suggest that the mother has developed diabetes; so called 'gestational diabetes'. This might require treatment with diet or even with insulin injections.

If the baby is not growing adequately, or is extremely small, this also requires careful monitoring, usually with ultrasound. Not all small babies are unhealthy, but if there is a suggestion that the baby is not receiving adequate nutrition through the placenta, this may be an indication for earlier delivery.

GENERAL HEALTH ADVICE

General health measures you can take include the following:
- Eat a healthy balanced diet.
- Look after your teeth; free dental health is available to pregnant women.
- Take a reasonable amount of gentle exercise.
- Concentrate on good posture to avoid back problems.

Most people today have a reasonably healthy lifestyle, which means that when they embark on a pregnancy no particular precautions or change of habits are required. This is particularly true of diet.

DIET

Those women who have a balanced diet and are not either very under or overweight should have no need to change their eating habits. there is no reason to greatly increase the amount of food eaten or to make substantial dietary changes. However, there is good evidence that folic acid (a B vitamin) may be beneficial in reducing the chances of having a baby with spina bifida and other neural tube defects (see page 152). All women planning to conceive are advised to take folic acid (0.4 micrograms) for one month prior to becoming pregnant and until twelve weeks of pregnancy.

Most mothers will gain up to about 12 kg (27 lb) in weight during a normal pregnancy. Often poor appetite and nausea in the first few months will mean that weight gain is usually steady throughout pregnancy until delivery. Excessive weight gained in pregnancy can be difficult to shed. Overweight mothers are also more prone to complications in pregnancy. For those who do find that they gain excess weight in pregnancy, some women find that breast feeding helps them to lose this weight when the baby is born, although they may retain some extra weight until breast-feeding has ceased. This extra weight will disappear without the need for dieting once you have finished breastfeeding.

Dieting in pregnancy is not advised, and a healthy and varied diet is recommended. For those who are very overweight there is an increased risk of certain obstetric complications, particularly high blood pressure, diabetes in pregnancy and problems at delivery. Therefore it is sensible to seek advice about a weight reduction diet prior to starting a pregnancy. In particular, the diet should be rich in calcium and iron. Skimmed and semi-skimmed milk contain just as much calcium as full-fat milk. Fresh fruit and vegetables and water can help with the constipation that troubles many pregnant women. Good sources of iron include leafy green vegetables, wholemeal bread, molasses, lentils, dried fruit, pulses and eggs, as well as red meat. Some foods, such as uncooked eggs, may be unsafe if eaten in pregnancy. Liver and soft cheeses should not be eaten, as they can cause listeriosis. Protein can be obtained from meat, fish, poultry, wholegrain cereals, beans and lentils, and low-fat dairy products. Vegetarians can usually get sufficient protein from their diet although vegans may be short on some nutrients and should consult their doctor for advice. Fresh fruit, fresh vegetables and cereals will all provide minerals and vitamins. Ask your midwife or dietician for more details.

EXERCISE

Physical and emotional preparation for childbirth is very important. By learning about what may happen, pregnant women can be better prepared in order to enjoy the experience of childbirth. Physical preparation is also useful. Most antenatal classes will offer the opportunity to take part in exercises that may help in childbirth. These are usually led by a trained physiotherapist and include limbering up and relaxation exercises. They can be learnt at the clinic and then practised at home. In addition to this, everyday sensible exercise is wise (see page 191).

SMOKING

The main advice given at pre-pregnancy counselling clinics relates to general health, especially concerning potentially harmful practices, particularly smoking. Maternal smoking increases by about one-third the chances of miscarriage and of delivering a small baby. It also increases the chances of the baby dying at or around the time of delivery and having major health problems in the first year of life. This is probably related not only to poor growth within the womb but also to the smoky environment after the baby is born.

Therefore there is always strong advice given to any woman who wishes to embark on pregnancy about giving up smoking, which is probably the factor that is of greatest benefit to the outcome of the subsequent pregnancy. It also has a knock-on effect of being beneficial for long-term health as lung cancer is now the biggest cancer killer of women in the Western world. Partner smoking should also be discouraged.

ALCOHOL

It is not thought that occasional or moderate consumption of alcohol is dangerous in pregnancy, but there is no clear information about an absolute safe level of alcohol consumption.

For this reason, pregnant women are advised to avoid alcohol, or to keep their consumption to a minimum, particularly in early pregnancy when most of the brain development occurs.

Heavy alcohol consumption in pregnancy is not advisable and can occasionally lead to abnormalities in the developing child and addiction to alcohol in the newborn baby. Alcohol crosses the placenta and so the baby is exposed to alcohol when the mother drinks.

DRUGS IN PREGNANCY

Many women will become pregnant whilst taking medication prescribed by their doctors. Others will develop medical problems while they are pregnant or after delivery and may need medication.

Pregnant women and their doctors are always concerned about the effect that any medicine may have on the developing child. Very few drugs are recommended for use in pregnancy. Occasionally this is because harmful effects on the baby have been demonstrated. More frequently, they are not recommended because the effects on pregnancy are not known. A drug which is known to cause serious abnormalities in pregnancies is called a teratogen. This does not mean that use of these preparations will always cause such serious problems, but these drugs should almost always be avoided.

Those women who take regular medication and plan to become pregnant (or who do not use contraception) should discuss this medication with their doctors. Often it is possible to switch to a similar drug that is known to be safer in pregnancy. In general, most drugs are best avoided during the early months of pregnancy, but it is not advisable to stop medication without discussing this with your doctor.

It may be impossible to know what is contained in drugs bought on the street. Crack cocaine is particularly dangerous in pregnancy and may lead to placental abruption (see page 168) as well as growth problems for the baby. If you have taken drugs and then find out that you are pregnant, you should consult your doctor or midwife for advice about the possible effects of these preparations on the developing baby.

MEDICATION FOR PSYCHOLOGICAL PROBLEMS

Many pregnant women find that previously diagnosed psychological problems improve during pregnancy. The most commonly used drugs are those for anxiety, including the benzodiazepines. These include such drugs as diazepam (Valium), chlordiazepoxide (Librium) and lorazepam (Ativan). There is a remote possibility that these drugs may cause problems in the baby if taken during the first three months of pregnancy. This finding has not been confirmed in all studies and if you were taking these drugs before you became aware that you were pregnant, it is very unlikely that your baby has been harmed. It is best to avoid taking them if you are breast-feeding as they transfer readily into your breast milk and thereafter into your baby. Other drugs, such as the barbiturates, are seldom used now and should not be taken by women who are pregnant or breastfeeding.

HAZARDS AT WORK

For the great majority of women, their working life is unlikely to impact on their pregnancy. However, certain jobs involving chemicals or contact with infections may be harmful in pregnancy. Women with concerns relating to these areas can seek advice from the occupational health or health and safety advisor.

There has been concern in recent years about the possibility of certain stresses at work or the use of electrical equipment, particularly video display units (VDUs), increasing the chances of miscarriage. However, at the moment we have no reason to believe that this is true.

TRAVELLING IN PREGNANCY

Since pregnancy is a normal and healthy condition, there is generally little reason to make changes in plans for travelling in most circumstances.

Because of the increased tendency for the blood to clot in pregnancy, it is wise to avoid situations where you may be sitting in cramped conditions without adequate leg room. If this does occur, simple muscle stretching exercises can help to maintain normal blood flow and to reduce the risk of blood clot (thrombosis).

Also, it is usually advised to avoid countries where there is a high risk of serious transmissible infections such as malaria. These countries include East and West Africa, Thailand and Papua New Guinea. Protection against malaria is advised for all those visiting areas where malaria is common, since preparations are available which do not appear to cause problems in pregnancy. Some of these preparations are thought to be safe in pregnancy. In addition those planning to visit a malarial area should take precautions to avoid mosquito bites, such as using insect repellent and wearing long sleeves and long trousers. However, if you need to be treated for malaria, then make sure you tell the doctor you are pregnant. Some drugs are not proven safe.

Some areas of the world require vaccination before travel, and some of these vaccines are best avoided in pregnancy. If you have to travel, however, seek professional advice. In some cases, the advice given may reflect where you intend staying, once you reach your destination, and what sort of accommodation you have.

It's worth knowing that walking and camping holidays in some warm, forested parts of Europe and Scandinavia are probably not advisable, as there is a risk of the disease tick-borne encephalitis in late spring and summer. Immunisation is not generally available for this.

AIR TRAVEL

Air travel is normally fine. In a pregnancy with complications, it may be wise to discuss any major travel plans with your midwife or doctor before making final arrangements. Many airlines do not permit pregnant passengers to fly if they are approaching their due date, and some forbid travel from as early as twenty-eight weeks. You may find that you are asked for a doctor's certificate confirming your fitness to travel, and confirmation of your due date. If you are thought to be at risk from giving birth prematurely, then you should also avoid air travel.

SOME TRAVEL TIPS:

■ Try and get an aisle or bulk head seat on the plane in order to get maximum leg room. Some airlines now let you pre-book your choice of seat in advance.

■ During a flight elasticated stockings may help varicose veins.

■ Always wear your seat belt when seated on a plane, and at all times in a car. The safest and most comfortable way to wear it is low around the pelvis and not straight across your bump.

■ The low level of humidity in most aircraft can cause dehydration. It may make the skin and eyes feel dry. The kidneys react to the dry atmosphere by conserving fluid, so drink plenty of non-alcoholic fluids.

■ On arrival, jet lag is best treated with small, frequent meals, and by avoiding drinks containing caffeine. Allow your body to adjust to local time gradually and naturally, sleeping when you feel the need.

■ Don't worry about the security screening checks in the airport. The devices used are not harmful to you or your baby.

■ Most women feel the heat much more when they're pregnant. If you are heading somewhere hot, pack clothing to keep you as cool as possible.

■ You are more at risk of thrush in pregnancy (an infection of the vagina and vulva, which causes itching, soreness and discharge), and hot, tight clothing such as shorts or trousers encourages it. So make sure clothing is loose and comfortable.

■ Take your co-operation card (with your midwife's and doctor's notes on) as it has important information, such as your blood group, which you may need in an emergency.

HOLIDAY EATING AND DRINKING

If you're not sure about the cleanliness of the water supply, drink bottled water only, after making sure the seal is secure. Boiled, filtered and chlorinated water can be used in an emergency. Short-term use of iodine-based purification tablets is safe on a one-off basis. Remember that salad vegetables in a restaurant or hotel will have been washed in tap water (if at all), and ice is certainly not safe in areas of poor hygiene. So don't drink diluted fruit juice, or iced drinks.

PREGNANCY IN OLDER WOMEN

The average age at which women in the UK give birth is gradually rising, as more couples delay starting a family until they have established careers and a home. In contrast, some couples may have had difficulty in starting a family at an earlier age and the first conception occurs only around or after their mid-thirties. However, there is a steady decline in female fertility with age, which becomes more marked in the late thirties. This is mainly due to a falling number of eggs that are capable of forming normal embryos.

It has been traditional in the past to consider that any woman over the age of thirty-five having her first baby as an 'elderly prima gravida'. Many such women attending the antenatal clinic are still given the impression that they are rather old to be having their first baby, but this is wrong and the expression is now out of date. In general, healthy women have healthy pregnancies, regardless of their age. Those women (of any age) who have medical problems preceding their pregnancy, such as high blood pressure, should seek advice from their doctor before conception (see page 162). In addition, diabetes of pregnancy (gestational diabetes) is more common in older mothers. In some centres all pregnant women will be screened for gestational diabetes and treated if necessary.

With increasing age, there is an increasing chance of having a baby with a chromosomal anomaly. This refers to Down syndrome and a few other rare chromosome abnormalities. There is no association between the instance of birth defects of unknown cause (e.g. spina bifida) and advancing maternal age. There is an increased risk of miscarriage and, to some extent, this is explained by the increased risk of chromosome anomaly. In these cases the anomaly is so severe that the embryo is not viable. For more information on the risks of Down syndrome and testing and screening procedures for this, see page 152.

Fibroids, although uncommon, are more likely to be present in the older woman. In pregnancy they may grow, shrink or remain the same. Rapid change in the size of a fibroid may cause pain. Unless they are situated in an unusual position, they do not cause trouble to the developing pregnancy. Ultrasound can be used to measure their growth. In the majority of cases, they do not interfere with the pregnancy or delivery and may need to be reassessed some time after the birth.

DELIVERY

In an uncomplicated pregnancy, there is no reason why delivery in the older woman should differ from that of any other pregnant woman

BREASTFEEDING

There is no evidence to suggest that older mothers are less able to breastfeed, and your midwife or doctor will encourage you to breastfeed your baby.

PRE-PREGNANCY COUNSELLING

Pre-pregnancy counselling can give advice to prospective parents prior to pregnancy, and help to optimise the health of the mother and baby during pregnancy.

This counselling may include general guidance concerning diet, lifestyle, the influence of illness or regular medication on a pregnancy, and problems relating to complications from a previous pregnancy which may have ended in the loss of the baby. The needs of every couple are highly individual and the pre-pregnancy counselling is geared to this.

Couples can seek advice from the family doctor or health visitor or consult a Pre-pregnancy Counselling Clinic. These clinics are associated with maternity hospitals throughout the UK. If necessary, they can make a referral to a specialist clinic should this be required.

HOW PRE-PREGNANCY CLINICS WORK

The GP may provide facilities for counselling, either themselves or by the Health Visitor. There may also be self-help groups locally which can give advice on specific subjects. The advantage of these groups is that they offer the opportunity of meeting other people with similar problems and who may be able to provide ongoing support.

Pre-pregnancy Counselling Clinics generally require a referral from the GP or from another hospital service. Some pre-pregnancy clinics send out a questionnaire asking about the specific problems of each couple in order to provide the most personalised service. It is important for the clinic to have as much information as possible about possible problems before the appointment. The clinics are usually run by medical and nursing staff with particular expertise and interest.

People who attend these clinics usually fall within four categories:

■ Women or couples wanting general health advice before embarking on their pregnancies
■ People with known medical disorders who wish to check the possible effects of their condition on pregnancy
■ If either parent has a health problem carried by the genes or has a family history of this, pre-pregnancy counselling might be helpful
■ Women with past obstetric problems who wish to discuss the possible reasons why their problems occurred and the chances of recurrence in the future.

KNOWN MEDICAL DISORDERS

Women who have had a diagnosis made of some form of medical disorder should seek advice about how their condition may affect a pregnancy. This is particularly true for those women who take regular medication, as it may be necessary to change medication prior to pregnancy. The conditions of particular concern are diabetes, epilepsy, renal disease, high blood pressure, endocrine disorders (such as thyroid disease) and women with a past history of blood clotting, particularly if they are on blood thinning (anticoagulant) therapy. Being pregnant may also affect the nature or pattern of the illness. Some common conditions improve in pregnancy and others

tend to get worse. If you have a known medical disorder, it is important to seek advice from your doctor, specialist or pre-pregnancy counselling clinic on how best to reduce any risks to you and your baby.

KNOWN GENETIC DISORDERS

Those couples who have a family history of an inherited condition, or have one themselves, may wish to seek advice before conception about the possibilities of passing it on to their children. Not all genetic disorders are hereditary, so there may not be an increased risk of these conditions recurring. Unnecessary worry may be avoided by having counselling prior to embarking on pregnancy. Tests can be carried out on both partners before conception, and the results can give a more accurate assessment of the risks of passing on a genetic condition. Those who are known to carry a genetic disorder may be able to have tests in early pregnancy to test whether the baby has been affected. The chances of genetic anomalies increase with the age of the mother. Tests are now available in pregnancy to indicate the chances that a baby carries common genetic anomalies such as Down syndrome, and these conditions can be diagnosed in pregnancy by tests such as amniocentesis and chorionic villous sampling (see page 152).

PREVIOUS OBSTETRIC PROBLEMS

Those women who have had problems in a previous pregnancy may wish to discuss these with their obstetrician or midwife. It may help to understand the cause of the problems and what can be done to reduce the chance of these problems recurring. Those who have a serious health problem that is likely to recur may be advised to stay in hospital for some of their pregnancy. For some women, a further pregnancy may be considered inadvisable because of the seriousness of their condition, and the possible effects that a pregnancy may have on their long-term heath.

Those women who have had recurrent (usually more than three consecutive) miscarriages may be offered tests to look for an underlying cause for miscarriage which may be amenable to treatment in a subsequent

pregnancy (see page 261).

Those women who had difficult or traumatic deliver should discuss the reasons why this happened and how it could be avoided next time. It may be that in a future pregnancy an elective caesarean section would reduce the problems.

Those who have had problems of thrombosis or blood clot in a previous pregnancy should seek advice concerning the need for blood-thinning drugs in a future pregnancy and the risks of a further thrombosis occurring.

COMMON CAUSES OF ANXIETY

Pregnancy is a normal event, but one which is accompanied by numerous changes in the body. Not all of these changes and adjustments are obvious and some may even be uncomfortable, but they are all normal. Not all pregnant women will experience these changes. Many women feel much happier and healthier in pregnancy than at other times. The common causes of anxiety have already been discussed and include backache, tiredness and sickness. Other symptoms which are less common may lead to problems and these are discussed more fully below. Most women experience no serious problems in pregnancy. However, some common concerns are discussed below.

VAGINAL DISCHARGE IN PREGNANCY

Vaginal discharges are of several kinds, some requiring treatment and others being perfectly normal and of no importance. To understand this, remember that the vagina, like the uterus, is very strongly influenced by the

female sex hormones oestrogen and progesterone. Oestrogen stimulates the tissues to mature and progesterone further develops them. This is most obvious in pregnancy, but changes occur in the lining tissues of the vagina and the cervix, as well as the uterus, during each menstrual cycle. These changes, caused by the hormone oestrogen, make the cells lining the cervix produce a thin, stretchy, slightly sticky mucus (rather like egg white) and this is most marked about two weeks before the period is due.

The cells that make up the lining of the vagina are arranged rather like bricks making up a wall. The top cells, which are thin and large, are constantly shed into the vagina, rather like leaves falling off a tree. In the vagina, they are acted upon by the helpful bacteria that normally live there to produce a weak acid (lactic acid), thereby preventing dangerous bacteria from growing in the vagina.

Thus the vaginal cells and the mucus add to the vaginal discharge. As well as this, some fluid seeps between the cells of the vagina to join the secretions there; this seepage is often increased during sexual excitement, anxiety, or sometimes if the woman is ill or emotionally upset.

The amount of normal vaginal secretions varies considerably just as the quantity of secretion in the mouth (saliva) varies. The secretions not only keep the vagina moist but also keep it clean. Sometimes, however, a vaginal discharge is a sign of infection.

NORMAL DISCHARGE IN PREGNANCY

A small quantity of thick mucoid vaginal discharge is usually present in early pregnancy and is often one of the earliest symptoms. It is usually clear, without an odour; it is not irritating or bloody and is much like the discharge that many women have prior to their menstrual periods. As pregnancy advances, this discharge often increases and may become quite heavy. Some women are more comfortable wearing sanitary pads during the last months of pregnancy for this reason.

Other than offending aesthetic sensibilities, the discharge should be of no concern. It is important to do the following:
■ Keep the genital area clean and dry
■ Avoid tight pants, jeans and leotards
■ Rinse the vaginal area after soaping during a bath or shower
■ Avoid exposing it to such irritants as deodorant soaps, bubble baths and perfumes.

ABNORMAL DISCHARGE IN PREGNANCY

Sometimes vaginal discharge is caused by bacteria that can cause infections. These infections are due to different organisms and are not serious, very common and can be treated easily.

If the discharge has a different odour to normal or is offensive, causes itchiness making you want to scratch, has a yellow-green colour, or is blood-stained, then this should be reported to the doctor.

VAGINAL DISCHARGE CAUSING INFECTION

The three main vaginal infections that are relatively minor that occur in pregnancy are:
■ Yeast infection (candida)
■ Bacterial vaginosis (BV)
■ Sexually acquired infections, such as chlamydia, Trichomonas (see page 127).

THRUSH

This is possibly the most common vaginal infection of all and one of the most irritating. It is caused by an organism called *Candida albicans* and no-one really knows why it occurs, although the fungus itself thrives because of the relatively high sugar content of the cells lining the vagina during pregnancy. It may be a new infection contracted during pregnancy or it may simply be a flare up of a dormant infection which has not previously caused any symptoms, for the thrush organism lives in the vagina innocently, and only causes a discharge due to some stimulus.

The main culprit is again the high levels of oestrogen and this is why thrush is common not only in pregnancy but also in diabetes.

It causes a thick, white, curdy discharge, often associated with intense irritation and redness around the vagina, and there is often a feeling of burning. This irritation may cause great distress and sometimes is so severe that it wakes women up during the night or prevents sleep. Because the urinary bladder is so near to the vagina it is not uncommon to experience urinary symptoms, such as frequency or burning while passing urine.

Thrush is easily recognised when the doctor examines the vagina because its appearance is quite characteristic, but sometimes a swab test is taken to confirm the diagnosis.

Treatment is usually by a pessary placed in the vagina and sometimes cream as well, which can be smeared around the entrance if there is soreness. Treatment for thrush can now be bought over the counter at your chemist.

RECURRENT THRUSH

Unfortunately thrush infections tend to recur, especially after pregnancy when the treatment can be more energetic. Hitherto treatment by mouth with a specific antibiotic has not been possible because this is not absorbed in the vagina but lately there is a useful drug (Diflucan) that can be used, although this is not commonly prescribed in pregnancy.

Your partner may harbour thrush but rarely has complaints. Sometimes thrush causes an irritation on the penis and, if so, treatment with a similar cream is all that is required.

One final point: there is no contraindication to having sexual intercourse during treatment with the cream and pessaries and, in fact, some doctors recommend this for the obvious reason that the partner will be treated at the same time.

TRICHOMONAS

This is an infection, also mild, and usually sexually transmitted, that is caused by a little organism that sits in the vagina and the male prostate gland. The sort of discharge that this produces is a thin, yellow-green discharge with a rather nasty fishy odour, though itching and irritation are not common. Again, the diagnosis is fairly simple on inspection and is confirmed by swab testing.

In most cases the infection will readily respond to a special antibiotic called

metronidazole (Flagyl) which should be given to the woman and her partner, although it is recommended that this treatment is not advisable in the early weeks of pregnancy. There are suitable alternative treatments that your doctor will advise.

BACTERIAL VAGINOSIS (BV)

This is a relatively new term coined for an old bacterial infection of the vagina. This infection is bacterial, very common, and again accompanied by a fishy odour. It is rather difficult to diagnose accurately but responds to the penicillin drugs or erythromycin which can be given in pregnancy.

This infection may have a role if the membranes rupture prematurely in late pregnancy and it is therefore important to treat this condition early on.

CHLAMYDIA

This is another bacterial infection that is sexually transmitted and the only symptom is a mild, irritating, usually yellow discharge which may go unnoticed. This organism is implicated when the membranes rupture (waters break) prematurely and some people feel there is an association between chlamydia infection and cot death babies. Two-thirds of babies born to infected mothers do contract the infection during vaginal delivery.

Chlamydia can be diagnosed both on inspection by the doctor and also by taking special swab tests. In the non-pregnant woman the antibiotic tetracycline is the best treatment, although this must not be taken in pregnancy because it may cause discolouration of the baby's teeth, and may also affect the way in which the premature teeth develop. There are, however, other good antibiotics that can be used instead, notably erythromycin.

BLOOD-STAINED DISCHARGE

Do not worry if you notice some blood smearing in the vagina as generally this is of no significance, but if it becomes anything more than just a stain then it should be reported to your doctor. Blood-stained discharge can be caused by some of the vaginal infections listed above because the vaginal walls become a little dry and irritated and bleed on contact. However, sometimes there are more important causes, such as blood coming from elsewhere in the pelvis.

CERVICAL ECTOPY (PREVIOUSLY CALLED EROSION)

One of the commonest causes of mild vaginal bleeding, especially after sexual intercourse or contact, is due to a cervical ectopy. The cervix is made of layers of cells where it penetrates into the upper part of the vagina. However, sometimes in pregnancy a sudden change can occur in the large, thick mucus-secreting cells that line the edge of the canal leading through the cervix. The cells now appear around the entrance to the canal to resemble pouting lips. This pouting of the cells is called an ectopy and is a normal event due to the presence of the hormone oestrogen.

It is common after pregnancy for this appearance of the cervix to persist although it does not need treatment unless a bloodstained or thick discharge continues. Treatment after pregnancy may not be needed. It usually consists of touching the area with an acid stick or hot wire called cauterisation and is a simple and effective treatment.

OTHER CAUSES OF BLOOD STAINING

■ Just occasionally poking through the cervix can be a little polyp, which is simply a little blood vessel on a stalk. It is of no consequence and usually does not need treatment although it is useful for the doctor to know that it is present as it may be the cause of a blood-stained discharge.

■ Again, it must be emphasised that simple blood staining is usually not significant but, if this turns into fresh bright bleeding, then this must be reported to the doctor immediately.

■ Later in pregnancy, or even as labour starts, a little blood-stained discharge is common and is one of the signs of impending labour. This is called the 'show' and is caused by a little plug of mucus that sits within the cervix guarding the entrance to the canal and preventing infection. When mild contractions start the mucus plug is pushed out and causes a little discharge or blood staining. It has no other significance.

■ Sometimes the discharge is watery as well and the woman may think that her waters have gone and the amniotic fluid around the baby has leaked through. Occasionally it is quite difficult to tell whether a watery discharge is being produced by the cervix (neck of the womb) or the waters around the baby, or even a small leakage of urine which can occur quite commonly. The doctor or midwife will be able to tell the difference so you should report it if you are worried.

BLEEDING IN EARLY PREGNANCY

Bleeding in the first trimester (first three months) of pregnancy occurs in about one-quarter of all pregnancies. Of these, not all will miscarry.

Bleeding before twenty-three to twenty-four weeks of pregnancy is called a 'threatened miscarriage'. The bleeding may arise from the cervix or from inside the uterus. If pain accompanies the bleeding, this suggests that a miscarriage may occur. The passage of tissue from the pregnancy makes this miscarriage inevitable. If pregnancy tissue is left behind in the uterus, this is called an 'incomplete miscarriage', and this tissue may need to be removed in a surgical operation. Pain in the first three months of pregnancy that is localised to one side of the abdomen with bleeding suggests that the pregnancy may be ectopic, (located outside of the uterus). This generally requires surgical removal.

Bleeding in early pregnancy may need to be managed in hospital, and should certainly warrant a visit to the GP. At the hospital an internal examination may confirm whether miscarriage is inevitable. This diagnosis will be made if the cervix is open. Miscarriage is often accompanied by heavy bleeding and pain. An ultrasound scan will indicate whether the fetus is still alive, although in very early pregnancy this may be difficult and the test will need to be repeated. However, sometimes the pregnancy is too early for this to be confirmed. A blood test may also be taken to measure the pregnancy hormone human chorionic gonadotrophin (hCG). This should double every 48 hours in a normal pregnancy. A level that is rising slowly may suggest an ectopic pregnancy. A falling level suggests a miscarriage.

■ If the ultrasound scan confirms that the fetus is alive and inside the uterus, then you will be advised to go home once the bleeding has stopped. Rhesus-negative women may require an injection of anti-D.

■ If the ultrasound scan reveals that a miscarriage has occurred but that tissue remains inside the uterus you may be offered surgery to remove this tissue, particularly if you are bleeding.

■ If the uterus is empty, this may indicate a complete miscarriage, or that the pregnancy is outside the uterus. Management in this situation will depend on other signs and symptoms, past medical history and perhaps the results of the pregnancy hormone levels.

BLEEDING IN LATER PREGNANCY

Bleeding in later pregnancy can arise from the placenta, particularly if it is low-lying in the uterus (placenta praevia), or if it starts to separate from the uterine wall (placental abruption). All bleeding in later pregnancy should be taken seriously and reported to the doctor or midwife. The baby's heart can be monitored and an ultrasound scan may be advised. Often no reason is found for the bleeding or else it is simply a sign that labour may be about to start. Heavy bleeding on its own or with pain will require a hospital visit.

HIGH BLOOD PRESSURE IN PREGNANCY

High blood pressure in pregnancy is often called pregnancy-induced hypertension (PIH) or pre-eclampsia. This is a complication of pregnancy which has been recognised for centuries. The condition is common and is occasionally serious. Pregnancy-induced hypertension is an increase in blood pressure in a pregnant woman who had a normal blood pressure before she became pregnant. If protein is also present in her urine, the condition is described as pre-eclampsia or pregnancy toxaemia. Although many steps in the process leading to the development of the condition have been identified and are understood, the initial cause is not yet known.

Pregnancy-induced hypertension will develop in five to ten per cent of women who are having their first baby. One-third of women with PIH will also have protein in their urine, ie they will have pre-eclampsia. Unless someone has previously suffered from PIH, the condition is unlikely to develop when having a second or subsequent baby. Although having an uncomplicated first pregnancy dramatically reduces the likelihood of developing PIH, a previous miscarriage has no protective effect.

WHO IS AT RISK?

Any pregnant woman who is due to have her first baby may develop pregnancy-induced hypertension. Some groups of women are at increased risk. These include:

■ Women with twin pregnancies
■ Women with a family history of PIH (in a mother or sister)
■ Women with diabetes
■ Women with a history of PIH in a previous pregnancy.

It is interesting to note that while smoking increases the risks of many of the complications of pregnancy, smokers are less likely to develop PIH than non-smokers. However, the severity of the condition tends to be increased if PIH does develop in a smoker.

TESTS AND SCREENING

At present, there is no accepted screening programme for PIH. However, several screening tests are being investigated, including blood tests, urine tests and special scanning techniques which measure blood flow to the placenta.

AVOIDING PIH

Restricting calorie, fluid or salt intake in pregnancy appear to have little or no effect on whether pregnancy-induced hypertension

(PIH) will develop, and neither does bed rest. However, if you are at high risk of developing PIH (see above) you may be given low dose aspirin from about 14 to 30 weeks.

SYMPTOMS OF PIH

You probably won't know if you have developed PIH. It usually occurs without any symptoms being present. Therefore it is vital that your blood pressure and urine are checked regularly by your midwife or doctor. PIH is found in most cases within a few weeks of the expected delivery date although it can develop earlier in the pregnancy. The time intervals between your regular blood pressure and urine checks will shorten as your pregnancy advances.

PREGNANCY PROBLEMS

It is very unusual for problems to result from PIH alone. However, if protein is present in your urine and your blood pressure is high, problems may affect both you and your baby. Although uncommon, these complications can be serious and therefore your pregnancy will be watched very carefully.

High blood pressure alone can occasionally lead to significant problems although pre-eclampsia may affect other organs such as the kidney, liver or blood.

The most common problem affecting the baby is prematurity since, in severe cases of pre-eclampsia, it is sometimes necessary to deliver the baby early. In addition, the blood supply to the placenta may be reduced in pre-eclampsia, causing your baby to grow slowly.

TREATMENT OF PIH

If you do not have any protein in your urine, your doctor may be happy for you to remain at home with regular blood pressure and urine checks, often by your community midwife.

However, if protein is found in your urine, you will be admitted to a hospital antenatal ward. This can be very frustrating for many women who feel completely well. It is difficult to estimate how long you would have to stay in hospital should you be admitted. PIH is a very unpredictable disease and the wellbeing of both you and your baby can alter very rapidly and precipitate treatment or delivery of your baby may be necessary.

While you are in hospital your condition will be monitored carefully:

■ The amount of protein in your urine will be measured accurately – this may involve you collecting your urine over twenty-four hours.

■ Blood and urine tests will check that your kidneys and liver are working well, and will measure the number of platelets in your blood. Platelets are one of the types of blood cells – numbers are reduced when pre-eclampsia is severe.

■ You will also be monitored, using ultrasound scanning techniques, to measure the baby's growth and wellbeing and regular heartbeat traces.

DRUG TREATMENTS

There are drugs that will lower your blood pressure without affecting your baby. However, these will not prevent the effects of pre-eclampsia on your liver and kidneys, and on the blood supply to your placenta. In view of this, many doctors only use drugs to lower blood pressure in women whose blood pressure has risen to unsafe levels. Once blood pressure control has been achieved, delivery of the baby is recommended.

DELIVERY OF THE BABY

If you have PIH without protein in your urine, you will probably be allowed to go into labour naturally. However, if you have protein in your urine you will be admitted to hospital and the possible delivery of your baby will be discussed on a day-to-day basis. If a definite diagnosis of pre-eclampsia has been made, your doctor is likely to recommend delivery when he or she feels that the baby would do well.

The mode of delivery will depend on how many weeks pregnant you are and how severe the PIH is. Therefore a caesarean section is not always necessary and you may be able to have a normal vaginal delivery. It may be recommended that you have an epidural in labour. Your anaesthetist may want to take a blood sample to check that your blood is clotting normally before you have an epidural.

If you are unfortunate to be one of the very small number of women who have severe pre-eclampsia, then you will be monitored extremely carefully throughout your labour. The priorities of your doctors will be to prevent your blood pressure rising to unsafe levels and to prevent eclampsia occurring. In this rare condition the woman has an epileptic fit, but you can be given drug treatment to reduce the likelihood of this.

AFTER THE BABY IS BORN

You will get better after your baby is born. Although PIH is occasionally found in the first few hours after delivery, the vast majority of women with PIH make a steady and uncomplicated recovery once their baby is born.

If you needed drugs to control your blood pressure while you were pregnant, then it may be necessary to continue these, but only for a matter of days or weeks rather than months.

When you go home with your baby, your doctor and community midwife will continue to check that your blood pressure is well controlled. You will probably have a hospital clinic visit to check that your blood pressure is normal and that your kidneys and liver are working normally. This usually takes place three months after the birth of your baby, as the normal changes of pregnancy have resolved by this time.

If your blood pressure was normal before you became pregnant and returns to normal after the birth of your baby, and the blood and urine tests taken three months after delivery are normal, then you are no more likely to suffer high blood pressure in later life than anyone else.

If you become pregnant again, you have a twenty-five per cent chance of developing PIH. In subsequent pregnancies it is often less severe and is found later in the pregnancy.

LESS COMMON PROBLEMS

The following problems are less common and the information is only relevant to a minority of women. However, if you should experience these difficulties it is important to have information which will allow you to understand what is happening and to ask relevant questions.

THROMBOSIS IN PREGNANCY

The body depends upon the supply of oxygen and nutrients that travel in the blood stream. The blood is pumped from the heart and speeds through the arteries to the tissues where it delivers its nutrients and, in return, washes out waste products. Blood returns rather more slowly through the veins to the heart having passed through the kidneys and lungs for removal of waste products and renewal of oxygen respectively. The nutrients are loaded on at the liver and delivered to the tissues. If any part of this flow system is blocked, then tissue damage follows. The commonest blockage is a clot, or thrombus, which forms in a blood vessel. During pregnancy this is most common in the veins damming back blood so that new flow into the areas is held back.

The commonest veins to allow clots in pregnancy are those in the leg in the back of the calf and in the pelvis draining from the uterus. A clot may occur because of:
■ Increased stickiness of the blood during and after pregnancy
■ A slowing of the circulation if the veins are compressed (as when the legs lie against a mattress for some time)
■ Minor damage to the lining of the veins may occur in the pelvis.

All these allow the liquid blood to solidify, become a gel and then a firm clot which blocks the vessel. Usually by-pass veins can carry some of the blood on so that the circulation is not completely stopped but tissues in the areas served by the vein are damaged and can lead to ankle swelling and a white leg after birth.

More serious is that some of the upper parts of these clots can break off and be carried in the blood stream of the veins up through the heart into arteries of the lungs. This, a pulmonary embolism, which usually causes chest pain and shortness of breath, can lead to very serious illness and needs immediate treatment in hospital.

A blood clot in the leg will normally show itself by causing the leg to become swollen, red and painful. If this should happen to you, then it is very important that you go and see your doctor immediately. You will be sent to hospital, where the flow of blood through the leg veins will be checked using ultrasound techniques. This is exactly the same as when ultrasound is used to scan your baby, and is not painful.

If a blood clot is confirmed, then you will be given special treatment to make the blood thin. This is known as anticoagulation and its aim is to prevent more clot formation and to try and make the clot that is present much firmer. This will be done by injecting a substance called heparin, which prevents blood clotting. Initially, it will be given by continuously infusing it into a vein, although after some days it will be possible to stop the continuous infusion and to give it by intermittent injection. If the blood clot is large and particularly if there is a pulmonary embolism, then occasionally treatment may be prescribed to dissolve some of the clots already formed. The anticoagulant treatment will be continued until about thirty-six weeks of pregnancy or immediately prior to labour. It will be recommenced after the baby is born as this again is a time when blood clots are more likely to occur. Anticoagulation is not given during delivery because of the risk of bleeding.

If you have had a clot in a vein or in the lungs in a previous pregnancy then you are likely to be given anticoagulants in each subsequent pregnancy, and when they will be started will be discussed with you when you attend the hospital for your booking visit. This is also true for women who have had clot while not pregnant, for example when on the oral contraceptive pill. Whether you are given anticoagulation and when it is started will depend if there was a particular factor which made it more likely for you to have a clot. These include some heredity disorders of clotting, which increase the chance considerably. Women with these problems are likely to be given routine anticoagulant treatment in any pregnancy.

RISK FACTORS
If you are a smoker then it is important that you try and stop as smoking will increase your likelihood of having a clotting problem. You should also eat a sensible diet. Other factors that make a clot more likely are operative delivery either by forceps or caesarean section, although in the main there is little that you can do about this.

AFTER PREGNANCY
If you have a clot in your leg during pregnancy then you will continue to receive heparin for a short interval after delivery. You will then be changed to warfarin which thins the blood effectively and can be taken in tablet form. It is then likely that you will continue on this treatment for some months. For those who have had a clot in a vein in the distant past but not in this pregnancy, then it is probable that no warfarin will be required.

For those who have a clotting episode for the first time, blood tests will be performed to check that there is no heredity disorder of the clotting pathways. These pathways are very complex and involve inter-reacting factors which allows very fine control of the system. However, people are born with very slight abnormalities of some of the proteins in the system, which gives them a tendency to clot. This is more likely if here are members of your family who have also had trouble with increased blood clotting.

If you are found to be one of these individuals, then it is likely that you will need to have blood thinning treatment if you have another baby and possibly after major operations, that is at times when clotting is more likely. All women who are found to have a predisposition to clotting should be seen by a haematologist (somebody who specialises in blood disorders) to discuss what it means. Since it also affects using the oral contraceptive pill and possibly hormone replacement therapy, then it is absolutely vital that the advice is well informed and correct.

However, with vigilant care by yourself and your doctors, further clots can usually be prevented or, if they do occur, can be treated properly before they give rise to a clot in the lungs.

MULTIPLE PREGNANCY

Twins are the most common multiple pregnancy, and approximately one in every eighty pregnancies is a twin pregnancy. Multiple pregnancy is more common in those who have a family history, and has a marked racial prevalence, being much more common in African women compared to white or Asian women. Twin pregnancy is also more common in older women.

Twins are either monozygotic (identical) or dizygotic (non identical). It may be possible to determine which kind of twins you are carrying by an ultrasound scan in early pregnancy. Otherwise, examination of the placenta after delivery usually provides this information. Non identical twins are no more alike than any other siblings, and may either be the same or different sex.

As well as in spontaneous conceptions, multiple pregnancy may occur as a result of fertility treatment. By law (in the UK), only three embryos can be placed in the uterus at the time of IVF (see page 241), and between a fifth and a quarter of these pregnancies are multiple. However, drugs that stimulate ovulation, such as clomiphene (see page 258) may lead to the development of many eggs which can, in turn, lead to twins and more rarely multiple pregnancies (such as triplets). These drugs should only be used with strict monitoring.

Many couples are delighted at the idea of twins. Others are anxious about how they will cope with the demands of a twin pregnancy and two tiny infants. A multiple pregnancy is considered 'high risk' and women with twins will usually be cared for by an obstetrician during their pregnancy. Certain complications, such as anaemia, high blood pressure and premature labour are more common in multiple pregnancy, and mothers will be monitored closely for these (see above). Because of the increased fetal need for vitamins and nutrition in multiple pregnancy, mothers are advised to take supplements of iron during their pregnancy. Normal activity is encouraged, but some women find a twin pregnancy more tiring than a singleton pregnancy, and must adapt their lives accordingly.

Preterm labour is more common in multiple pregnancy, with triplets even more than twins. At term, the majority of twins are both head down ('cephalic'), and most women opt for vaginal delivery. However, breech presentation is more common in twins, and your obstetrician may advise delivery by caesarean section if the first twin is breech. In the rare event of triplets, caesarean section is commonly advised. Many hospitals have special clinics, particularly for women with multiple pregnancies. Here you will be able to discuss all your concerns with the obstetrician and midwife as well as meeting other mothers in a similar situation.

MEDICAL CONDITIONS

For many women having a baby is very important even if they have an underlying medical condition which will increase the risks for them and their babies. Many of these conditions are rare but often the women concerned have difficulty in obtaining information which is why they are covered in some depth in this chapter.

The first condition to be discussed is asthma, which is becoming much more common as we tend to take less exercise and live in a polluted environment.

ASTHMA

If you have asthma, pregnancy is the ideal time to think about your general health and to make sure that your asthma is well controlled. Women with asthma should be leading normal and active lives, and there is no reason why your asthma should prevent you from having a normal pregnancy and a healthy baby. Too many people suffer unnecessarily with their asthma, either because they do not realise that they have it or because they (and sometimes their doctors) think that it is acceptable for an asthmatic to wake up wheezing and coughing at night, or to feel breathless during normal daily activities.

Asthma is common in young people, so it is also common for asthma to affect pregnant women. it is said to occur in about one in 100 pregnancies but, because it is often undiagnosed, this is probably an underestimate. There are over 10,000 babies born in the UK each year to mothers who have asthma.

No woman should decide not to have a baby just because she has asthma, since asthma is usually not affected by pregnancy and there are no long-term effects of pregnancy on asthma.

About three-quarters of all pregnant women feel a little breathless at some time during their pregnancies. This may be due to pregnancy hormones which make them breathe more deeply. Therefore, if you feel breathless while you are pregnant it does not necessarily mean that your asthma is getting worse.

What will make your asthma worse is suddenly to decrease your asthma treatments when you are pregnant. Many women, thinking that their treatment may be harmful to the baby, stop using their inhalers or tablets, or are reluctant to take additional treatment when they are pregnant. In fact, poorly treated asthma might be more dangerous for you and your baby than the medication used to control and treat it.

The important message is that the treatment of asthma is harmless to your unborn baby, but if under-treated, severe asthma might be detrimental. The right advice and treatment can make you feel healthier and can help you to have a successful and fulfilling pregnancy.

WHAT IS ASTHMA?

Your body needs oxygen in order for the various body systems to work. The two lungs act rather like balloons which are blown up when you breathe in and go down when you breathe out. Their job is to transfer the oxygen from the air that you breathe in to the blood, so it can be transported to and used by different parts of the body.

The breathing tubes (bronchi) carry air into and out of the lungs. In asthma, these are irritable with a tendency to narrow, making it more difficult to breathe in and out.

Women with asthma usually have repeated episodes of wheezing and shortness of breath or coughing. Sometimes there are clear provoking trigger factors, such as pollen, dust or fur, that set off these attacks which may be made worse by colds and chest infections, exercise and emotional upsets. Asthma is a very variable condition – some people have only occasional mild attacks whereas others need long-term inhaled treatment and tablets to keep them well.

HOW IS ASTHMA TREATED?

The treatment of asthma in pregnancy is the same as for a non-pregnant woman. None of the drugs routinely used in the treatment of asthma have been shown to be unsafe during pregnancy, but severe asthma that is left untreated or is poorly treated could be dangerous to both a pregnant woman and her unborn baby.

Asthma treatment can be divided broadly into two types:
1 Treatment used to prevent attacks
2 Treatment used to relieve the symptoms of asthma if an attack does occur.

Nowadays it is thought that if someone with asthma needs to use a reliever medication more than once or twice a day, then they should, in addition, be taking a preventer. If they are already doing so, then the dose of the preventer needs to be increased. Modern treatment of asthma is based very largely on medication that is inhaled (breathed in) rather than taken by mouth as tablets or capsules, although drugs in this form can sometimes be useful as an addition to inhalers.

RELIEVER TREATMENTS

Reliever inhalers, such as salbutamol and terbutaline, dilate (open up) the bronchi. They are quick and effective and will relieve the symptoms of coughing, wheezing and breathlessness within a few minutes. If you have asthma, you should always carry your reliever inhaler with you.

PREVENTER TREATMENTS

The most common inhaled preventer drugs are beclomethasone, budesonide and cromoglycate; nedocromil is also used. These medications must be taken regularly (morning and evening) if you are to benefit from them. They work by preventing the inflammation in the bronchi which causes asthma attacks. Unlike the bronchodilator (reliever) inhalers described above, which take effect immediately, you will notice no immediate improvement after taking your preventer inhaler. However, this does not mean that it is not working. It will only begin to work after two or three days and does not reach its maximum effectiveness for longer than this.

OTHER TREATMENTS

There are other treatments for asthma. Your doctor will advise on which treatments are best for you. Make sure that you discuss with your doctor all your different asthma treatments and that you understand how each is to be used. Most commonly, problems arise because people do not understand that their preventer

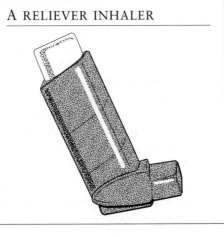

A RELIEVER INHALER

Left: Inhalers may be required by women with asthma. The same drugs are used as for women who are not pregnant.

medications need to be taken regularly rather than just when symptoms are present. There are some drugs that should be avoided while you are pregnant, including the following:

■ Certain antihistamines, sedatives and sleeping tablets may cause sedation in the baby

■ One particular antibiotic called tetracycline causes permanent discoloration of the baby's teeth

■ Cough medicines containing iodine can harm the baby's thyroid gland

■ Also, never take medicines that have been prescribed for someone else.

ARE THERE ANY RISKS TO THE BABY?

Provided your asthma is well controlled and correctly treated, there is no increased risk for your baby.

BEFORE PREGNANCY

If you are asthmatic and planning to become pregnant, it is a good idea to discuss it with your family doctor or respiratory physician (chest specialist) first. He or she will be able to answer many of your questions and concerns, and will make absolutely sure that you are receiving the best possible treatment for your asthma.

ANTENATAL CARE

When you attend the booking-in clinic, you should tell the doctor or midwife that you have asthma and what medication you are taking. Mention again any sleep disturbance or other symptoms you are experiencing. If you are not already attending an asthma clinic, this may be organised for you, or you can ask to see a specialist if you are concerned about your asthma.

SMOKING

Smoking is bad for your health at any time, as it increases the risk of heart attacks, strokes

and especially lung cancer. If you are asthmatic, smoking will make your asthma worse. Long-term smokers may develop chronic bronchitis which is a disease similar to asthma but, unlike asthma, the narrowing of the bronchi is not reversible.

TRIGGER FACTORS

Avoid definite trigger factors for your asthma, e.g. feather pillows, contact with domestic animals or smoking.

BAD AND PROLONGED ATTACKS

There is no point in putting on a brave face and convincing yourself and your doctors that you have your asthma under control if you do not. Very rarely, even with all the correct treatment, asthmatics need to go into hospital. Don't wait until you are gasping for breath, particularly when you are pregnant. A closer check can be kept on you and your baby in hospital if you are having a bad or a prolonged attack.

LABOUR AND DELIVERY

There is no reason why you should not have a normal vaginal delivery. It is unusual for asthma to get worse during labour, perhaps because the body produces hormones which are natural steroids and similar to the treatment that many women receive on a regular basis to help prevent asthma worsening.

PAIN RELIEF

You may choose from the same range of pain relief, including epidural anaesthesia, as somebody without asthma. Entonox (gas and air) can be used safely.

INDUCTION OF LABOUR

Sometimes it is necessary to induce labour, This is usually done either with vaginal pessaries (containing prostaglandins) or by infusion of a drug called oxytocin, which makes the uterus contract. Certain prostaglandins can make the bronchi narrow, bringing on an asthma attack so this form of induction is not usually used if you are asthmatic.

AFTER THE BABY IS BORN

It is important to continue your asthma treatment after your baby is born, although with other things on your mind it may be more difficult to remember to use your inhalers regularly.

BREASTFEEDING

Neither asthma nor the drugs used to treat it should prevent you from breastfeeding. The amount of these drugs secreted from your bloodstream into your milk is very small and they are not detrimental to your baby.

WILL YOUR CHILD DEVELOP ASTHMA?

Asthma is partly an inherited (genetic) disease, and the risk of any child developing asthma is about four per cent. If either the mother or the father has asthma or eczema, the risk is about ten per cent. If both are affected, the risk may be as high as thirty per cent.

However, even if your child does develop asthma this should not prevent him or her having a perfectly normal childhood. Although your own childhood may have been disrupted and been made miserable by asthma, nowadays the outlook for children with asthma is very different. Over the last thirty years, very effective treatments have been developed, so we now expect asthmatic children to lead normal lives and join in all sports and childhood activities.

DIABETES

Diabetes in pregnancy used to be a serious

problem but now it is easier to control and monitor. Most diabetic mothers do well in pregnancy but it is important that there is good liaison between the mother and the medical staff throughout. Diabetes affects about one in a hundred women who have it before the pregnancy starts, and another one in a hundred will develop it during pregnancy but it will go away afterwards. Generally, it is the women in the older reproductive age group who are more likely to have diabetes. However, mothers who are diabetic for the first time in pregnancy may need only a specific diet rather than insulin treatment.

WHAT IS DIABETES?

The condition is due to a lack of insulin made by the pancreatic gland in the abdomen. The amount of insulin in the blood stream increases when sugar is taken in during a meal and keeps the level in the blood reasonably constant. Diabetics either cannot produce insulin at all or need more to keep the sugar level constant than the pancreas can produce. In diabetics, blood sugar levels are uncontrolled and rise rapidly after a meal, dropping to low levels between meals. This leads to a spill over of sugar into the urine, which will be noted after the urine is checked in the antenatal clinic. Blood sugar levels may be checked also after a meal to reveal the condition.

ANTENATAL CARE

If you know that you are a diabetic you will probably attend a special clinic and can get advice before pregnancy about what you should be doing. A tight control of diabetes by rigorous attention to the dose of insulin and the carbohydrate intake before pregnancy reduces problems. It is sensible to attend a hospital for antenatal care and the obstetrician there will probably consult with a diabetic specialist so that both are involved with the pregnancy. Your family doctor will also be kept well informed about any changes in the way your diabetes is being looked after.

MONITORING DURING PREGNANCY

Pregnancy can make the control of diabetes more difficult because many of the hormones produced by the placenta tend to increase the blood sugar, and therefore blood testing should be applied more rigorously. The mother's diet must allow for the growth of the baby, and you will almost certainly require an increase in insulin doses to compensate for this. If you have had diabetes for some years you will know about glucose sticks for testing the blood sugar levels, and these should be used in pregnancy. If you are newly diabetic you will need to be shown the self-testing techniques. After the baby is born, you will return remarkably quickly to your previous insulin requirements and so the dose should be watched very carefully in the first few days after delivery.

It is likely that you will be seen much more frequently at the antenatal clinic and assessed carefully as pregnancy advances. If all goes well then a vaginal delivery may take place, but should there be any problems, it may be better to elect for a caesarean section.

AFTER THE BIRTH

The babies of diabetic mothers are often plumper but their weight is related to the carefulness of the control of the diabetes during pregnancy. Your baby will need careful examination and observation after delivery to ensure that no after-effects of the diabetes affect your baby in the first few days of life. There is no reason why a diabetic mother can-

not breastfeed. For those who are insulin-dependent diabetics, it does mean that the balance between insulin and the carbohydrate in the diet must be watched very carefully. If you were diabetic for the first time in pregnancy, the problem should resolve after the baby is born. It is likely to recur in a future pregnancy and possibly when you are older. If you are overweight for your height and build dieting may help considerably to relieve the problem.

EPILEPSY

Epilepsy is found in about one young women in a hundred. The severity varies considerably with some women having fits only very infrequently, while others are less well controlled. As with many medical problems in young women, if a pregnancy is planned then it is worth discussing what you can do to help get the best outcome both for yourself and your baby before the pregnancy starts. Most large hospital units hold pre-pregnancy clinics where this sort of advice can be obtained. Your own doctor can refer you to one of these at an appropriate time.

ANTI-EPILEPTIC TREATMENT

Drugs taken to prevent epileptic fits can affect the baby in the very early stages of pregnancy. however, the drugs will often have an effect prior to the women herself knowing that she is pregnant. It should be stressed that the chance of the baby having any sort of malformation is very small, even with high doses of medication.

If you are an epileptic on treatment and you know that you wish to become pregnant then you might wish to discuss with your doctor the possibility of changing to one of the safest anticonvulsants such as phenytoin, which is associated with the least risk of an effect on the baby. On the other hand, if you have not had a fit for a very long time, then it may be possible to stop the drugs altogether. It is most important if you are having regular epileptic fits that you keep taking your medication as the effects of the fits themselves can be far worse for the baby than the drugs themselves.

THE PREGNANCY

In pregnancy the frequency of fits seems to be the same as before for most epileptic women, however, in some rare instances the rate may increase. Part of the reason for this is that because of changes in the body chemistry, you may require more anticonvulsant medication. It is likely that your doctor will check the levels of the drug in your blood from time to time. Frequently repeated epileptic fits can occur very rarely, but are more likely if treatment is not adequate.

It is important for you to take extra folic acid (4 mg tablets) in pregnancy. This vitamin is needed for your baby's development and its absorption is altered by taking anti-epileptic medication. Extra folic acid can help prevent certain malformations in the baby, such as spina bifida.

THE BIRTH

There is no reason why you should not have a normal delivery and your chances of having a caesarean section will be the same as for women without epilepsy. However, vitamin K will be given to your baby at birth. This is a vitamin that is concerned with the clotting of the blood, and again its level in the body can be affected by the anti-epileptic drugs. It is possible that you will have been already given an injection of vitamin K during your pregnancy.

Generally, you will be able to go through pregnancy safely, but you will need extra attention and looking after. Most doctors would recommend that you do not travel on holiday or business too far away from where medical help can be obtained.

HEART DISEASE

Most women with some form of heart disease will be able to have normal pregnancies and healthy babies. Heart disease can be congenital (you are born with it) or it can be acquired. In congenital heart disease the person is born with a defect in the structure of the heart, such as an abnormal hole between two of the chambers. Some of these defects are very minor but others are serious enough to require treatment, which is usually an operation performed in childhood. Following corrective surgery, the heart may be almost normal, or may still have a slight defect.

The acquired heart disease most likely to affect women wishing to have children is rheumatic heart disease. This is caused by rheumatic fever, usually contracted in childhood and now very rare in the UK. It damages one or more of the heart valves, leaving them narrowed or leaky.

Maternal heart disease affects about one in 100 of all pregnancies in the UK.

The incidence of congenital heart disease in pregnancy is increasing, as the women with more severe defects who underwent corrective surgery as children are now able to have children themselves. The advent of heart and lung transplantation has meant that women with the most severe forms of heart and lung disease are now reaching child-bearing age in good enough health to have successful pregnancies.

WILL HEART DISEASE PREVENT YOU HAVING CHILDREN?

Most women with heart conditions lead full

and active lives, and are able, sometimes with the help of drugs or surgery, to have children safely. If you are able to have children, there is no evidence to suggest that pregnancy or childbirth will shorten your life, whether you have either congenital or rheumatic heart disease. Therefore there is no reason to suspect that, having given birth, you will not be around to care for your growing child.

However, there are a few heart conditions in which pregnancy could endanger a mother's life. If you have any of these conditions you may be offered sterilisation or, if you do become pregnant, your doctor will probably recommend that you have a termination.

Women with artificial heart valves usually have near normal heart function and most have successful pregnancies.

RISKS TO THE BABY

There are two risks to consider:
■ How the growth and development of your baby will be affected by your heart condition
■ Whether your baby is likely to be born with a heart defect.

The babies of mothers with rheumatic heart disease tend to be a little lighter than usual, but otherwise are completely normal.

If you or your partner have congenital heart disease, your baby is twice as likely to have a congenital heart defect as a baby with parents not affected by heart disease, i.e. a risk of about two to four per cent. This risk varies with different types of heart disease.

Most cases of congenital heart disease in the baby can now be diagnosed by ultrasound in the first half of pregnancy. If a defect is discovered that would not be amenable to surgery in infancy, termination of the pregnancy can be considered if you feel this is appropriate for you.

WHAT TO DO BEFORE BECOMING PREGNANT

It is most important, if you have any form of heart disease, that you seek medical advice before becoming pregnant. This allows detailed assessment of your individual condition, the risks of the pregnancy to you and your baby, and consideration of any alteration in drug therapy that may be required.

In women without heart disease, pregnancy leads to an increase in the amount of circulating blood in order to supply the placenta and the growing baby. The heart has to beat faster and do about forty per cent more work. If there is some pre-existing weakness in the function of the heart, it may not be able to cope with the additional demands of pregnancy.

For some women who may have no symptoms, pregnancy carries a risk of developing fluid on the lungs (pulmonary oedema) and therefore they may be advised to have heart surgery before becoming pregnant.

SPECIAL ANTENATAL CARE

Ideally, as a pregnant woman with heart disease you will attend a combined clinic, where you can see both an obstetrician and either a cardiologist or a doctor who specialises in medical problems in pregnancy. Whatever the arrangement, close supervision is required and frequent visits may be arranged – sometimes once a week. This is to enable the doctors to:
■ Keep a close watch on how your heart is coping with the extra demands put on it by pregnancy
■ Detect any abnormal heart rhythms
■ Check that your baby is growing normally.

You may be sent for extra blood tests or extra ultrasound examinations. You may be given drugs to treat any heart failure, high blood pressure, rhythm disturbance or anaemia that develops. If any signs of heart failure do develop, you will be asked to come into hospital where a closer check can be kept on you and your baby.

SYMPTOMS TO WATCH FOR

Many of the symptoms of heart disease occur in normal pregnancy but this is not a reason to dismiss them, especially if you have heart disease.

■ You should report any breathlessness, especially if it is getting progressively worse. This could be a sign that you are becoming anaemic or that your heart is not pumping as well as it should.

■ You should also tell your doctor if you feel faint or light-headed, if you experience palpitations or if you develop any pain in your chest.

■ Any infection will increase the risk of problems, particularly if it involves the heart itself, so it is important to treat it promptly. Tell your doctor if you develop stinging or burning when you pass urine (dysuria), as this may indicate a bladder infection.

MEDICATIONS DURING PREGNANCY

Some women with heart disease need permanent treatment with drugs. These may be to:

■ Control an abnormal heart rhythm (antidysrhythmics)

■ Thin the blood (anticoagulants)

■ Control high blood pressure (antihypertensives)

■ Control heart failure (diuretics).

The most common drug in the first group is digoxin, which is also the most tried and trusted in pregnancy. Provided that the level of digoxin in your blood is right for you, it will not be harmful to your baby. There is also some evidence suggesting that women taking digoxin have earlier and shorter labours. Many of the other antidysrhythmics, antihypertensives and diuretics are also safe during

pregnancy, but if you are taking any drugs, you should check with your doctor as they may need to be changed or the dose altered.

If you have an artificial mechanical heart valve, you will need long-term anticoagulation (blood thinning), which is usually with warfarin treatment. During pregnancy it will be replaced by heparin, given into the veins by a drip or under the skin by injection, since warfarin can adversely affect the mother and baby. Warfarin may lead to an increased chance of having a baby with an anomaly and also, if taken at the time of delivery, will increase bleeding problems in both yourself and your baby. Consequently, it is unusual for a pregnant woman to receive warfarin except between twelve and thirty-two weeks. However, this risk has to be balanced against the risk of a blood clot, which is particularly dangerous if you have an artificial heart valve. Most doctors recommend that if you have a mechanical heart valve, you continue to take warfarin in pregnancy.

After the baby is born the heparin can be restarted, and once the risk of bleeding in the mother is not so high, the warfarin can be reintroduced about one week later.

LABOUR AND DELIVERY

In most cases, a normal vaginal delivery is possible, although if an early delivery is thought to be safer for you or your baby, then a caesarean section may be performed.

PAIN RELIEF

You will be watched very closely during labour, and may have various monitors and drips attached. You will be offered the same range of pain relief as a woman without heart disease, but you may be encouraged to have epidural anaesthesia. This relaxes the blood vessels so that the heart does not have to work so hard.

SECOND AND THIRD STAGES OF LABOUR

In order to prevent too great a strain being put on your heart while pushing during the second stage of labour, forceps may be used to deliver the baby more quickly. To help the delivery of the placenta (afterbirth), most women are given a drug to help the uterus contract as the baby's shoulders appear. If you have heart disease you may be given an alternative or no injection at all.

ANTIBIOTICS IN LABOUR

If you have structural heart disease, you will probably have been told of the importance of taking antibiotics when you go to the dentist or have even a minor operation. The same can apply to childbirth, whether you deliver vaginally or by caesarean section. This is to prevent infection in the heart which is a particular risk if you have an artificial heart valve, if you have a forceps delivery, if your waters break long before your baby is born, or if you have had previous episodes of infection. Which antibiotics you get, when you get them, and for how long, will depend on the hospital's policy and on your particular circumstances. However, most women with rheumatic or congenital heart disease will be given antibiotics during labour.

POSTNATAL CARE

The effects of pregnancy on women with heart disease are still present for some time after delivery. In fact, the risks of blood clots and infection are higher. Therefore you will also be closely monitored after your baby is born. Your medication may be altered again and you may be kept in hospital for a little longer than is usual. Like all newborn babies, your baby will have a thorough examination by a paediatrician, checking particularly for any heart problems.

BREASTFEEDING

Almost certainly, you will be able to breast-feed. Most of the drugs given to pregnant women with heart disease, including warfarin, are not detrimental to your baby if small amounts cross over from your bloodstream via your milk.

HOW TO HELP YOURSELF

■ It is very important that you get plenty of rest.

■ You should eat a sensible, balanced diet.

■ You should try to avoid putting on too much weight as this will place an additional burden on your heart.

■ It is vital that you attend all your antenatal appointments.

■ You should report any new symptoms to your doctor or midwife and discuss any anxieties or worries that you may have, so that you can receive the support to allow you to enjoy this very special time.

KIDNEY DISEASE

If you are a woman with a kidney disorder who is considering a pregnancy or is already pregnant, you will need information about the effects of your disease on pregnancy. During pregnancy, the kidneys undergo considerable change with up to seventy per cent increase in size and blood flow, and fifty per cent increase in filtering capacity – alterations that will not be noticeable. However, changes in the rest of the urinary tract in pregnancy are more obvious.

■ It is common to pass urine more often.

■ It is common to occasionally need to rush to the toilet.

■ You are more likely to pass urine at night and to accidentally leak urine. These changes will settle down when pregnancy is over.

KIDNEY TESTING IN PREGNANCY

If you have a kidney disease, the function of your kidneys will need to be checked by a set of kidney tests throughout pregnancy. How often they are performed and the type of tests depends on the severity and type of the kidney disease.

■ A dipstick test is used to detect protein, sugar and/or blood in a urine sample at each clinic visit. This is only a rough test and often gives false results due to contamination. A positive result suggests that other tests should be carried out.

■ Urine culture and microscopy is used to screen for infection and will need to be performed monthly, especially if kidney infections are happening frequently.

■ Blood tests are usually performed every one to two months to check kidney performance.

HOW TO COLLECT A SPECIMEN

When a urine specimen is requested, it must be collected properly to avoid contamination and a false result. Only a small amount will be needed.

1 Ensure that you are clean and dry.
2 Start to pass urine.
3 While passing urine, catch a small amount in a receiver.

If a twenty-four hour sample is requested, forgetting to add just one sample when you pass urine will give an erroneous result.

1 Set a time to start the collection (usually 8 or 9 a.m.).
2 Empty the bladder and discard the urine.
3 Collect all urine passed for twenty-four hours – if any is not added, it will cause a false result.
4 Empty the bladder at the same time the next day and add this last sample to the collection.

KIDNEY DISEASE IN PREGNANCY

The effects of kidney disease on pregnancy will depend to some extent on how severe the disease is. The severity can be graded according to:

■ Tests of kidney function, including a test to measure the level of a substance called creatinine in the bloodstream. As a rough guide, the higher the level, the more severe the kidney disease.

■ Some problems of pregnancy, such as high blood pressure may be worse in those with kidney disease.

QUESTIONS YOU MAY ASK

When contemplating a pregnancy, there are several questions you may wish to ask:

■ Is the chance of a successful pregnancy poor?
■ Will pregnancy make my kidney disease worse?
■ Will my kidney disease make it difficult for me to bring up a child?

Ask your family doctor, kidney specialist or gynaecologist for pre-pregnancy advice. By understanding what you can expect from a pregnancy, you can decide for yourself whether the risks are worthwhile.

RISKS IN PREGNANCY

The degree of risk ranges from a very small risk in mild disease to a high risk in severe disease. When pregnancy is successful, there does not appear to be any long-term effect on the baby. There are a few kidney diseases that can be inherited by the baby and again pre-pregnancy advice should be considered. The risks of kidney disease are:

■ Poor growth of the baby
■ Loss of the baby prior to birth
■ Premature birth.

PROBLEMS IN PREGNANCY

■ The kidney disease may worsen with deterioration in kidney function.

■ Your blood pressure may become raised and perhaps need treatment.

■ Pre-eclampsia, a condition that is found only in pregnancy and disappears soon after delivery, is much more common in women with kidney disease and occasionally means that the baby needs to be delivered early. Common features of pre-eclampsia include high blood pressure and protein in the urine which lead to impaired growth of the baby.

■ Pregnancy makes the kidneys more prone to infection, which may further impair kidney function.

■ Anaemia is common in women with kidney disease and may be made worse by pregnancy. **Note:** The more severe the kidney disease, the more common the complications and the greater the chance of your baby being delivered prematurely.

MONITORING IN PREGNANCY

You will be looked after by the obstetrician, kidney specialist, family doctor and your midwife who may visit you at home. The aim is to identify any complications early on and to decrease any risk to you and your baby. As a result, the more severe the kidney disease, the more often you will need to be seen at the hospital. The overall aim is to treat women with kidney disease as normally as possible.

LABOUR AND DELIVERY

Most women with kidney disease will deliver normally. However, since there is a greater chance of your baby being born early, a very close watch will be kept on you during pregnancy and labour.

URINARY TRACT INFECTIONS AND PREGNANCY

A kidney infection (pyelonephritis) is the commonest kidney problem to arise in pregnancy.

This is probably because the flow of urine from the kidney to the bladder becomes more sluggish, making it easier for a urine infection to spread to the kidneys. Usually there is pain over one or both kidneys as well as a high temperature, fever, shivering and vomiting. In severe infections, hospital admission will be needed. A high temperature can lead to the early onset of labour and prompt treatment minimises any risk to you or your baby.

Some types of kidney infection need special consideration.

■ **Chronic pyelonephritis** is a term used for the recurrent kidney infections, perhaps on and off since childhood, that often result in some kidney damage. The number of infections may increase in pregnancy, and early detection and treatment are therefore necessary.

■ **Lower urinary tract infections** can be classified in two types:

1 An infection which has no symptoms and is detected by routine testing (asymptomatic).

2 Cystitis which is a symptomatic bladder infection with lower abdominal pain and burning on passing urine.

It is important that these infections are treated before they progress to a kidney infection.

■ **Repeated urine infections** in pregnancy, which have been proven by urine culture and microscopy, will often need further assessment four months after the birth of your baby to look for an underlying cause.

Note: All urine infections should be proved by sending a sample for culture and microscopy and treated promptly, especially if you already have a kidney disease.

DIALYSIS AND PREGNANCY

It would be unusual to fall pregnant if you are undergoing dialysis. However, contraception should not be forgotten as a pregnancy may have serious implications. The risks to the mother and baby are the same as in severe kidney disease. Dialysis is also more difficult and needs to be performed more often, which again increases the risk to the baby. If you are on dialysis, you should not risk getting pregnant. It would be better to wait until after a successful kidney transplant.

CONDITIONS REQUIRING SPECIAL CONSIDERATION

In most cases of kidney disease, the likely outcome of pregnancy depends almost entirely on the severity of the disease rather than the type of disease. there are a few exceptions to this rule and conditions such as polyarteritis nodosa, systemic sclerosis and systemic lupus erythematosis require special consideration. If you are uncertain about your kidney disease and want to know whether it is the best time or even safe for you to fall pregnant, ask your doctor for pre-pregnancy advice.

KIDNEY TRANSPLANT AND PREGNANCY

If you have had a kidney transplant and want a baby, it is important that you wait until the time that is the least risk to you, your transplanted kidney and to the baby. Your fertility may improve after transplant as your general health improves and contraception should not be forgotten until you are ready to fall pregnant. Pregnancy does not appear to increase the risk of rejecting a kidney transplant either during or after a pregnancy.

SICKLE CELL DISEASE

Sickle cell anaemia is an inherited disease producing painful crises and anaemia in both men and women. It is especially common in

people of African, Asian and Middle Eastern ethnic origin. It varies considerably in its severity, both between sufferers and at different times in an individual's life. Sickle cell disease tends to get worse in pregnancy and leads to problems with both mother and baby. Specialised medical care is required and this often involves the use of blood transfusion.

PRE-PREGNANCY ADVICE

If you have sickle cell disease then it is important to discuss things with your doctor before becoming pregnant. There may be existing health problems which could complicate your pregnancy and it is an opportunity to discuss any previous pregnancy. You can ask your family doctor or the local hospital haematology clinic for advice. A referral can be made to the obstetrician who will be supervising your pregnancy.

You can arrange for your partner to have a blood test to check whether he has sickle cell disease or any other inherited blood disorder.
■ If he has sickle cell disease too, then all your children will also have the disease.
■ If your partner is a carrier for sickle cell disease then half of the children born will have sickle cell disease.
■ If he does not have either condition then all the children born will be carriers for the disease, that is they will not be affected themselves but may pass the disease onto a child in the future.

If you are a carrier of sickle cell disease, then this is known a having 'sickle cell trait'. Whether your children will be affected depends on whether your partner has the disease, the trait or is unaffected.

Women with sickle cell trait usually have completely normal pregnancies, although there is a slightly increased risk of urinary tract infections and anaemia.

ANTENATAL CARE

As soon as your pregnancy is confirmed, an appointment will be arranged for you to attend the hospital antenatal clinic. At this stage, you may choose to have tests to determine the genetic make-up of the baby early on in pregnancy. As a result, it can be predicted whether the baby will have sickle cell disease or not. This is usually performed by chorionic villus sampling whereby a small piece of placental tissue is taken away for testing at around twelve weeks of pregnancy. The test results are usually available in about a week, and thus a decision can be made as to whether the pregnancy is to be continued.

Other techniques, such as amniocentesis and fetal blood sampling, can be performed and will give the same information. The type of test offered will depend on your local hospital.

Ultrasound scans will be taken throughout the pregnancy. An early scan may be done to confirm the pregnancy and another at eighteen to twenty weeks to check that the baby is developing normally. As women with sickle cell disease are likely to have smaller babies than other women, scans are performed every two to three weeks from twenty-eight weeks to monitor the growth of the baby.

CONCERNS IN PREGNANCY

There are several problems associated with pregnancy and sickle cell disease. Therefore, as well as seeing doctors in the antenatal clinic the haematology doctors are usually involved, too.

■ A sickle crisis is the main problem and this seems to be more common in pregnancy. The usual precautions of keeping warm and guarding against infection are necessary.

■ There is in an increased risk of infections in pregnancy, especially urinary tract infection. Regular urine testing for this will be performed.

■ Blood pressure problems are also more likely, and this is checked at every clinic attendance.

■ Anaemia is a common problem in women with sickle cell disease, especially in pregnancy. Folic acid is given to help prevent this; the normal dose is 0.4 mg.

■ Visual problems may worsen, and a referral to an eye doctor may be necessary.

■ The doctors in the antenatal and haematology clinics will advise as to whether blood transfusions are necessary in the pregnancy.

Because of the various complications that are possible, antenatal check-ups are more frequent than the usual arrangements for routine antenatal care.

BLOOD TRANSFUSION IN PREGNANCY

This can sometimes be necessary in pregnancy either to correct anaemia or to reduce the amount of abnormal sickle blood in the circulation. Anaemia is common in all women who are pregnant but is more common in women with sickle cell disease as you tend to be anaemic anyway. Blood transfusion is safe and all blood is screened for viruses, including human immunodeficiency virus (HIV) and hepatitis. An ordinary blood transfusion corrects anaemia and will reduce the amount of sickle blood in the circulation. An exchange transfusion removes some of the woman's own blood before transfusing new blood. This has the effect of reducing the abnormal sickle blood faster.

Benefits of transfusion:

■ Reduces risk of sickle crises
■ Corrects anaemia
■ Improves tiredness
■ May improve oxygen supply to the fetus.

Risks of transfusion:

■ Blood antibody formation
■ Infection
■ Discomfort and inconvenience
■ Transfusion reactions.

SICKLE CRISES IN PREGNANCY

If you should have a crisis it will be treated in the same way as at other times. You will be admitted to the antenatal ward. Pethidine or morphine are the most commonly used drugs to relieve the pain. Blood transfusion is not necessary to treat a crisis, but a crisis in pregnancy often indicates that you will need a blood transfusion in time.

LABOUR AND DELIVERY

You can have the same pain relief in labour as other women – gas and air (Entonox), pethidine and epidural. Along with adequate pain relief, it is important to keep warm and have adequate fluids. This involves a drip and having fluid given into a vein.

If everything has gone normally during the pregnancy and labour, then you will be encouraged to have a normal delivery. If a caesarean section is needed, this is usually best performed under an epidural anaesthetic.

After your baby is born it is still important to maintain adequate fluid intake by a drip and to keep warm and mobile. Heparin may be given to you by injection to prevent blood clots (see above).

INFECTION IN PREGNANCY

TOXOPLASMOSIS

This is a common infection by a parasite that causes very little in the way of symptoms. By the age of thirty, about thirty per cent of the population will be infected. Roughly speaking, there is about a ten per cent chance of catching toxoplasmosis for every ten years that you live.

For healthy adults and children, there are no risks associated with this infection, but there is a risk when a pregnant woman catches toxoplasmosis. The mother herself is not at risk but the unborn child may be. This is because the fetus has an underdeveloped immune system and is more likely to be affected by an infection.

HOW IS THE INFECTION CAUGHT?

The original source of the infection is the cat and the parasite is passed on in its faeces. Once a cat becomes infected, it probably continues to pass the parasite for about three weeks. After that time, the cat will not normally be a source of infection again. However, in soil, the cat's faeces may remain infective for as long as eighteen months. Apart from humans, other animals, such as sheep and pigs, can catch toxoplasmosis by contact with infected soil. If contaminated lamb or pork is then eaten by humans and if the meat is raw or undercooked, the infection can be passed on. Fresh fruit, lettuce, vegetables and unpasteurised milk (especially goat's milk) can also be a source of infection.

SYMPTOMS

Generally, the effects are very mild. Symptoms may include a mild fever, swollen glands (particularly in the neck), tiredness, headaches, aching joints and a sore throat – symptoms that can be very similar to common viral infections, such as 'flu or glandular fever. Many people have no symptoms at all and are unaware that they have been infected.

THE UNBORN CHILD

What happens to an unborn baby during pregnancy depends on when the mother becomes infected. If the disease is caught early in pregnancy, particularly the first three to four months, the infection is less likely to pass through the placenta, but if it does happen, then it can lead to miscarriage or damage to the baby in the womb. Infection at this time can cause fluid to collect in the brain (hydrocephaly), scarring of the brain (which could lead to epilepsy), mental retardation and damage to the sensitive part of the back of the eye (chorioretinitis) which can result in partial or total blindness. If the infection is caught in the latter part of pregnancy – the last three months – then the baby may not suffer any symptoms and may be born apparently completely healthy but may then develop symptoms, especially eye damage, many months or even years later.

Assuming that there are about 700,000 births per annum in the United Kingdom and a rate of infection of about two per thousand pregnancies, some 1,400 women every year could develop toxoplasmosis whilst pregnant. Of these, perhaps up to forty per cent will show evidence of infection transmitted across the placenta, and of these about ten per cent will have severely affected infants. Though the exact numbers are not known, it has been estimated that about 400 to 500 babies would be infected every year, of whom forty to fifty would have a severe infection.

TESTING FOR TOXOPLASMOSIS

Antibodies to toxoplasmosis can be detected in the blood in the same way that it is possible to detect antibodies to rubella (German measles). If they are present, it means that either there has been an infection in the past and you are immune or that you have a current or recent infection. If there are no antibodies present, it means that you have never had the infection and are therefore not immune. Repeat testing throughout pregnancy would then be required to detect an acute infection so that suitable treatment can be started without delay. This would involve testing about seventy to eighty per cent of pregnant women a number of times throughout pregnancy. Not enough evidence is available at present to support the introduction of these tests on a routine basis throughout the United Kingdom.

Blood tests become positive about three weeks after becoming infected. If you would like to be tested, you can ask your family doctor to take blood samples in the surgery or you may be referred to your hospital or antenatal clinic to have the test done there.

However, the tests only identify an infection in the mother, and only abut forty per cent of infected mothers will pass the infection on to their babies. After careful counselling you may be offered a test called amniocentesis which is described on page 153. The diagnosis is made by being able to identify the parasite in either the baby's blood or in the amniotic fluid (the fluid in which the baby lies).

AVAILABLE TREATMENTS

If you are shown to have had an infection you may be given an antibiotic called spiramycin (which can only be obtained from hospitals). Giving this drug will reduce the risk of passing the infection from the mother to the baby by about sixty per cent. If your baby is subsequently shown to be infected, then more powerful antibiotics are given as a four-week course alternating with a two-week course of the spiramycin. These drugs cannot be given in early pregnancy because they affect the developing baby and may harm it in some way. After diagnosis, the antibiotics have to be taken for the reminder of the pregnancy.

IS TERMINATION OF PREGNANCY ADVISABLE?

If the test is carried out in the first twelve weeks of pregnancy and the result confirmed by a Toxoplasma Reference Laboratory is positive, you may wish to consider termination of pregnancy. The alternative is to commence spiramycin and wait for tests to see if there is fetal infection and then commence other antibiotic treatment if these prove to be positive.

IF THE BABY IS INFECTED

If your baby is found to be infected when it is born, then treatment with antibiotics will be required for about the first year of life. This is thought to reduce the risk of further damage by about sixty per cent but unfortunately will not reverse any damage already present.

To ascertain whether your baby has been infected, a blood sample can be taken from the umbilical cord at birth – this is not dangerous for the baby. It is sometimes necessary to test another blood sample from the baby when it is one to two weeks old.

AVOIDING INFECTION

If you are pregnant, you can help avoid infection by:
- Not eating raw or undercooked meat
- Washing your hands thoroughly after handling raw meat
- Washing kitchen surfaces and utensils after contact with raw meat
- Washing fruit, vegetables and lettuce thoroughly before consumption
- Always wearing gloves for gardening and washing your hands after touching soil
- Not drinking unpasteurised milk, especially goat's milk

- Not emptying cat litter trays. If this is unavoidable, gloves should be worn and the hands washed thoroughly afterwards
- Disinfecting cat letter trays with boiling water for five minutes, preferable every day
- If you have a pet cat, there is no need to get rid of it just because you are pregnant, but do not forget the precautions (above) that are required to avoid infection if you have a cat.
- If you live on a farm, you may be at risk but, again, it is just a matter of being sensible and taking precautions. Toxoplasmosis infection is quite common in sheep and there is a risk of human infection when handling an infected lambing ewe or the afterbirth or its newborn lambs, or handling the contaminated clothes of another person involved in lambing. Thus pregnant women on a farm should not handle lambing ewes or bring newly-born lambs into the house. If this does happen, make sure that you shower and wash thoroughly, especially your hands, after contact with a lambing ewe. Ask someone else to launder any contaminated clothing.

At present, there is no vaccine to protect you against toxoplasmosis, and it is unlikely that there will be one in the near future.

WILL FURTHER PREGNANCIES BE AT RISK?

It is believed that an acute infection during one pregnancy will not affect any subsequent pregnancy. Women are advised, however, not to become pregnant until at least six months after the onset of the acute infection. This time interval will allow the infected mother to build up antibodies to protect the newly conceived fetus. This may not apply to women whose immunity is affected by certain drugs, such as steroids, or who have an infection, such as AIDS. If you have any worries, you should seek advice from your doctor.

OTHER INFECTIONS

GERMAN MEASLES (RUBELLA)

It is now very rare for women to have German measles while pregnant, since an immunisation programme has meant the infection has become much less common. The immunisation programme was started as it has been known for a long time that being infected with German measles in early pregnancy can lead to abnormalities in the baby. This is because the virus which causes the infection can pass through the placenta. The result of this infection varies considerably, and ranges from death of the baby, birth of the baby with active infection or congenital anomalies. The incidence of damage also varies from one epidemic to another, and may be as much as fifty per cent in some instances.

An important feature is that the effects on the baby vary very much according to the stage of pregnancy. If the mother has the infection during the first eight weeks of pregnancy, then the baby may be born with a cataract (this is when the lens of the eye becomes opaque) or heart problems. If the infection is between eight and twelve weeks' then deafness may occur. On the other hand, probably a quarter of the babies that have been exposed to German measles whilst they were in the uterus may be born apparently normal and not show any problems until after two or three years.

DIAGNOSIS

Most doctors will find German measles difficult to diagnose because it is often very mild and may not always be associated with a characteristic rash. The best way to be certain is to do special blood tests, as soon as possible, after the infection. It is possible to tell if there has been a recent infection or if a mother is not immune (resistant to infection with German measles).

If infection is proven in early pregnancy, then termination of pregnancy can be offered to those who wish it.

AVOIDING INFECTION

Immunisation with a vaccine against German measles is now standard for girls over the age of fourteen. When you book into the antenatal clinic one of the blood tests that will be carried out will be to check for immunity to German measles. If it is not present then vaccination will be offered after your baby is born and you will need to avoid becoming pregnant again for at least one month. If you are not immune to German measles, then you will be told of this and advised to avoid contact with anyone who is known to have this infection. It is now becoming very rare and it is hoped that it will be eradicated altogether.

CHICKENPOX

This is one of the few infections where the virus will actually pass through the placenta. It does not cause abnormalities in the baby, but may lead to the baby developing the infection itself, although this is very rare indeed.

Very rarely, mothers who have chickenpox in pregnancy can get serious complications including a particular sort of pneumonia which can make her very ill. Also, a high temperature in pregnancy can lead to problems, with early delivery of the baby. If you think you have had chickenpox then blood tests can be carried out to see if this is the case, but it should not cause you too many problems.

CYTOMEGALOVIRUS

This is a virus which is found in many animals and in the western world most individuals will be resistant to the infection before the age of thirty five. It can cause an illness somewhat like glandular fever and very rarely can lead to infection of a baby inside the womb, which may be associated with problems of the nervous system resulting in mental retardation. Unfortunately there is no effective treatment for the problem and no known way of preventing it.

Although other infections can occur, it is very unusual that there are adverse affects on the baby. Sometimes if it produces a very high temperature, this can lead to problems, but overall the afterbirth provides a good barrier between mother and baby preventing transfer of infection.

AVOIDING STRESS AND STRAIN IN PREGNANCY

Pregnancy is not an illness and the role of the obstetric physiotherapist is largely to promote good health in pregnancy, adjustment to the physical changes and to minimise the impact of physical stresses and strains which may occur. In some regions, the obstetric physiotherapist may be available to offer advice and support before and after pregnancy. For those who do not have access to these specialists, information is given in the appendix about contact numbers for information about local services and further advice.

From early pregnancy hormonal changes cause the ligaments and muscles to become more elastic. These changes help in adapting to carrying the baby and for labour, but an increase in joint laxity can cause pain in and around any joint. The spine, pelvis and legs are particularly at risk. In contrast, stiff joints may improve in pregnancy.

POSTURE

As the uterus grows in size during pregnancy, the muscles of the abdomen and back change in length and this can lead to poor posture. Prolonged poor posture can lead to back pain, nerve entrapment and muscle weakness.

STANDING

Pregnant women should aim to stand with equal weight on each foot. Weight on the soles of the feet should be evenly distributed towards the heels and under the balls of the feet, especially the big toes. The pelvis should be over the arches of the feet, not in front. Lift the head towards the ceiling using the trunk muscles around the ribs, the shoulders will pull back as the spine elongates and pressure will be taken off the lower back, plus you will look 2.25 kg (5 lb) lighter.

SITTING

When sitting, many pregnant women are helped by using some sort of lumbar support in the lower back. The support could come from a rolled up towel or jumper. Roll the support and put elastic bands at the end to keep it in shape. Make the roll to fit the curve of your back; too big will cause an increase in the curve, too small and curve maybe lost completely. Correct back support will also encourage the neck to be in a good position and could decrease or prevent neck pain as well as back pain. Sitting with legs crossed is not a good idea; it strains the back and pelvis and impedes circulation.

When driving, place the seat so that the legs are comfortably bent. Avoid separating the thighs getting in and out of the car; swing both legs in and out together.

SLEEPING POSITIONS

When sleeping flat on the back, the natural curves in the body should be supported. One pillow under the head should be sufficient. It should be pulled into the neck and clear of or over the shoulders – not under the shoulders as this bends the upper back forwards and could lead to upper or lower back problems. The lower back should be supported by a mattress, soft enough to mould to the natural contours of the body. If you have a mattress so firm as not to support the contours of your body, then you will need one, two or more pillows under your thighs which will flex the hips, relax the muscles from in front of the spine so the lower back rests on the mattress. Try to avoid pressure under the backs of the knees and make sure the heels are in contact with the mattress and not in mid air.

This position is only possible up to approximately thirty to thirty-two weeks of pregnancy, by which stage the baby is a sufficient weight to restrict the flow of blood back to the heart. If the blood flow into the heart is reduced then the output will be reduced. This means that less oxygenated blood will reach the baby and your organs, so you will become light headed, dizzy and/or nauseous. If you are awake you will automatically turn on your side or even sit up. If you are asleep you

CORRECT POSTURE – STANDING

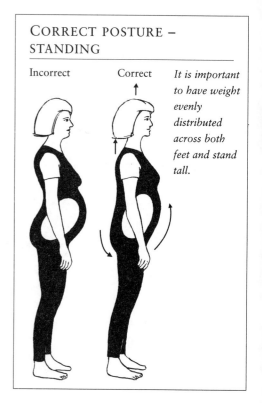

Incorrect   Correct   *It is important to have weight evenly distributed across both feet and stand tall.*

CORRECT POSTURE – SITTING

Correct back support is important when sitting.

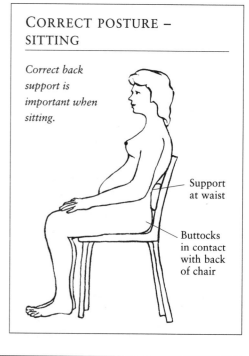

Support at waist

Buttocks in contact with back of chair

will wake up so that you can turn on to your side and not do any harm.

In later pregnancy sleeping on a wedge of pillows may be more comfortable than just putting pillows under your head and shoulders or trying to sleep sitting up because of breathing difficulties or the regurgitation of acid.

BED MOBILITY AND MOVING FROM LYING TO SITTING

When lying in bed, avoid turning over by twisting in the middle, aim to roll over like a log so that the shoulders, hips and bent knees move at the same time. When getting out of bed, use your hands on the bed to push you up while dropping your legs over the side of the bed (see diagram overleaf).

SITTING TO STANDING

To stand up, move the pelvis to the edge of the bed. Place the stronger leg close to the bed and the other just in front, both hip width apart. Place hands on the bed and push straight upwards, try not to rock and lean forward. When sitting in a deep soft chair, move the pelvis to the edge, sit forwards, then using the arms of the chair, push up as above. Reverse the process to sit down.

LIFTING

Most people know to bend the knees to keep the back straight when picking things up from the floor. But it is not easy to do unless the legs are one walking step apart so that the front foot is firmly on the ground and the back heel

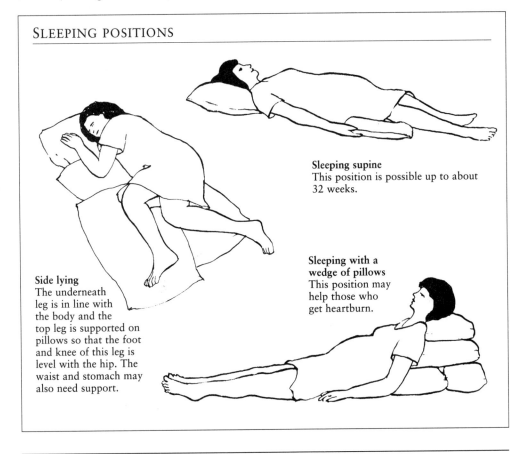

SLEEPING POSITIONS

Side lying
The underneath leg is in line with the body and the top leg is supported on pillows so that the foot and knee of this leg is level with the hip. The waist and stomach may also need support.

Sleeping supine
This position is possible up to about 32 weeks.

Sleeping with a wedge of pillows
This position may help those who get heartburn.

can rise off the floor. This way you are stable and can get down low enough. If the feet are side by side you will be on the balls of the feet and unstable. Bending the knees to use the legs and not the back should be done at all levels, as when picking up a cup from a coffee table, lifting a baby out of a buggy, lifting a pile of clean clothes off the ironing board and picking things up from the floor.

Lifting with a bent back and half bent knees is just as bad as straight knees and may lead to disc problems.

CARRYING

If you cannot avoid lifting heavy things, then even out the weight equally on each side, so as

---

GETTING OUT OF BED

These steps should be followed when getting out of bed or off a chair.

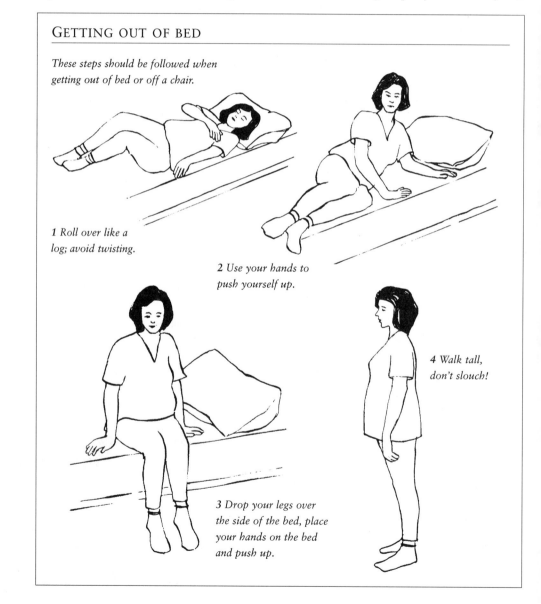

1 Roll over like a log; avoid twisting.

2 Use your hands to push yourself up.

3 Drop your legs over the side of the bed, place your hands on the bed and push up.

4 Walk tall, don't slouch!

---

not to cause strain on one side of the body, try this with a baby as well as with shopping. Do not carry children on your hip.

IRONING

Stand at an angle to the board with the opposite foot in front. Have the board slightly lower than waist height. As you rock forwards and back, bending and straightening your front knee, your body weight will help to get the creases to come out quicker! Standing square to the board causes twisting of the spine and you will tend to lean forwards from the waist to press on stubborn creases.

VACUUMING

Put the lead over one shoulder, hold the handle with both hands and press the elbows into the sides. Place one leg in front, rock forwards and back and the body weight will move the cleaner across the floor. Holding the handle with one hand twists the spine and you will also tend to lean forwards.

HOUSEHOLD TASKS

For jobs close to the floor e.g. making beds, loading the washing machine, gardening and so on, it is much better to go on one knee and have the other leg up. You can lean forward from the bent hip, keeping the back straight. With both knees on the floor there is still a tendency to lean over from the waist. To mop up spills go on to all fours. Wash the far side of the bath while you are still in the bath as the water is draining out. When out, bend down onto one knee at an angle and close to the bath to clean the near side. Do all kitchen jobs sitting if possible.

REST

Rest is particularly important in pregnancy, especially if you are not sleeping well and are

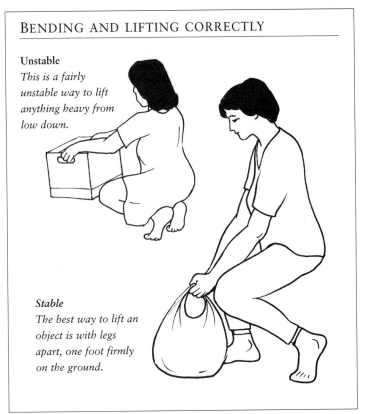

BENDING AND LIFTING CORRECTLY

Unstable
This is a fairly unstable way to lift anything heavy from low down.

Stable
The best way to lift an object is with legs apart, one foot firmly on the ground.

still working or looking after other children. You can rest lying down or sitting with plenty of back support and legs up. The whole leg should be supported and not just the thighs and heels, otherwise the knee ligaments can be over stretched, producing more joint movement and even pain. Lying in the bath for a short time can be very relaxing, but not for longer than 20 minutes. Your rounded posture could cause back pain. If you need heat to reduce pain, lying down with a hot water bottle would be better.

BACK PAIN

If the back pain is worse at night and you are very stiff the next morning, ice may be better to reduce the pain than heat. Use a bag of frozen peas covered in wet kitchen towel and placed over the painful area. Make sure that it is in good contact, and that there is no air gap between the skin and the wet kitchen towel. Maintain contact for ten minutes. Repeat every two hours to reduce inflammation and to reduce pain. If the skin is sensitive apply a thin layer of olive oil or vegetable oil first, before the ice pack. Crushed ice cubes in a wet cloth are better, although messy and not as convenient as frozen peas. Use the ice plus the following exercises and your normal activities of daily living to distract yourself from the pain during the day and use your pain relief in the evening and at night to more effect. If night pain is bad, take two paracetamol half an hour before bed. Have another two handy in case you wake with pain four hours later. You can take the normal adult dose in 24 hours but if the pain continues for more than three or four days, go and see your GP, midwife or obstetrician.

MAINTENANCE OF LOWER BACK MOBILITY

In order to prevent the lower back muscles from becoming short and tight the following exercises should be performed throughout pregnancy two to three times per day, first thing in the morning preferably before getting out of bed, last thing at night before sleep and thirdly if the back feels stiff at any point during the day or on return home from work.

PELVIC TILT

The lower abdominal muscles (i.e. below the belly button) should be drawn in first and held in place while the buttocks are squeezed and the pelvis tilted upwards, so that the lower back flattens into the support. This position should be held for ten seconds while continuing to breathe normally but if this is difficult, begin with a five second hold. Repeat five times gradually increasing to ten at one go.

The same exercise can be done rhythmically; as soon as the pelvis has been tilted the movement is released and immediately re-performed, and repeated for between 30 seconds and one minute.

The slow hold will help to maintain or improve the strength of the abdominal muscles, thereby helping to maintain correct spinal posture and joint mobility. The rhyth-

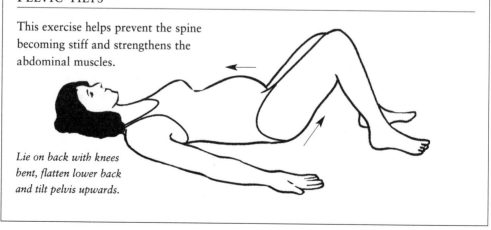

PELVIC TILTS

This exercise helps prevent the spine becoming stiff and strengthens the abdominal muscles.

Lie on back with knees bent, flatten lower back and tilt pelvis upwards.

mical contractions assist joint mobility and aid the reduction of back pain.

If pelvic tilting is attempted for the first time late into the pregnancy, the lower spine may be very stiff and it may be necessary to stretch out the lower back muscles first, to allow the movement to take place.

Pelvic tilt can also be performed against a wall: lean against the wall with your feet 30–45 cm (12–18 in) from the wall and hip width apart. Bend at the knee, sliding down the wall. Draw in lower abdominal muscles, tilt the pelvis forwards to press the small of the back into the wall. Begin holding for five seconds, breathing normally and gradually increase to ten seconds. Make sure that the head and shoulders are in contact or as close to the wall as possible. Release the pelvis slowly, then straighten the knees. Begin with five repetitions and increase to ten.

LOWER BACK MUSCLE STRETCH

Lying on your back, raise one leg and hold the bent knee. Slightly separate the legs around the 'bump' and slowly pull the knees towards the chest. The stretch should be felt in the lower back. A stretch should be uncomfortable not painful while being per-

formed and the discomfort should ease on release. The stretch should be held for fifteen seconds, then released, and repeated twice at one go. This is performed twice a day. If pain is produced and lingers then stop. Once the lower back muscles have been lengthened sufficiently to perform a pelvic tilt, then frequent regular tilting of the pelvis should be enough to maintain lower back mobility. Should the range of movement of tilt reduce for whatever reason, then again perform the stretches first. These can be done on a wedge of pillows.

PRONE KNEELING

Care must be taken not to sag with gravity so that the lower back becomes compressed. Start with a flat back, then lower the head towards the floor, rounding the shoulders forwards and arching the back like a cat, drawing in the lower abdominal muscles at the same time. Hold for five seconds, breathing normally. Return to a flat back. Gradually increase the hold to ten seconds and repetitions from five to ten at one go.

SIDE LYING

This is the least helpful position but may be

PELVIC TILT EXERCISE

1 Pull up the pelvis and make an arched back, like an angry cat.

2 Relax only to neutral; flat back increases the curve into the opposite direction, which can cause backache.

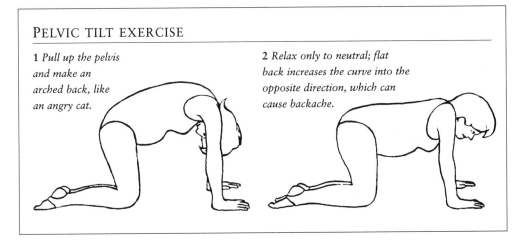

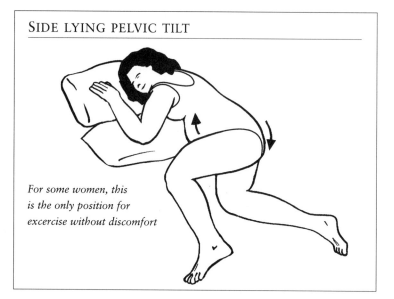

SIDE LYING PELVIC TILT

For some women, this is the only position for exercise without discomfort

PELVIC TILT SITTING

If back is just stiff, this position may work. Roll pelvis backwards to straighten lower back; using abdominal muscles, pull pelvis forward.

the only position you can exercise without discomfort. Perform as above, drawing in the lower abdominal muscles first, rounding the pelvis forwards so that the lower back straightens or even flexes and keep the rest of the spine still. Hold as before. Release slowly taking care not to push the pelvis backwards. Progress as above. If possible repeat on both sides and not just the favourite or most comfortable side.

SITTING

This is possible if the back just feels stiff. If pain is present, it may be impossible to do since there is more compression through the joints in sitting than in any other position.

Keeping the upper trunk still, let the pelvis roll backwards so that the curve in the lower back straightens. Using the abdominal muscles, pull the pelvis forward. Hold and repeat as above or perform rhythmically.

PELVIC FLOOR EXERCISES

The value of pelvic floor exercises is as follows:
■ To restrict the loss of strength, maintain or improve the muscle strength during pregnancy, and to reduce the risk of stress incontinence in late pregnancy
■ To be aware of the pelvic floor muscles so that tension and relaxation can easily be recognised especially the release of tension in the pelvic floor muscles during the pushing

stage of labour (second stage)
■ Pelvic floor exercises can be performed within an hour of delivery. The sooner the pelvic floor muscles are moved the quicker the reduction in swelling to decrease the pain and the sooner the circulation is increased to help healing
■ Postnatally to aid the return to the pre-pregnancy state or better
■ Strong pelvic floor muscles support the

abdominal contents so as to help prevent uterine, bladder and bowel prolapse.

PELVIC FLOOR MUSCLES

There are various muscles making up the muscular bowl of the pelvic floor, but the aim of the pelvic floor exercises is mainly to shorten and lift the deep levator ani muscles. Imagine the muscles can move up and down like a lift and that in pregnancy the pelvic floor is stretched with the increase in weight. The effect of the hormones is to move the lift from the ground floor down to the lower ground.

After a caesarean section the muscles have to be exercised to bring them back up to ground level and after a vaginal delivery the muscles have to be brought up from the basement.

In any muscle there are slow and fast twitch muscles fibres. In the pelvic floor, the slow are responsible for the continuing support of the pelvic contents and the fast give rapid support during coughing etc. Just as a marathon runner trains differently from a sprinter, there are different exercises for pelvic floor.

1 A SLOW TWITCH MUSCLE CONTRACTION
This should begin by gently squeezing the back passage, then in stages lifting the vagina then the front passage and finally the whole lot together, holding at the top (initially for a few seconds) then releasing slowly. Rest for five seconds. Repeat this five times.

If you have difficulty locating the pelvic floor muscles, imagine you are trying to stop from passing wind, holding in a tampon, and trying to stop from leaking urine while coughing with a full bladder, all at the same time. You can actually try to stop the flow of urine mid-stream to locate the muscles. Try this once every two weeks and do not repeat it

again once you are able to do it, as this could cause kidney problems.

If you have difficulty feeling any movement in the pelvic floor you can try gently and slowly pulling in the lower stomach muscles (below the waist) and slowly squeezing the buttocks together, imagining the pelvic floor muscles are lifting up and backwards, towards your lower back. Once you can move the pelvic floor muscles by themselves, stop using the stomach and buttocks.

2 A FAST TWITCH MUSCLE CONTRACTION
This is performed by lifting the pelvic floor muscles as fast as a blink, releasing immediately and fully back to the starting position. Repeat this ten times.

These two exercises should be repeated six to ten times daily, roughly an hour apart.

Sub-maximal exercises or bracing involve lifting the pelvic floor muscles through a third of their range and bracing them at that position during coughing, sneezing, bending, running for a bus, lifting and so on. They can also be performed by holding the muscles at part way up while doing the washing up, walking etc., gradually increasing the hold.

Strength and endurance of the slow twitch muscle fibres are improved by gradually increasing the hold at the top from a few seconds to twenty seconds, from five seconds' rest to no rest between the five repetitions, in all positions, six to ten times daily. This could take six months, but once able to do this, a maintenance programme of holding for twenty seconds, five repetitions once daily for life would suffice.

A sub-maximal contraction should gradually be increased up to fifteen minutes. This time allows for locating the toilets in a strange place, getting there, waiting and undressing, whilst still controlling the urge to void.

SPORT AND EXERCISE IN PREGNANCY

Women are encouraged to continue their physical activities as normal for as long as they feel able and well. Activities should be stopped if there is pain, dizziness, nausea or excessive tiredness.

The usual precautions should be taken, that is, not to exercise on a full or empty stomach, loose clothing should be worn and plenty of water to hand. Women who do not normally take exercise are not advised to take up strenuous exercise, but could use the stairs instead of lifts, walk briskly ten minutes every day, try swimming or cycling on an exercise bike or go to antenatal exercise classes.

Set exercising should be done two or three times per week; once is not enough, the body forgets the exercise and also changes can occur in a week and joints could be damaged.

Yoga and relaxation benefit everyone. Being aware of the position of joints, tension in the muscles and the pattern of breathing

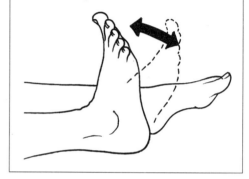

FOOT AND ANKLE EXERCISES

Moving the feet up and down helps blood flow in the leg veins.

can aid sleep in pregnancy, can increase the natural response to your body in labour and can help with control in the hectic postnatal period.

ABDOMINAL EXERCISES

Pelvic tilting can be continued throughout pregnancy. Drawing in the lower abdominal muscles, below the waist and holding for ten seconds, ten times two to three times daily independently of the pelvic floor muscles. Curl ups and twisting to alternate sides in late pregnancy is restricted due to loss of range of movement in the spinal joints and should not be forced. However working within the available range, without strain or pain so as not to increase the separation of the abdominals is permitted. If there is a history of late closure of the abdominal muscles from a previous pregnancy then do not do these exercises after 16 weeks into this pregnancy.

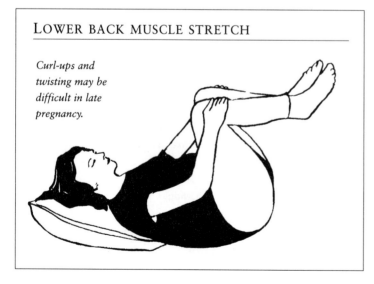

LOWER BACK MUSCLE STRETCH

Curl-ups and twisting may be difficult in late pregnancy.

COMMON PHYSICAL PROBLEMS OF PREGNANCY

Swollen feet and/or varicose veins can be controlled by avoiding standing still, sitting cross-legged and wearing tight knee socks and helped by activity, sitting as discussed earlier or half sitting with legs supported, wearing ankle socks, tights or stockings and doing foot and ankle exercises.

Swelling in the hands with pins and needles and/or pain can be helped by hand exercises and sometimes ice over the inner wrist. If this does not help, seek a referral to a physiotherapist.

Rib pain at the back or front of the chest with or without radiating pain around the chest wall may be helped by the following exercise:

1 Sit unsupported. Reach the arm on the side of the chest pain up the ceiling. Place the hand of the other side into the chest wall at the level of the pain on the opposite side.

2 Lift the spine to the ceiling and lean away from the painful side pushing the hand into the chest wall acting as the pivot to the movement. This way the joints and soft structures on the side of the pain are stretched. Hold for fifteen seconds. Repeat twice, when necessary.

LESS COMMON PROBLEMS OF PREGNANCY

Symphysis joint dysfunction can present as pain in the lower abdomen or as groin pain and is usually worse with activity especially stairs, getting in and out of the bath and car, turning over in bed and standing on one leg to get dressed, etc. Rest is the order of the day, followed by a referral to a physiotherapist and avoiding all the pain producing activities.

The physiotherapist will teach you specific exercises, maybe mobilise other joints of the pelvis and lower back, and maybe issue elbow crutches and/or a belt to stabilise the pelvis.

Hip pain can be due to pregnancy induced osteoporosis and should be made known to your midwife, GP or obstetrician immediately for further investigations and referral to a physiotherapist.

Any pain that does not resolve after following the postural advice and carrying out the routine exercises regularly needs further attention from a physiotherapist. Your GP, midwife or obstetrician can refer you to a physiotherapist and depending on your geographical location maybe to a specialist obstetric physiotherapist.

Chapter eleven

CHILDBIRTH

The experience of childbirth will be different for every woman. This chapter aims to try and dispel some of the myths, provide information about normal childbirth and to explain a few of the more common problems that some women may encounter. Many of the problems are little more than a variation on normality, requiring careful explanation rather than provoking anxiety.

ADVANCE PREPARATION

Many women find that their experience of childbirth is enhanced by knowing what to expect in advance. Excellent sources of information are antenatal clinics and classes run by community or hospital midwives. There is also the local NCT (National Childbirth Trust) which will provide groups for support, exercise and information before and after the birth. There are a multitude of publications on the subject of childbirth written from the perspective of the mother, the midwife and even the child. The best advice is often to read widely, listen carefully to all the advice and then come to your own conclusions.

The baby is born as a result of 'labour'. This is where uterine contractions cause the cervix to dilate and allow the passage of the baby through the pelvis.

Many women ask how they will know that labour is starting. Signs that labour may be starting may include:

■ A 'show'; usually mucus mixed with old blood
■ Loss of fluid (waters breaking)
■ Painful, regular period-type pains (contractions)
■ Fresh bleeding is not a normal occurrence, and this should be reported to the midwife.

There is great variability in the speed of labour between women, and between first and subsequent labours. It can be disappointing to learn that labour has only progressed to one or two centimetres after many hours. This is important in softening the cervix to prepare for the birth.

THE START OF LABOUR

Mild, irregular contractions are normal throughout the second half of pregnancy. For most women labour starts spontaneously with a slow increase in the frequency and intensity of contractions. This generally occurs around forty weeks after the first day of the last menstrual period (LMP).

The baby is 'due' any time from thirty-seven to forty-two weeks after the LMP. This is also known as 'term'. About ten per cent of women deliver early or 'preterm' (before thirty-seven completed weeks). About five per cent will go beyond forty-two weeks. Pregnancies continuing beyond forty weeks are sometimes called 'post-term' or 'post-dates'.

NORMAL PREGNANCY AND LABOUR

THE WATERS AND LABOUR

Usually women experience painful contractions for some time before the waters break. When the waters break the contractions may get stronger and more frequent. In some women (approximately eight per cent) the waters break before labour starts but the majority will nonetheless go into labour within twenty-four hours. At term, it is usual to advise encouragement of labour when the waters have been broken for more than twenty-four to forty-eight hours and labour has not started. This is because there is a small risk that the baby may become infected once the waters have broken and it is likely that repeated vaginal examination will be avoided. Labour is often induced using a chemical (prostaglandin) gel inserted vaginally or with an oxytocin drip (see below).

When the cervix is already dilated and labour needs to be induced, this can be done by breaking the waters and thus stimulating contractions. If labour is established but progress is slow and the waters and membranes are intact, then once again the waters can be broken and this may accelerate labour by an average of one to two hours. Once the waters are broken, contractions may feel more painful and some women require extra pain relief at this time.

THE STAGES OF LABOUR

Labour is conventionally divided into three stages. The first two stages reflect changes in the dilatation (opening) of the cervix. The first stage of labour is defined from the onset of regular contractions until full (10 cm or 4 in) dilatation of the cervix. The second stage is from full dilatation until delivery of the baby. The third stage is the delivery of the placenta (afterbirth). The first stage can be further divided into the 'latent' and 'active' phases. The latent phase describes the time starting with the onset of regular uterine contractions and the start of the active phase. During this time the cervix becomes thin (effaced) and softens. In the active phase of labour, the cervix progressively dilates. Length of labour varies. The normal rate of cervical dilatation for a women having her first baby is approximately 1 cm (^{1}/$_2$ in) per hour.

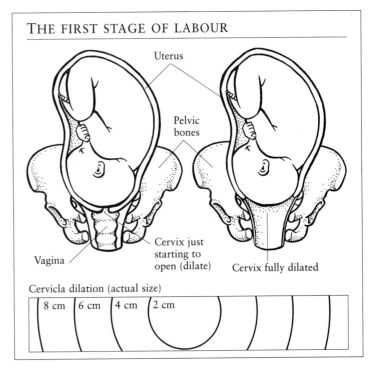

THE FIRST STAGE OF LABOUR

Uterus

Pelvic bones

Vagina

Cervix just starting to open (dilate)

Cervix fully dilated

Cervicla dilation (actual size)

8 cm	6 cm	4 cm	2 cm		

UTERINE CONTRACTIONS

These are responsible for creating an efficient mechanism of labour and a propulsion force for delivery of the child. Each contraction develops slowly, reaches its peak and then subsides. With each, the uterine muscles shorten and then elongate, but not quite to their length before the contraction. There is therefore a degree of shortening of the muscles which helps propel the baby out of the uterus.

During the active part of the first stage of labour and in the second stage of labour, the uterine contractions are usually at their strongest and most frequent, occurring commonly three to four times in ten minutes and lasting for up to fifty seconds, with the uterus relaxing in between. During the second stage of labour, the urge to push adds considerably to the uterine force, almost doubling the pressure on the baby as the mother pushes down with the abdominal and diaphragmatic muscles.

THE BONY PELVIS

This can be considered as having three levels, each continuous with the other.
1 The inlet, shaped like an ellipse, is wider across than front to back.
2 The mid-cavity, which is circular, has equal diameters from front to back and across.
3 The outlet, again shaped like an ellipse, has its front to back diameter wider than the across diameter.

The distance from the inlet to the outlet is approximately 10 cm (4 in).

The bony pelvis is lined at the side by layers of muscle with the bladder in front, the rectum or lower end of the bowel behind, and the uterus or womb in the middle. The floor of the pelvis at the outlet consists of two strong muscles which slope downwards from behind to form a gutter shape.

THE BABY'S HEAD

To negotiate the pelvis, the baby's head usually presents its smallest possible diameter. This is the so called 'occiput anterior' position, with the head tucked into the chin (flexed) and the baby facing towards the mother's back. Uterine contractions help to ensure that this optimal position occurs.

At the same time, the pelvic side walls press on the head, causing it to change shape, or mould, and become smaller through the over-riding of the bones of the baby's head at the points of juncture or suture lines. This further reduces the presenting head diameter by about half a centimetre.

THE MECHANISM OF LABOUR

In early labour, the head presents to the inlet of the pelvis facing sideways. As it descends, the leading point of the head (the crown) is pushed against the downward sloping pelvic muscles and is rotated forwards so that the head is looking backwards. With continuing pressure from above, the top of the head appears first and the baby is born looking back or down. Occasionally the head will rotate backwards and the baby will deliver looking up and forwards. This is called the 'occiput posterior' position, and may lead to a more difficult labour because the baby's head takes up more room in this position.

During labour, an area of swelling (the caput) may develop over the leading part of the head. This, along with the moulding, can cause the baby to look rather strange at birth but the swelling soon goes down.

THE SECOND STAGE OF LABOUR

The second stage of labour starts when the cervix is fully dilated. For the average-sized baby at term, the cervix will be fully dilated when it is 10 cm (4 in). However, for a much smaller or premature baby, it may be possible for delivery to start without the cervix being fully dilated. The second stage ends with the delivery of the baby.

Full dilation of the cervix will usually be accompanied by descent of the baby's head, stimulating strong contractions and an urge to push in the mother. The exact cause of this urge to push is uncertain, and it usually occurs with full dilatation of the cervix.

However, if a woman starts to push before full cervical dilatation this may cause the cervix to become swollen. If this occurs, pushing may be discouraged. Alternatively, the cervix may be fully dilated with labour into the second stage for some time before the urge to push develops.

Because of the shape of the pelvis the baby's position will change during its descent from the abdomen through the cervix and out through the vagina. The force of the contractions, and the shape of the muscles of the pelvic floor help in this process.

STRESS TO THE BABY DURING THE SECOND STAGE

During the height of a contraction the blood supply from mother to baby is likely to be reduced. In between contractions, the uterus is relaxed and the placental and umbilical blood flow and oxygen supply will return to normal. The baby's oxygen reserves are restored and it can prepare for the next contraction.

THE SECOND STAGE OF BIRTH

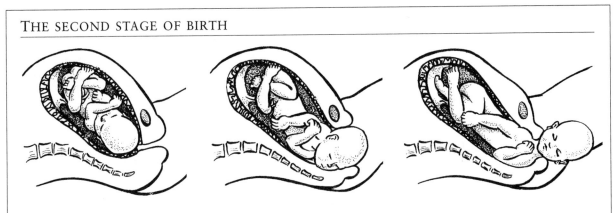

When the cervix becomes fully dilated, the head descends through the pelvis and the baby is born.

This is helped by the combination of uterine contractions and the mother's 'pushing'.

MONITORING IN LABOUR

During labour the condition of the mother and of the baby will be monitored by a midwife. Ideally, a midwife will always be with the labouring woman.

The mother may be monitored by testing her pulse, temperature and blood pressure. The number, apparent strength and duration of uterine contractions will be assessed. The psychological state of the labouring woman is also very important, and the midwife will act to provide support and encouragement, following on from information given by her colleagues at antenatal classes.

All babies are monitored in labour, although the method varies. These aim to assess the rate and pattern of the heart-beat and the colour of the waters (liquor). In particular, the reaction of the baby to uterine contractions will be assessed, because this is the time when the baby may be under stress.

The baby may be monitored continuously or intermittently. The choice of monitoring will depend on the wishes of the woman. She and her caregivers may take into account the history of the pregnancy (and perhaps of any previous pregnancy), the stage of labour, any complications of labour and the policy of the unit if the mother delivers in hospital.

Intermittent monitoring can be performed simply by listening to the baby's heart with a special earpiece or by using electronic fetal monitoring devices. This is usually a trumpet-shaped device (Pinard stethoscope) or a Doppler device which uses ultrasound to record the baby's heart beat. This may be done every ten to fifteen minutes in the first stage of labour or after each contraction in the second stage of labour. The colour of the fluid lost through the vagina can be checked visually. Continuous monitoring of the fetal heart uses electronic devices, either strapped around the mother's abdomen or attached to the baby's head by means of a small clip. The clip monitor may be advised if the baby is to be continuously monitored and it is not possible to do this via the abdominal device. An additional strap on the abdominal device can also help to time the uterine contractions. This is the 'cardiotocograph' or CTG. This is widely used in maternity units throughout the UK although the benefits are still controversial. Although some women find its use threatening, this is not true for all.

The normal fetal heart rate is between 110 and 160 beats per minute, but this is expected to vary over time, and accelerations in the heart rate are a sign of fetal well-being. Dips or 'decelerations' may sometimes be an indicator of distress, depending on their frequency, duration and timing with regard to contractions.

In normal pregnancy there is no good evi-

Below: A normal CTG indicates that the baby is not stressed at the moment.

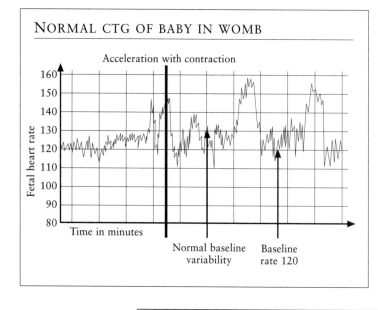

NORMAL CTG OF BABY IN WOMB

Acceleration with contraction

Fetal heart rate: 160, 150, 140, 130, 120, 110, 100, 90, 80

Time in minutes

Normal baseline variability

Baseline rate 120

dence that continuous monitoring of the fetal heart rate is beneficial to the mother or her baby. In uncomplicated pregnancy and labour, intermittent monitoring of the baby's heart rate is the choice of many women and their midwives. This approach has been shown to avoid some caesarean sections performed because of anxiety about temporary changes in the heart rate trace when it is recorded continuously. Intermittent monitoring also allows for greater freedom of movement. However, if the pregnancy and/or labour is thought to be 'high risk', continuous monitoring is likely to be advised. Similarly, if circumstances change during the labour, for example, meconium is passed by the baby, the midwife may advise that monitoring is continuous. In addition, those women who decide to have an epidural for anaesthesia will need to be monitored continuously, as the epidural may lead to sudden changes in blood pressure which can affect the oxygen and nutrition supply to the baby.

Antenatal classes are a good time to ask about the policy of your midwife or hospital unit regarding fetal monitoring in labour, as there is a great deal of variation around the country.

BABY BECOMING DISTRESSED

This is suggested by abnormalities in the fetal heart rate and/or by the passage of fresh meconium by the baby. Sometimes, these observations tend to falsely indicate distress, and additional information can be obtained by taking a small sample of blood from a cut on the baby's scalp, taken through a metal tube placed in the vagina. This procedure can be uncomfortable, and the obstetrician may recommend an epidural for pain relief. If the results from this test are reassuring, the labour can safely continue. However, this test may need to be repeated as long as the heart rate remains abnormal.

PAIN RELIEF IN LABOUR

A variety of techniques and medications are available to help women with the pain of labour. Whether you decide to use some or any of these methods is completely your own choice. Many women find it helpful to explore the options before labour, so that they can make an informed decision on the day.

DRUG-FREE METHODS

Many pregnant women are keen to use pain control techniques which will not interfere with the progress of their labour. Some popular drug-free methods include massage, aro-

matherapy and using a warm bath. These techniques provide sufficient pain relief for many women in labour, and may improve the experience of childbirth for women who wish to try them.

TENS
In this form of pain relief small electric pads, which are connected to a small obstetric pulsar device, are taped to the mother's back. These small pulses of electricity are designed to block the sensation of pain from contraction. By holding and operating the pulsar, the mother can give herself small amounts of elec-

tric current as needed to help cope with the contractions. TENS can be used right through the second stage of labour as it does not appear to impair the urge or ability of the mother to push.

TENS machines can be hired from a midwife or direct from the manufacturers. This method is most effective when used from the start of labour. It has the advantage of not affecting the baby or the mother's alertness in labour. The dose and frequency of electrical pulses can be controlled and the mother is free to move around. TENS machines are not designed to eliminate the pain of labour but to reduce it to a manageable level.

ACUPUNCTURE

This is an ancient form of therapy which involves the insertion of very fine, sterilised needles into the body along invisible energy channels or 'meridians'. Acupuncture is believed to work by releasing calming messenger chemicals in the brain. It is also sometimes used to try to induce labour.

AROMATHERAPY

The use of essential oils derived from plants is thought to stimulate the natural healing process. The oils are either massaged into the body, inhaled, added to a bath or used in a compress or burner. Advice from a qualified aromatherapist is recommended.

HOMOEOPATHY

These remedies are derived from natural substances and aim to treat the whole person, mentally, physically and emotionally. They should only be used in pregnancy and labour after advice from a trained homoeopath.

REFLEXOLOGY

This is based on the belief that areas of the foot relate to areas of the body and that by massaging these parts of the foot, the body can be treated. There is some evidence that reflexology in labour may reduce the number of epidurals needed and shorten the length of labour.

RELAXATION

Relaxation techniques can help to control the perception of pain so that tolerance of contractions is increased. Mental and physical relaxation using yoga, controlled breathing, positive attitude and massage may all help. National Childbirth Trust antenatal groups and active birth classes both teach relaxation techniques.

WATER

In the same way that warm water can ease period pains, it may provide relaxation and pain relief during labour.

DRUG METHODS

ENTONOX

This is a common form of pain relief during labour. It is a fifty per cent mixture of nitrous oxide and oxygen (often called 'gas and air'). Normal air contains twenty per cent oxygen, so if you have Entonox you will be breathing in twice the normal amount of oxygen. Entonox reduces the contraction pain and does not cause loss of consciousness. However, if breathed in for too long, drowsiness and confusion may result. As it takes about thirty seconds for Entonox to act, and inhalation, which can be either from a face mask or through a mouth tube, should be commenced early in the contraction when it is starting to develop. Once a contraction begins to wear off, you should stop breathing the Entonox in order to stay alert between contractions.

PETHIDINE/DIAMORPHINE

These are 'opiate' pain killers and are given by injection into a muscle. Because of the tendency for these type of drugs to cause nausea, they are generally given with an anti-sickness drug. The efficacy of these medications varies between women. Pethidine has a variable effect on pain but usually causes you to be less aware of your surroundings. This is, for some women, one of the more unpleasant side effects of the drug. Diamorphine (heroin) is not available in all units, since it is a drug of addiction. It is an extremely effective pain killer, although it also leads to decreased awareness. Pethidine can be administered by midwives, unlike other opiate drugs, which gives it a wider use.

These drugs are avoided in the second stage of labour (full dilatation of the cervix) because of its possible depressant effect on the baby's breathing if given too soon before birth. However, should the second stage occur unexpectedly soon after opiates have been given, the effects can be reversed to some extent by an injection to the baby and the sleepy infant can be awakened. Some feel concerned that there may be an increase in drug addiction in the child, but the evidence for this is not conclusive.

EPIDURAL

Epidural anaesthesia uses drugs injected around the spinal nerves in order to numb the lower half of the body during labour. This is a popular method of pain relief, particularly for women having their first baby. Because there is some evidence that an epidural can slow down the progress of labour if it is inserted too early, and may increase the chances of an instrumental (forceps or vacuum) delivery or even a caesarean section, many doctors and midwives encourage labouring women to wait

until labour has established before considering an epidural.

The epidural will be inserted by an anaesthetist. In some centres, low dose epidurals are given which may allow you to retain some muscle power and sensation in her legs whilst still relieving the pain of the contractions. This is sometimes called a 'mobile epidural'. When an epidural is used, the fetal heart rate will need to be continuously monitored.

When the cervix is fully dilated, it can be very helpful to have some sensation in order to improve the efficiency of pushing. Most women find it difficult to push effectively when they are quite numb and they do not have control over their abdominal muscles.

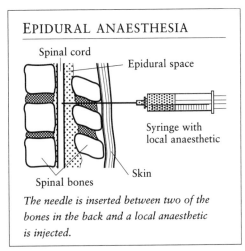

EPIDURAL ANAESTHESIA

Spinal cord

Epidural space

Syringe with local anaesthetic

Skin

Spinal bones

The needle is inserted between two of the bones in the back and a local anaesthetic is injected.

PERINEAL INFILTRATION

As the baby's head crowns, the stretching and thinning of the skin between the front and back passages (the perineum) can cause considerable discomfort. Sometimes the perineum will need to be cut (an episiotomy). Prior to this, the perineum should always be infiltrated with local anaesthetic to deaden the area. Occasionally, a midwife will suggest infiltration of the perineum with local anaesthetic to reduce this discomfort.

ASSESSING THE PROGRESS OF LABOUR

A midwife will assess the progress of labour by a combination of carefully watching the labouring woman for changes in her contractions and breathing, noting whether she has pressure in the vagina or rectum and noting the fetal heart rate. Intermittent vaginal examinations to assess the degrees of cervical dilatation will be carried out.

If the midwife feels that labour is progressing slowly because of poor uterine contractions, she may advise starting a drip containing oxytocin, a synthetic version of the female hormone that stimulates uterine contractions. In hospital births, this drip is often used in induced labour and in women having their first baby, particularly those who choose to have an epidural for pain relief. It is less commonly used in those women who have had one or more babies before, and then at a weaker dose. This is because the uterus may respond to this drug with very strong contractions. Similarly, it must be used with care when a woman has previously had a caesarean section, because of the small risk that very strong contractions may cause the scar to rupture.

When the woman feels the 'urge to push', the midwife may advise a vaginal examination to ensure that the cervix is fully dilated. Pushing on an incompletely dilated cervix may sometimes lead to swelling of the cervix, and occasionally even to tears. In this case, pushing would be discouraged. An epidural may even be advised in order to diminish the strong urge to push.

Not all labouring women will feel the urge to push as soon as the cervix is fully dilated, particularly if they have an epidural. In this case, the midwife may often advise waiting until the head descends with good contractions, and then encourages active pushing so as not to overtire the mother.

Active pushing can be hard work for the mother, and she will benefit from support and encouragement in the labour room as well as good contractions. In between contractions the midwife will encourage slow and regular breathing and relaxation.

It is not possible to predict how long pushing will need to continue before delivery. It is usually quicker in those women who have had a baby before. During active pushing, the midwife will review the situation and ensure that progress is being made. If she feels that delivery is not imminent, she may then discuss the possibility of assisted delivery, using the vacuum (Ventouse) or forceps.

POSITION OF THE MOTHER

Most women will adopt a number of different positions in labour, as they find most comfortable. There is no one position which is 'correct' for all women. Those women who have specific plans for delivery, such as on all-fours, squatting on the floor or in the bath, should discuss this with their midwife in advance to ensure that she is comfortable with this arrangement.

The only position which is actively discouraged is for heavily pregnant women to lie flat on their back, as the pressure of the uterus may compress the major blood vessels in the mother and cause her to feel faint.

THE BIRTH OF THE BABY

With pushing, the baby descends through the cervix and down the vagina. Since the rectum (back passage) is directly behind the vagina, it is not surprising that many women feel pressure in the rectum which feels like an imminent bowel movement at this time.

With each push the head may advance less than a centimetre. After the contraction, it may then slip back a short way. Eventually the head 'crowns' as the top of the baby's scalp emerges through the vaginal labia and no longer recedes between contractions. As the head crowns, the midwife may advise the woman to stop pushing and instead to pant slowly through the mouth. This technique helps to ensure a slow delivery of the head and to protect the perineum from tearing. Once the head delivers, the shoulders normally quickly follow and then the rest of the body is delivered onto the mother's abdomen.

CROWNING OF THE HEAD

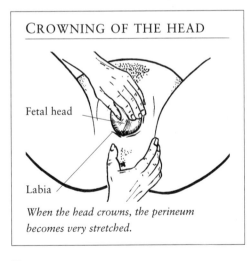

Fetal head

Labia

When the head crowns, the perineum becomes very stretched.

EPISIOTOMY

An episiotomy is a cut made from the vaginal opening into the skin and muscle tissues around it. It might be advised when the mid-wife or doctor delivering the baby feels that the tissues of the vaginal opening are resistant and are preventing the baby from coming out. Also, if they feel that a large tear is about to occur, an episiotomy may prevent a tear that might extend to the rectum or anus, potentially causing long-term problems. When the delivery is assisted using the forceps or vacuum cup (Ventouse), an episiotomy is often required.

Episiotomy is not performed as a routine procedure, and it is usually very hard to predict before the moment of delivery when it might be required. More women have episiotomies with their first vaginal delivery than with subsequent deliveries. A woman in labour may wish to ask her attendant about their personal episiotomy rate. The chances of a woman needing an episiotomy may be less with a more experienced midwife in attendance.

Before any cut is made anaesthetic is needed, local infiltration is usually very effective.

Repair of the episiotomy is carried out following the third stage of labour (see below), once the placenta has been delivered. The repair is usually carried out by the midwife who delivered the baby, using absorbable sutures, which do not need to be removed.

EPISIOTOMY

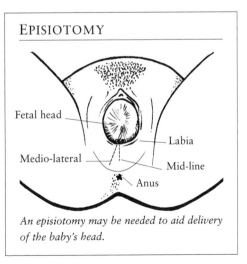

Fetal head

Labia

Medio-lateral

Mid-line

Anus

An episiotomy may be needed to aid delivery of the baby's head.

DELIVERY

In a healthy pregnancy and normal delivery, the baby can be handed directly to the parents if they wish. However, since newborn babies can lose heat very quickly, it is important that they are kept warm. Direct skin-to-skin contact between the mother and baby is encouraged.

In the womb the baby will have breathed in the amniotic fluid surrounding it. After birth, a series of intricate changes occur which allow him/her to breath air. During this transition it is not uncommon for the baby to cough up some fluid and mucous. During a vaginal birth, the squeezing of the baby's chest as it passes down the vagina helps to expel some of this fluid. Babies born at caesarean section may not have this chest compression, and hence continue to bring up some fluid from the chest for a short time after they are born. This is a temporary problem, but may mean that the baby needs to be admitted to the Special Care Baby Unit for observation.

ASSISTED DELIVERY

Sometimes there may be difficulties or complications in labour that necessitate an assisted delivery. The majority of babies are born without help from medical staff, but some require assisted delivery using either obstetric forceps or a Ventouse.

Assisted delivery may be indicated when the baby appears to be distressed (as indicated by the baby's heart rate and/or the passage of meconium), when the second stage is delayed (usually if the baby is not about to deliver after one hour or so of active pushing) or if the mother is too exhausted to push any more and asks for help.

Very occasionally an instrumental delivery will be planned with the mother in advance. This may arise when active pushing is thought to be potentially hazardous for the mother; for example, if she has a history of brain haemorrhage.

FORCEPS DELIVERY

Many women have a great fear of forceps delivery, believing that it will harm them or their baby. Obstetric forceps are designed to fit around the baby's head and to guide it out through the vagina. These days, forceps are only used when the baby can easily be delivered vaginally. In addition, the forceps are sometimes used to turn the baby's head around to a more favourable position for vaginal delivery if failure to progress is diagnosed. Some women may find it helpful to get to their feet or on hands and knees prior to a forceps delivery being recommended. This may stimulate progress.

Analgesia is very important. If an epidural is already sited, it can be topped up. Otherwise, an epidural or spinal anaesthetic may be inserted. However, this takes time to work and if the doctor decides that it is better not to delay the delivery, then a local anaesthetic may be used to numb the area.

THE VENTOUSE (VACUUM EXTRACTOR)

This instrument is commonly used as an alternative to forceps for delivering babies in the second stage of labour. It can also be used to turn the baby's head around. A metal or plastic cup is inserted into the vagina and

VENTOUSE

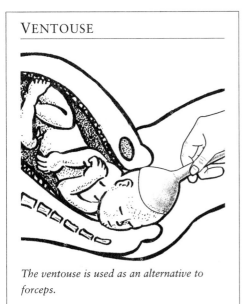

The ventouse is used as an alternative to forceps.

fitted on to the baby's scalp. A tube joins the cup to a suction machine so that a gentle vacuum can be created. After a few minutes, when the suction cap is firmly attached to the scalp, traction is applied during contractions with the mother pushing.

With the vacuum extractor the scalp skin that is sucked into the cup remains raised above the rest of the head. The French call this bump a 'chignon', which means hair-bun. After delivery this bump of skin soon flattens. However, it leaves a visible mark for some days. This is less prominent with the plastic cup than the metal one, but the metal cup is more suitable when the baby needs to be turned.

IS INSTRUMENTAL DELIVERY HARMFUL?

Any instrument can cause harm if it is used inappropriately or without sufficient care. Vacuum and forceps deliveries are only performed by highly trained and skilled personnel, and only in clearly specified circumstances. If your obstetrician does not feel that an instrumental delivery can be safely performed and the baby needs to be delivered immediately, he or she will advise you to have a caesarean section.

The forceps and the vacuum cup can cause minor abrasions. Most of these injuries amount to bruising, although sometimes (particularly with the metal cups) the uppermost layer of the skin can peel as well. Compared with forceps the vacuum extractor is associated with twice as many 'lump-bruises' (cephalhaematoma) on the head. On the other hand, the forceps are twice as likely to leave temporary marks on the baby's face.

The vacuum extractor is also associated with an increased risk of small bruises at the back of the eye (retinal haemorrhages). These disappear very rapidly, however, and are not thought to result in any long-term effects. Serious injuries to babies are fortunately extremely rare and, with careful attention to the rules of vacuum delivery, should not occur.

An episiotomy (cut) is not always needed. If the perineal skin is stretching adequately it does not need to be cut. However, there are some situations where a cut is necessary. It is often very difficult to predict whether an episiotomy will be required before delivery of the baby.

Pain relief is needed for an instrumental delivery. For those who already have an epidural sited, this can be topped up. Otherwise, the usual options would include infiltration of the perineum or an injection to block the nerves that cover this area. Instrumental delivery particularly the vacuum method, requires active pushing to be effective. For this reason the forceps may be used if the mother is unable to push.

THE THIRD STAGE OF LABOUR

This relates to the delivery of the placenta (afterbirth) and it starts as soon as the baby is born, with the separation of the placenta from the wall of the uterus. It finishes when the placenta has been delivered, which usually takes only a few minutes, if this stage is actively managed.

Active management of the third stage of labour means that the cord is cut immediately after delivery of the baby, an injection (usually syntocinon) is given and the placenta delivered by gentle traction on the umbilical cord. These techniques are designed to promote early contraction of the uterus and hence to minimise blood loss. Postpartum haemorrhage, bleeding after delivery of the baby, can be sudden and severe, and active management of the third stage of labour has been shown to reduce the incidence of this.

Some mothers choose to have a 'physiological' third stage, where the placenta is allowed to separate without drugs and the cord is not cut until it finishes pulsating. Natural separation of the placenta may take several hours, although it can occur within twenty minutes and is aided by putting the baby to the breast. For most women this will be perfectly safe, but because of the small increased risk of bleeding with this approach, it is important to discuss these plans with the midwife before labour.

After the placenta is delivered, the midwife will continue to make regular checks for an hour or so to make sure that the uterus is properly contracted and there is not excessive blood loss.

PROBLEMS IN THE THIRD STAGE

These may occur when the uterus fails to contract or the placenta does not separate from the uterine wall. If the placenta does not separate, it may need to be 'manually removed' under anaesthetic. If the womb fails to contract, the large blood vessels which have been supplying oxygen and nutrition to the baby will continue to bleed. This must be controlled, and the uterus can be massaged or drugs used to promote contraction. Very rarely, the placenta is difficult to separate from the wall of the uterus, a situation known as placenta accreta. This problem is more likely to occur when previous pregnancies have been delivered by caesarean section.

Rarely, bleeding may arise from a tear in the uterus or vagina. Repair of this will require good pain relief, and may need to be performed in the operating theatre.

If there is heavy blood loss, a blood transfusion will be advised. Blood used for transfusion in the UK is always screened for viruses such as hepatitis and HIV. For smaller amounts of blood loss, iron tablets are usually sufficient to make up for the loss.

PRETERM LABOUR

All babies born before thirty-seven weeks gestation are classified as premature. However, with modern neonatal care, most babies born after thirty-two to thirty-four weeks do very well. Those born before thirty-two weeks may have more problems, mainly relating to immaturity of the lungs, and require longer specialised care in the Neonatal Unit.

A diagnosis of preterm labour may be made if the waters break or if there are painful regular contractions before thirty-seven weeks. Very occasionally, the cervix dilates without pain or ruptured membranes. The management of this situation will depend very much on how advanced the pregnancy is and whether there is any sign that the baby is distressed. If the waters break before term without any sign of infection, it may be advised that the pregnant woman is admitted into hospital to await events. It is likely that vaginal examination will be avoided in this instance and if it is necessary, great care will be taken with sterility in order to avoid infection. However, if there are any signs of infection inside the womb, such as a high temperature, or offensive vaginal discharge, labour will usually be induced following administration of appropriate antibiotics.

When uterine contractions occur before term, the onset of labour can sometimes be delayed using a drip containing a drug which counteracts uterine contractions. Very occasionally, an obstetrician will advise the insertion of a suture (stitch) into the cervix to try and prevent it opening up.

Sometimes when the waters or membranes break early in pregnancy, provided that the hole is not too big it may seal off and the pregnancy can continue. In some circumstances, the production keeps up with the drainage but labour does not start for hours, days or weeks. Antibiotics may be advised, but it remains unclear whether they are helpful in all circumstances.

Under normal circumstances, when the waters break it usually means that labour will begin soon if indeed it has not already begun before the membranes rupture. However, the waters may not break until late in labour.

In the majority of cases the cause of preterm labour is unknown. Some women will be at increased risk because of complications in their present or previous pregnancies. These include previous preterm birth, multiple pregnancy (twins and triplets, etc.) and early rupture of the membranes (breaking of the waters). Pregnant women who are known to have these risk factors will receive more careful attention in their pregnancies, but there are no reliable ways of preventing preterm labour.

Very premature delivery (i.e. before twenty-eight weeks) is uncommon but of great significance as these babies are likely to need help with breathing, feeding and keeping warm. The outlook for premature babies has improved dramatically over the past decade, and continues to do so. The great majority of babies born after thirty-two weeks will survive (over ninety per cent) with little in the way of long-term effects. Babies as young as twenty-three weeks have been known to survive, but the more premature the baby, the higher the possibility of breathing difficulties and other serious complications. In addition, a proportion of premature babies go on to have long-term disabilities. This also relates to the degree of prematurity.

Special care baby units are today very good at not only keeping these tiny babies alive but also looking after the whole family in terms of keeping them informed and offering general support and reassurance.

An important advance in improving the outcome for premature babies has been the introduction of steroid injections for the mother before delivery (steroids of the same type are produced by all humans at times of stress). These appear to be safe for the mother and baby, and help to mature the baby's lungs. Immature lungs are the main complications of prematurity. Two injections twelve hours apart are usually given to women in preterm labour.

PROLONGED PREGNANCY

About five per cent of women do not go into spontaneous labour by forty-two weeks. Sometimes this is because the stage of the pregnancy has not been correctly calculated. This is one of the reasons that those women who are unsure of the date of their last period are encouraged to have a scan early in pregnancy. Pregnancy continuing after forty-two weeks is associated with a very slight increased risk in stillbirth. Although doing a trace of the baby's heart rate and doing a scan to look at the amount of fluid around a baby are helpful in identifying a baby already in trouble, these tests can not always detect if a particular baby is at risk. For this reason, many midwives and doctors recommend induction of labour at between forty-one and forty-two weeks.

INDUCTION OF LABOUR

This describes the process of trying to artificially bring on labour. Once labour has started, it may not then need any further artificial stimulation.

Induction of labour is advised when the obstetrician feels that it is better for the baby to be outside than inside the uterus. Post-term pregnancy is one reason for induction. Other reasons may include:

■ Raised blood pressure
■ Diabetes
■ Reduced rate of growth in the baby
■ Too little amniotic fluid.

Some women may request induction if they have lost a baby in a previous pregnancy or sometimes to fit in with their domestic arrangements. This can be discussed with a senior doctor, but it is important to remember that induction of labour is not without potential risk, and some doctors may be reluctant to advise 'interfering' in an otherwise perfectly normal pregnancy. In addition, induction of labour is not always successful, and failed induction often leads to caesarean section.

The mode of induction depends on various factors, including the number of previous pregnancies and the condition of the cervix (the neck of the womb). As a general rule, induction is quicker and easier in those who have had vaginal deliveries before, and when the cervix has already started to soften and dilate. Induction can be more prolonged in women having their first baby, and may be associated with higher risk in those who have previously had a caesarean section, because of possible weakness of the uterus.

In general, if you are being induced you will be admitted to hospital for the induction in the evening or early in the morning. A doctor or midwife will do an internal examination to assess the condition (ripeness) of the cervix and give it a 'Bishop score'. This assesses the dilatation, consistency and position of the cervix. The higher the Bishop's score, the greater the likelihood of achieving vaginal delivery.

If the cervix is 'ripe' and already dilating, it may be possible to break the waters and start labour. This would be performed during an internal examination on the labour ward. The examination can be uncomfortable, and you may decide to have pain relief (such as gas and air) during the process.

If the cervix is not 'ripe' some prostaglandin gel can be placed in the vagina which acts on the cervix to soften it and get the labour started.

Prior to either of these procedures the well-being of the baby will be assessed by studying the pattern of the heartbeat to ensure that all is well. The midwife will also ensure that this is done when the labour ward is not too busy, as this gives her the best opportunity to explain what she is doing and to give you time to ask questions.

Reactions to the prostaglandin gel are very variable. Most women will find that the cervix begins to soften and dilate with minimal uterine contractions although this may take many hours and require up to three applications of the gel given at approximately four- to six-hourly intervals. Very occasionally, women will react strongly to the gel with powerful contractions which lead rapidly to delivery. These contractions may cause distress to the baby and are very painful for the mother. This is the reason why monitoring will be continued for at least one hour after the gel is inserted. Paradoxically, some women will have little or no change in their cervix following insertion of the gel. The gel may have a more rapid effect in those who have had children before. Some obstetricians avoid using prostaglandin when a previous delivery has been by caesarean section. In the future, other drugs may be available to induce labour which have a more consistent effect on the cervix.

It may take two or three doses of gel before the cervix has ripened enough for the membranes to be ruptured or the labour to get going.

Induction of labour is not always successful. Failed induction is more likely in women in their first pregnancy when the cervix is firm and tightly closed at the start of induction. Labour may also be difficult to induce earlier in pregnancy. This is one reason why you may be advised to have a caesarean section if the baby needs to be delivered prematurely because of complications in the pregnancy.

After the membrane rupture a drip containing the drug syntocinon may be needed to get the contractions going. This is a drug which is similar to a hormone which women produce naturally and will make the pregnant uterus contract. In general, if you are being induced you will be advised to have the baby's heart rate monitored electronically throughout your labour.

IS INDUCTION MORE PAINFUL?

Induction is often more painful than a spontaneous labour as there is not always the slow build up of contractions in a relaxed home environment that you would expect with a normal labour. Also, some women feel that contractions brought on by oxytocin are more painful than spontaneous contractions.

BREECH PRESENTATION

Breech presentation is when the baby's bottom or feet are in the mother's pelvis, rather than the head. Up to one-third of babies lie bottom first at thirty weeks but by term all but five per cent will have turned to being head first. If the baby is noted by your midwife to be bottom first at thirty-six weeks (or later) a scan will be advised in order to confirm the presentation. The scan may also estimate the baby's size and where the legs lie in relation to the bottom. If the pregnancy has been otherwise uncomplicated, the doctor may offer to try and turn the baby around; this is known as External Cephalic Version (ECV).

EXTERNAL CEPHALIC VERSION

ECV is a procedure where the doctor tries to manipulate the baby into a head first (cephalic) position at about thirty-seven to thirty-eight weeks. Prior to performing this procedure a heart rate trace of the baby will be performed. Some obstetricians use a drug to relax the womb. This is usually an inhaler, similar to that used by asthmatics. The ECV itself is a little uncomfortable as the doctor pushes the baby's bottom out of the pelvis and then encourages your baby to do a somersault. If the baby is manipulated into the cephalic position there is about a ninety per cent chance of it staying there. An ultrasound scan may be performed before and after the procedure.

ARE THERE ANY RISKS WITH ECV?

ECV can be so uncomfortable that it has to be abandoned. The main risk of ECV is that the waters can break or labour can start and therefore it is not usually done before thirty-seven weeks. There is a small risk of injuring the uterus or causing distress to the baby and the procedure is therefore done in the hospital and the baby's heart beat is monitored electronically during and afterwards to ensure that the baby is well.

POTENTIAL PROBLEMS WITH BREECH PRESENTATION

Although breech presentation is a normal variation, the decision about how to give birth may be a difficult one for some women, especially if this is their first baby.

Some doctors and midwives have been concerned that the vaginal delivery of a baby by the breech may be more traumatic for the baby. However, the evidence for this remains

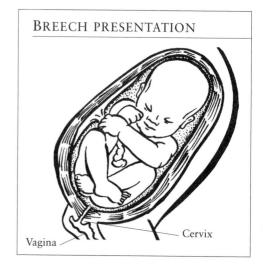

BREECH PRESENTATION

Vagina — — Cervix

unclear. The major concerns relate to the passage of the baby's head through the cervix in labour. When a baby delivers head first, once the head is through the rest of the baby will almost always follow. In a vaginal breech delivery, there is concern that the head is not delivered until the body of the baby is out. If there is difficulty with the delivery of the head, this may result in potentially serious delays during delivery. The option of caesarean section, available when the head is stuck during a cephalic (head first) delivery, may not be available when the body of the baby has already delivered during a breech labour. Similarly, it is not possible to use the ventouse to deliver a breech baby, and the forceps cannot be applied if the head has not descended through the cervix.

For those women who are considering a vaginal breech delivery, additional information about the size of the baby, the size of the mother's pelvis and the position of the baby's legs in relation to the body may help her to make her decision in consultation with her doctor and midwife. However, none of these measurements are a guarantee of a successful vaginal breech delivery, and in many hospitals up to fifty per cent of women who attempt vaginal breech delivery will end up having an emergency caesarean section. This figure may be lower in those women who have had successful vaginal deliveries in the past.

Because so many breech babies are born by caesarean section in the UK, many midwives and doctors are less experienced than they were at vaginal breech delivery. Those women who wish to have a vaginal birth with a breech baby should discuss this with their midwife and doctor.

WHY SOME BABIES ARE BREECH

Reasons for breech presentation include the following:
■ Twins
■ The shape of the womb or of the pelvis
■ Too much amniotic fluid
■ First baby
■ Fourth (or greater) baby.

In the past, a small percentage of breech babies was found to have serious abnormalities. This is much less common since ultrasound is widely available to pick up these patterns at an early stage of pregnancy. Obstetricians are usually involved in the care of women with a baby presenting by the breech. Some advise that all women with breech babies are delivered by caesarean section whereas others feel that if great care is taken in assessing factors such as the size of the baby and mother prior to delivery, and the delivery itself is performed by an experienced attendant, then it is quite safe to give birth vaginally. Breech babies will usually have special hip checks by the paediatrician after birth.

DELAYS IN LABOUR

A delay in the progress of labour may be diagnosed when the neck of the womb does not open at the normal rate. If there are no problems with the mother or the baby, the mother may wish to consider resting and awaiting events. Some labours do 'stop and go'. However, the midwife or doctor will examine the woman and may recommend that uterine contractions be stimulated to become more effective by the use of a hormone (oxytocin) in a drip. If labour does not progress in the presence of good uterine contractions, then the doctor will usually advise that the baby be delivered by caesarean section.

The majority of women will go through labour and have their babies with minimal intervention from medical staff. However, things do not always go according to plan, and it is worth being aware of common problems that may occur in labour so that they will be less alarming if they do happen.

CAESAREAN BIRTH

Caesarean birth (section) is the abdominal delivery of the baby by operation involving cutting into the uterus and extracting the baby under anaesthetic. The name 'caesarean section' derives from the Roman Law introduced in the reign of the Caesars and not, as is commonly thought, to the delivery of the infant Julius Caesar.

REASONS FOR CAESAREAN BIRTH

In the UK, the number of babies delivered by caesarean sections has been gradually rising over the last fifteen years, and up to one-third of all babies are delivered by caesarean in some hospitals. Caesarean sections are carried out either 'electively', as a planned operation, or as emergencies.

ELECTIVE CAESAREAN

These will be planned with the mother during her pregnancy, and are usually scheduled for thirty-eight weeks of pregnancy or later. When the mother has had two or more caesarean sections in the past a repeat section is usually advised. This is because of the small risk that the scar on the uterus may be put under excessive strain during the contractions of labour, a situation which is more likely following induction or acceleration of labour. If the scar were to open during labour, this would put the mother and baby at risk. When a 'classical' (cut made up and down in the uterus) caesarean has been performed in a previous pregnancy, the mother will generally be advised that all subsequent deliveries should be by caesarean section, as the scar from this operation is more

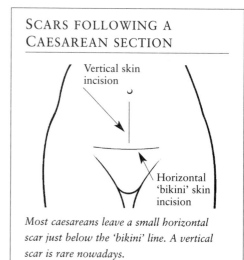

SCARS FOLLOWING A CAESAREAN SECTION

Vertical skin incision

Horizontal 'bikini' skin incision

Most caesareans leave a small horizontal scar just below the 'bikini' line. A vertical scar is rare nowadays.

likely to break down. One previous 'lower segment' caesarean section is certainly not now considered to indicate that all subsequent deliveries should be by caesarean, depending on the reason for the previous caesarean. If it is likely that the problem will recur, a further caesarean may be advised. Nowadays, the majority of women who have had one previous caesarean section decide to try for a normal delivery in their next pregnancy and are successful.

When the placenta is lying in front of the baby, so called 'placenta praevia' a caesarean is needed for delivery. In these circumstances labour contractions are likely to lead to bleeding which may be heavy.

In addition, some women choose to have caesarean sections if the baby is in the breech position, particularly if the baby is large and it is their first pregnancy. Some women request a caesarean delivery because of anxieties about labour, or problems in previous deliveries. These concerns should be discussed with the obstetrician during pregnancy and arrangements made which can allay these concerns.

Elective caesarean sections should not be carried out before thirty-eight weeks of pregnancy as there is a small risk that the baby will have breathing difficulties which may be serious. These are less common in the more mature baby.

EMERGENCY CAESAREAN

Many caesareans are performed as emergency procedures. An emergency section can be carried out either before labour has started or, more commonly, in labour. Prior to labour, emergency section may be advised where there is evidence of any danger to the baby or to the mother.

In labour, common reasons for advising caesarean section are when there is a marked delay in the progress of labour or if there are changes in the fetal monitoring which may indicate that the baby's oxygen supply is reduced.

Emergency caesarean section can be a frightening experience for the mother and her partner. However, the results from this operation are generally good and skilled staff are always on hand in the labour ward to act immediately if necessary. Caesarean section is only performed with the permission of the mother and the decision will always be discussed with a senior doctor, usually a consultant, although the caesarean section will commonly be performed by the registrar on duty,

In order to clarify 'what went wrong', many couples find it helpful to go through the events after the caesarean and to be clear about the reasons why the operation was advised and the implications for future pregnancies. This can also be done at a later time, by arrangement.

THE ANAESTHETIC

The caesarean section operation is carried out under one of the following anaesthetics:
■ Epidural anaesthetic
■ General anaesthetic.

The great majority of elective and emergency caesarean sections are now carried out under 'regional' anaesthetic, this refers to spinal or epidural anaesthesia. The woman is then awake during the operation, although numb from the chest down, her partner can be present and the couple can take some active participation in the delivery

A minority of caesareans are carried out under general anaesthetic. This may be advised in an extreme emergency, where there is very heavy bleeding or where regional techniques are not possible or safe. Some women request general anaesthetic, often because they are anxious about being awake during the procedure. In many cases, the anaesthetist will recommend regional anaesthesia because it is usually so much safer for the mother. In addition, there is less nausea after regional anaesthesia, and an epidural can be run continuously for a short time postoperatively for pain relief.

EPIDURAL AND SPINAL ANAESTHETICS

This takes about ten minutes to insert and a further twenty to forty minutes to become fully effective. Tests are carried out to make quite certain that the anaesthetic is working perfectly before the operation starts. These techniques mean that you can be fully awake during the operation and yet feel no pain, although some do experience some discomfort.

An unwanted effect of these spinal and

epidural anaesthetics is that the legs become numb and you are unable to move them. This will last for as long as the epidural is running and will take two to three hours to wear off afterwards. However, residual side effects are uncommon, and epidural or spinal anaesthesia is an unusual cause of long-term back problems.

GENERAL ANAESTHETICS

For those women who are advised or elect to, have a general anaesthetic, the modern general anaesthetic agents and techniques are very reliable and safe. The anaesthetist will want you to breathe oxygen through a mask which you can hold yourself for a few minutes. You will then be given an injection through the drip and sleep occurs within a few seconds.

HOW LONG DOES A CAESAREAN SECTION TAKE?

The anaesthetic can take up to 40 minutes in the case of an epidural, or three minutes in the case of a general anaesthetic. The skin preparation and draping of the abdomen with sterile drapes can take two or three minutes. Once the obstetrician has actually started the operation it may only take three or four minutes to actually deliver the baby. In those instances where the mother is awake, the baby is immediately shown to her and skin to skin contact encouraged. The obstetrician repairs the abdomen which may take twenty to thirty minutes.

POSTOPERATIVE RECOVERY

Most women who have had a caesarean section stay in hospital for about five days after the operation. The recovery time is usually slower than following a normal delivery, and it may be several weeks before you are able to go about all your normal activities. In addition, some car insurance companies forbid driving for up to six weeks after a caesarean section, although driving should be safe when you are able to do an emergency stop without pain.

The scar in the abdomen will usually be a small transverse scar placed just below the top of the pubic hair line and it is likely to fade over time. It is very rarely that a vertical scar is necessary, and the obstetric indications for this are exceedingly rare; but if there is already such a scar from some previous operation then the obstetrician may use this incision again. Some women tend to produce thick 'keloid' scars; this is more common in Afro-Caribbean women.

Each time a caesarean section is performed the operation may become slightly more technically difficult. This is because of scarring that inevitably occurs as the tissues heal. The chances of bleeding or damage to the womb and bladder at the time of the operation are increased with repeated operations. Also, the uterus may become weaker after repeated operations. This is the reason for advising caesarean section after two or more previous caesareans.

RECOVERING FROM A CAESAREAN BIRTH

During the first twenty-four hours the pain from the incision will usually be controlled by a continuing epidural, if you had this for the operation, or by an infusion of strong pain killer controlled by the patient. A catheter will have been inserted into the bladder before the operation, and this may be left in for the first day or until the woman is mobile. Eating and drinking are started gradually from several hours after the operation, depending on whether regional or general anaesthesia were used. Before this, fluid will be supplied by a drip into a vein on the arm.

Wind pains may occur as the bowels gradually start to work again.

Breastfeeding should start normally after a caesarean section, but the mother may need help in picking up the baby in the initial stages.

The wound should be fully healed within six weeks, but infection of the urine or the wound is quite common, even when antibiotics are given routinely at the time of the operation. Although you may walk to the toilet on the second or third day, moving normally takes longer and you will need more rest than a woman who has had a normal vaginal delivery. If you get an ache at the end of the day at home you have probably done too much, and should take it easy for a few hours. Movement is encouraged in order to lessen the chances of postoperative complications.

HOME BIRTH

Home births used to be the norm in Britain but are now relatively unusual with only about two to three in every hundred deliveries occurring at home. About half of these are 'accidental' when labour has come on suddenly and the woman is unable to get to hospital, and the other half have chosen to have a home delivery.

HOME VERSUS HOSPITAL DELIVERY

At a home birth, the labouring woman has the familiarity and security of her own home, perhaps a more relaxed environment and the opportunity to have family and friends around who can join in the experience of labour.

Those women considering a home birth should discuss this with their midwife. In general, if there have been problems in this or previous pregnancy, or if problems are predicted she will advise against a home birth. Two midwives will be allocated for the delivery, and your general practitioner will usually be on call also. Your antenatal care can be monitored by the family doctor and the practice midwives, and arrangements can be made if problems arise in labour and you need to be

BIRTH IN WATER

Some women find that immersing themselves in water during labour is an effective method of pain relief, and some also chose to give birth in water, usually in a specially designed birthing pool. Not all hospitals have a birthing pool, so if you plan to have a water birth in hospital, ensure that the equipment is installed and is functioning. It is also possible to hire these pools for use at home or in a maternity unit.

In most hospitals, use of the birthing pool is only advised for those with uncomplicated pregnancies and labours. Continuous monitoring of the baby is not possible underwater, so those who are advised to have this form of monitoring would be advised not to use the birthing pool.

Although many women who have used water immersion during labour find that it greatly enhances their experience of childbirth, the effectiveness of water in reducing the pain of labour and the safety of water birth continue to be areas of controversy.

transferred to hospital care. The frequency of this varies, but in about five per cent of home deliveries a transfer during labour is required.

The potential disadvantages of home birth relate to unpredictable hazards that can arise (although these are rare), even though the pregnancy may have been completely normal. The main concerns relate to uncommon but potential risks such as sudden heavy bleeding, usually after delivery and to the need for helping the baby to breathe in the first few minutes of life if it does not do so spontaneously. In both these cases, expert help and equipment would be needed and it is not possible to have the level of support at home that is available in hospital. In these circumstances emergency services may need to be summoned from the local hospital, but there will inevitably be a delay before these arrive.

Home birth is a controversial area in obstetrics and opinions vary widely about whether it is to be recommended and about its safety. Women having home delivery are carefully selected and are those where a problem in pregnancy is very unlikely. However, occasionally problems will occur which are much less easy to deal with at home, as described above. Obstetricians are keen to avoid serious problems where possible and many feel that the risk for the mother is increased. It is difficult to obtain statistical evidence to support or refute the argument, as major complications are rare and numbers extremely small. It is important to come to your own decision, based on the best evidence available and on your particular circumstances. There is little strong scientific evidence about the comparative benefits of home and hospital birth, and there are potential advantages and disadvantages for each. You may wish to weigh the risks of hospital birth against the risks of home birth.

THE POSTNATAL PERIOD

The concept of a long 'lying-in' period, when the new mother was confined to bed and cared for by hospital staff or at home by female relatives, has completely gone. Research shows that lying in bed can be detrimental to health. Now, women are encouraged to get out of bed as soon as possible after giving birth, and are discharged home within a few hours, a day or, at most, forty-eight hours after a normal birth.

Having a new baby is often a tiring experience. Some women may chose to stay in hospital longer, particularly if they do not have support at home. The assistance of midwives in establishing breastfeeding is also a reason

why some women choose to stay for a few extra days.

In order to keep healthy during this postnatal period, adequate sleep and a good diet will boost your energy levels. Plenty of roughage and water are important to avoid constipation. You can do this by eating whole grain cereals, vegetables and fruit that are a good source of natural fibre. Some women have painful haemorrhoids (piles) following delivery and require cream or suppositories.

Some women have difficulty controlling the passage of wind after delivery. A smaller number cannot control their bowel movements or are incontinent of urine. Women who have had a forceps or vacuum delivery are more likely to have bruising, soreness, urinary or bowel symptoms. These symptoms tend to improve over the next three months, but should be discussed with a specialist if they persist. Pelvic floor exercises (see pages 198 and 229) may be helpful.

BREASTFEEDING

Breastfeeding is best for both you and your baby. When a baby is put to the breast immediately after birth it helps the womb to contract. The milk the baby gets initially (known as colostrum) is also full of antibodies to help protect the baby from infection as well as being a perfect balance of nutrients which give it a good start in life.

Breastfeeding is a pleasurable experience; it brings you close to your baby and it is also flexible, since it does not require the making-up of bottles. Initially, you and your baby have to adjust to each other but with help any initial difficulties quickly pass and it is then possible to relax and enjoy the closeness breastfeeding brings.

Breastfeeding helps you to lose weight as well as being contraceptive (but only if you fully breastfeed, including at night). It may also protect women from getting breast cancer in the future.

Breast milk is best for your baby. Protection from infections such as gastroenteritis will continue and breast-fed babies are ten times less likely to develop this unpleasant stomach bug than bottle-fed babies. It also offers some protection from breathing problems such as asthma and bronchitis. It may also lower the risk of developing insulin-dependent diabetes.

It would be unrealistic to say that all mothers and babies establish breastfeeding

COMFORTABLE FEEDING

You will spend a lot of time feeding your baby. Make sure you have enough support for your body and legs and that the baby is raised high enough so you are not leaning forward.

easily, as the breasts can get sore around the third day when the volume of milk in the breasts increases. However, with the help of the midwife or health visitor, and self-help such as using warm compresses before feeding to soften the breasts, these initial discomforts can be overcome.

If your baby is in special care, milk can be expressed from the breast using a special pump and given to the baby until it is ready to suck.

There are very few women who are advised not to breastfeed, one example being those who are HIV-positive. Drugs often pass into the breast milk, but this is rarely a problem. If you take regular medication, talk about these issues with your doctor or midwife, who will give you the information you need and, if necessary, find an alternative medication.

THE LOCHIA

The lochia (postnatal vaginal discharge) is lost from the uterus after birth. Bright red initially, it becomes pinky brown, then brown and eventually tails off to nothing. Many books say this process will be completed within ten to fourteen days but women often find that extra activity (including sexual intercourse) may cause a brighter red loss for a few days, and some that it takes at least six weeks for the lochia to cease.

Normal lochia is a light to moderate loss (no clots) and does not smell offensive. If the lochia is smelling and the uterus is tender, then this may indicate an infection needing antibiotic treatment. Occasionally, a piece of placental tissue can be left inside and cause heavy or persistent bleeding or an infection. This may need to be removed in hospital.

SECONDARY POST PARTUM HAEMORRHAGE

This is excessive blood loss occurring more than twenty-four hours after delivery, usually due to a retained piece of placenta and/or an infection inside the uterus. After a few days there may be a sudden blood loss accompanied by cramping pains in the lower abdomen. Sometimes a piece of placenta is expelled at this time and the bleeding abates, but sometimes the retained tissue has to be removed under anaesthetic. As secondary haemorrhage may occur after leaving hospital it is important to report any excessive bleeding to your doctor or community midwife.

POSTNATAL CARE

The midwife has a statutory duty to attend women during the postnatal period, a period of not less than ten and not more than twenty-eight days after the birth. Many new mothers, especially those with their first baby, find this extremely helpful and reassuring. At each visit the midwife may check the following:
■ The baby's umbilical cord. She will take a blood test (heel prick) for the baby to test for an important metabolic disease (phenylketonuria, PKU) between the seventh and tenth days

■ Your perineum to see that it is healing well
■ Your breasts for signs of infection or cracked nipples and any wounds.

She can also answer any specific questions about the postnatal period and care of the baby.

The six week postnatal check may be arranged at the midwife, GP or hospital clinic, depending on local policy and the circumstances of the pregnancy. This is an opportunity to ensure that all the normal postnatal changes have occurred, and to ensure that screening tests such as cervical smears are up-to-date. In addition, many women wish to discuss returning to normal activities, such as sexual intercourse. This is also a good time to confirm or rethink decisions about a method of contraception which were made during pregnancy. A vaginal examination is not usually performed unless there have been problems with pain or discharge.

The doctor will also ask how you are feeling. The transition to motherhood with the awesome and lifelong responsibility for a tiny infant can be overwhelming for some women, especially those who experienced poor parenting themselves.

PUERPERAL DEPRESSION

The 'baby blues' that can affect up to fifty per cent of women on the third or fourth day after birth, are usually transient. These mood swings are thought to be related to the changes in hormonal levels after the birth. They are not linked with later depression from which as many as ten per cent of women suffer.

The symptoms of depression are less clear-cut, because of the broken sleep and fatigue of new parents, but screening questionnaires such as the Edinburgh postnatal depression score can be used by health visitors and doctors to identify women who are becoming depressed. Counselling and support will help many but anti-depressant drugs can prevent the depression from becoming chronic and affecting the development of the baby in subtle ways. The importance of friends as well as family to support the new parent(s) has been realised and groups set up in some parts of the country help women who are isolated from their families or have none.

About one women in 500 develops a severe mental illness in the first month after delivery, but fortunately in most areas there are specialist mother and baby units where they can be treated successfully, without being separated from the baby.

DIFFICULTIES WITH THE BABY

The vast majority of women will have a live healthy baby at term (thirty-eight to forty-two weeks of pregnancy). Sadly, about one woman in a hundred still leaves hospital without a live baby and coming to terms with such a loss is difficult, although professionals are well trained today to support parents in this situation than some years ago, and specialist support groups (such as the Stillbirth and Neonatal Death Society, SANDS), provide counsellors who have themselves lost a child.

If your baby is premature or sick, it may require special or neonatal intensive care. Today even very small babies have a good chance of survival, although their time in the intensive care unit can be very stressful for the parents. Breastfeeding can be established successfully even if the baby is very premature as long as you learn to express milk to keep lactation going and this milk (EBM) is the best for the baby.

Once the baby comes home it will need more warmth, more frequent feeds and is more susceptible to infection until the baby reaches the weight of a normal full-term baby (six to seven pounds). The first time you go out, leaving the baby with even the most trusted baby sitter (often your own mother), you will feel anxious. Later, if you return to work it can be a wrench leaving your baby with another person, but after the postnatal period life goes on, enriched and more complex. Enjoy it and your baby, because they grow up so fast.

GETTING YOUR BODY BACK TO NORMAL

Hormonal changes in pregnancy revert back to prepregnancy levels at three to six weeks after childbirth. Joints and ligaments take between four and six months to return to normal strength.

All women need to rest for the first three to six weeks, but those women who have had muscle and joint problems in pregnancy may need more rest in the first four to six months to allow the ligaments to recover. Avoiding heavy lifting during the months when the trunk and pelvic muscles are repairing, while continuing to strengthen these muscles with abdominal and pelvic floor exercises, may help to avoid back problems and prolapse in the future.

REST

It is important to try and sleep during the day if you are up at night with the baby. If you can not sleep, rest lying down by practising a relaxation technique or listening to calming music but not watching TV or reading. If you can, unplug the telephone and restrict visitors to certain times to allow for rest.

POSTURE

Trying to maintain a neutral spine and pelvis is more important now, since there is less support for the lower back. The pressure from the growing baby keeping the abdominal muscles taut provided support for the lower back in pregnancy. After delivery there is no pressure from the baby and the muscles are slack and not taut, therefore now there is more risk of damaging the lower back. All the previous rules of good posture and advice apply (see page 191).

FEEDING THE BABY

Whether breast or bottle feeding you should be sitting well supported with a lumbar roll and pillows or cushions under your arm and the baby. These will raise the baby to breast level for good eye contact and stop you rounding down to the baby or having to keep your shoulder in an elevated position. With breastfeeding you can also lie on your side; this is useful if you are resting in the afternoon or throughout the night and gives the back a rest.

NAPPY CHANGING

STANDING

Choose a surface of approximately waist height. This will allow for eye contact without bending from the waist and rounding the back. If a surface is below waist height one knee on a chair or one foot slightly raised will allow you to bend forward from the hip keeping the back straight.

KNEELING

If the surface is well below waist height i.e.. the bed or settee, then kneel at an angle with one knee on the floor and the other leg with the hip bent and the foot flat on the floor. Again this allows you to lean forward from the hip, keeping the back straight.

SITTING

Do not sit on the bed / settee and twist to one side. Only sit on the floor with legs apart if you can lean forward from the hips, keeping the back straight, otherwise you will lean forward from the waist with a rounded back. Do not kneel on the floor, sitting back on the heels, as the only way to lean forward is from the waist with a rounded back.

EXERCISES

Exercises should be begun as soon as possible after delivery. It is better to take pain killers and be mobile than to avoid movement because of discomfort. Early mobility will prevent complications, particularly for those women who have had a caesarean section.

BREATHING EXERCISES AFTER DELIVERY

Breathe in through the nose, hold for two counts, release the air through the mouth making sure all the air is out of the lungs. Then a bigger breath can be taken in the next time. As the air is breathed out pull in the lower abdominal muscles below the waist. Repeat this five times at one go. It maybe more comfortable to perform this exercise with the legs slightly bent and soles of the feet resting comfortably on the mattress.

COUGHING

Deep breathing may stimulate a cough, and the following support should also be tried for sneezing, laughing and vomiting.

If you have had a caesarean section, place one hand flat over the wound with the other hand on top. Just rest the hands there, do not push yet. Then at the same time as the cough is performed momentarily press hard inwards to prevent the build up of pressure pushing the abdominal muscles out and pulling on the stitches. There will be some discomfort, but less than without support. The stitches will not be broken, but the secretions must be cleared to prevent a chest infection or pneumonia developing.

With perineal stitches, place one hand over the pad and push upwards momentarily as the cough is performed; this will stop everything from being forced downwards. The other hand can support the abdomen if necessary.

FOOT AND ANKLE EXERCISES

With the knees straight, quickly and firmly move at the ankle pushing the foot up and down so that the calf muscle acts to pump the blood up to the trunk. Repeat continuously for twenty to thirty seconds. Do not curl the toes, this can cause cramp. The ankles can also be turned in a circle one way and then the other, if preferred. Repeat at least ten times in each direction, every hour during the day. This aids circulation when walking is restricted, and helps to prevent blood clots from forming. It also helps to reduce swelling in the lower legs and prevent cramp.

PELVIC FLOOR EXERCISES

Pelvic floor exercises can be performed immediately post caesarean; they will encourage circulation into the pelvis which will aid healing of the wound and help to remove swelling, and therefore reduce the pain. They should be repeated ten times fast and five times slowly, every waking hour or at least a minimum of every time the baby is fed i.e.. approximately six times daily. Pelvic floor exercises should be performed immediately after vaginal delivery. For the same reasons. If these are painful, they can be delayed for the first few days after delivery:

RHYTHMICAL PELVIC FLOOR EXERCISES

Slow and gentle pelvic floor exercises can be performed immediately after delivery. Squeeze the pelvic muscles and lift them up slightly, releasing slowly. Repeat in a rhythmical pattern and continue for thirty seconds to one minute. The gentle movement will be enough to make the muscles move and not increase the pressure on the swelling causing more pain, but will encourage an increase in circulation to aid healing and reduce the swelling already there, in turn reducing the pain.

Repeat rhythmically for thirty seconds to

one minute every waking hour until the normal protocol of pelvic floor exercises can be performed.

If haemorrhoids are present outside the body, perform the rhythmical pelvic floor exercises only until they reduce. Holding a contraction could make them worse. If pelvic floor exercises cannot be performed because of pain, then a small ice pack consisting of ice cubes or a frozen sachet of normal saline in a wet paper towel should be applied to the swelling for ten minutes every two hours. This has a pain relieving effect as well as helping to reduce the swelling. Pelvic floor exercises after the application of the ice pack maybe easier to perform. pelvic floor exercises may be easier to perform while sitting in a warm bath. Always dry the perineum thoroughly by patting gently and replacing the sanitary towel with a clean dry one.

Pelvic floor exercises should be done between six and ten times a day for four to six months, until the collagen is back to normal strength.

PELVIC TILTING

Begin half lying or lying, with knees bent. Perform as before. Hold for ten seconds. Repeat five times, hourly while in hospital. The mobility will increase circulation, aid healing and reduce swelling and pain. Rhythmical pelvic tilting will ease back pain. Gentle toning of the abdominals will help prevent back strain. Repeat ten times, three times daily at home.

CURL-UPS

Women who have had caesareans should wait two to three days before beginning this exercise. Perform the curl-ups lying with knees bent.

Repeat the pelvic tilt, hold this position, breathe out as the head and shoulders curl up and slide hands towards knees. Release immediately. Repeat five times, hourly while in hospital.

If the abdominal muscles bulge outwards, do not use the arms and just lift the head only;

POSTNATAL EXERCISES – CURL-UPS

Straight curl-up
Pull your tummy in and tuck your chin in. Slowly lift your head and shoulders while stretching your hands towards your knees as far as you feel comfortable. Then slowly uncurl making sure that you make no sudden jerks or movements

Side curl-up
As straight curl-up but stretch your right hand towards your left knee. Slowly uncurl, then repeat the exercise with your left hand towards your right knee.

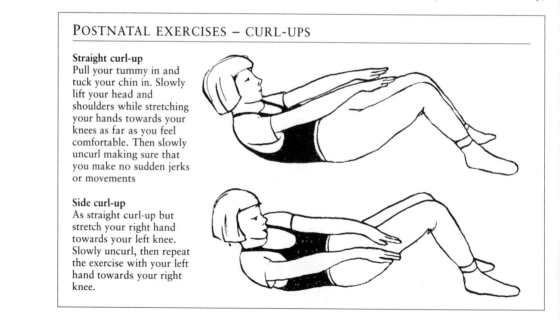

if the muscles still bulge outwards, then stop. Continue with the pelvic tilting only for two more days, then try again, with head only, progressing to using the arms as the muscles strengthen and remain flat.

This exercise can be progressed further by holding at the top for a few seconds, whilst breathing, before releasing. Repeat ten times, three times daily.

CHECKING FOR SEPARATION OF THE ABDOMINAL MUSCLES

Lie on the back with knees bent. Place, width-ways, the middle three fingers of the hand you use for writing, approximately 2 cm (1 in) above the belly button. Perform a pelvic tilt and then a curl-up as in the previous exercise. Do not worry if the stomach muscles bulge. As the abdominal muscles are shortened the long muscles running from the top to the bottom of the abdomen, (the recti) will tend to close the gap and the tense edges of the muscles felt on the sides of the fingers. The muscles may squeeze the fingers so that one, two or all fingers will have to be removed. Some women have no gap, the average gap is two fingers and up to four fingers is acceptable. If at ten days the gap is still four fingers with exercising, then extra

attention from a physiotherapist is needed.

You may have this checked for you by a physiotherapist in hospital or your community midwife. If you are unsure and no one is able to check the gap, self refer to a postnatal exercise class run by a physiotherapist or obtain a referral from your community midwife or GP.

The recti have closed if the tip of the finger fits tight between the edges of the muscles or if there is a small gap with a 'solid floor' and the finger does not sink into soft tissue. An average two-finger gap will close in approximately two to three weeks, longer if the gap is bigger or the exercises not performed as instructed. Only when the gap is closed and curl-ups performed without bulging should gentle oblique abdominal exercises begin, usually from three weeks onwards.

DIAGONAL CURL-UPS

Start by lifting the shoulder in a diagonal and reaching the hand to the opposite thigh. Lift, breathing out and lower immediately, repeating ten times to each side, once daily. Progress by holding for a few seconds before releasing as well as lifting higher and moving the shoulder further into the diagonal. Breathe out lifting up; in and out while holding; and breathe in while lowering.

HIP HITCHING

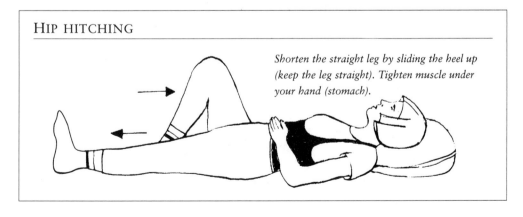

Shorten the straight leg by sliding the heel up (keep the leg straight). Tighten muscle under your hand (stomach).

HIP HITCHING

Lie on the back with one leg bent. Push the straight leg away from the body, then using the muscles of the waist to hitch the hip into the body, shortening the straight leg. Repeat this ten times with each leg. Breathe throughout, as at rest. Progress to both legs straight and simultaneously push one leg away from the body, while hitching the opposite hip into the body. Repeat ten times.

KNEE ROLLING

Lie on the back with both knees bent. Place hands onto the ribcage, keeping the elbows on the support. Roll both knees to one side letting the hips follow by twisting the spine but leaving the elbow and shoulder in contact with the support. Now draw in the lower tummy muscles and breathe out as you lift the knees back to the mid line position. Repeat to the other side. Repeat five times to each side. Progress by slowly increasing the number of repetitions to each side.

Better results will be obtained, the slower the knees are lifted to the mid-line position.

LIFTING

Do not lift anything heavier than the baby. As your pelvic floor and abdominal muscles return to normal and as the baby increases in weight, you will gradually be able to lift heavier things. Therefore it is important that you have help in the first three weeks with all your household tasks plus shopping. Get help with toddlers or young children especially with walking them to nursery or school. If you are able, gradually begin to undertake household activities but get help setting up the ironing board, getting out the vacuum cleaner and still get help lifting toddlers, walking them to school and large amounts of shopping, right up to four months. It can take up to six months for the pelvic floor and abdominal muscles to regain their strength to support the body fully, longer if you are breastfeeding.

DRIVING

After delivery, you should feel competent to hold the car in a straight line should you need to do an emergency stop, as the seat belt will press hard into the abdomen, otherwise you may be responsible for causing an accident and not avoiding one.

After a caesarean section, it is advisable to check your insurance policy. Some policies say you may drive, after an abdominal incision, 'when your doctor says you are fit'. Other policies say no driving for eight weeks after an abdominal incision. If you drive outside these clauses you maybe financially liable if you are involved in an accident.

SWIMMING

This may be resumed as soon as the recti gap has closed and the lochia (blood loss like a period) has completely stopped, i.e. normal clear vaginal discharge, or after your six-week postnatal check has occurred, which ever you prefer.

KNEE-ROLLING

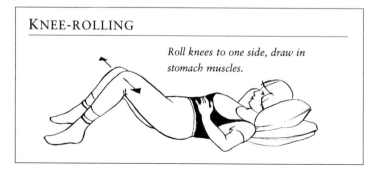

Roll knees to one side, draw in stomach muscles.

POSTNATAL EXERCISE GROUPS

Begin as soon as you are able if a physiotherapist is running the group. Often other groups begin after your six week postnatal check, if run by your local gym, leisure or adult education centre.

GOING TO THE GYM

If you are used to exercise, once the recti have closed, you can get aerobic exercise from a static exercise bike. You can also lift or push light weights. The lowest weight must be used and increase the sets of repetitions. Have the gym manager check your posture if there are no mirrors available. You must not strain and breathe out forcibly with the weights, as this increases the pressure in the abdomen and pushes down on the pelvic floor muscles and out on the abdominal muscles.

Do not begin brisk walking on the treadmill until after six weeks and start with ten minutes, gradually increasing. Do not row or use the stair master for four months.

With rowing the back is flexed, stretching the ligaments and possibly causes the spinal discs to move backwards. The stair master causes uneven pressure on the pelvis which could result in sacroiliac joint problems.

Should you try rowing or stepping and back, pelvic or leg pain is produced, you should stop and try again after the baby is six months old. Should problems occur after six months you should obtain a referral to a physiotherapist.

SPORT

Any activity which includes bouncing up and down, such as tennis, net ball, squash, badminton, plus low impact or step aerobics, should not be commenced until four months after the birth. Doing a progressive floor exercise regime including pelvic floor exercises and aerobic exercise on the bike or swimming should allow the muscles to return to their normal strength to support the back and pelvic content. Beginning sport before four months could result in back or urinary and pelvic floor muscle problems.

If you performed these sports two to three times per week right up to the time of delivery, you maybe able to return earlier i.e. with a half full bladder, legs apart, can you jump up and down and cough without leaking urine, and have not suffered any backache for two weeks after your six week postnatal check.

Repetitive high impact sport, such as jogging, aerobic and step classes, trampolining, etc., should not be performed until six months postnatal, which is the latest that collagen has been recorded to return to its normal strength when not breastfeeding.

These are only guidelines. If you are used to performing sport or exercise at a high level, then seek individual advice from on obstetric physiotherapist.

POSTNATAL DEPRESSION

Balance rest and exercise. Fatigue progressing to exhaustion can lead to depression. If you feel you may be depressed talk to your community midwife, health visitor or GP. They can offer practical help and advice and refer you for further professional help, if necessary.

Chapter twelve

INFERTILITY

About one in six of all couples have some problem getting pregnant and that includes some trying for a second or subsequent baby. Here, we explain some of the main problems and what can be done to overcome them.

HOW LONG SHOULD IT TAKE TO CONCEIVE?

Getting pregnant can be a matter of chance. Like trying to throw a six with a dice, you may be lucky first time, but there is no guarantee you will succeed, even after lots of attempts. Out of all the couples who manage to conceive without any medical help, about seventy-five per cent of them (three out of four) manage it within six months of having regular sexual intercourse without contraceptives. After a year, the figure is ninety per cent. Another five per cent manage it within two years and the rest may succeed after two years of trying.

Many couples who have been trying for a year or two to become pregnant are normal and healthy, without any underlying fertility problems. They go on to conceive in time, without any help.

WHEN SHOULD YOU SEEK HELP?

If you have been trying for a baby for a year or more and have been having regular sexual intercourse (about two or three times a week), it is a good idea to see your family doctor as a first step. He or she can do some very basic tests and, if none of these show any specific cause for the delay, the chances are you will conceive within the next year. There is no real need to move on to any more specialist tests until after that further year, unless you are a woman over thirty-five. Fertility starts to decline from this time onwards, and women of this age do not have much time to lose. For these women, there is a strong case for moving on to these specialist tests after a year of trying to conceive.

When you decide to be referred to a specialist, most clinics prefer people to present as couples rather than as individuals. This emphasises the joint nature of fertility problems and allows the two partners to understand more of what the other will go through during the process. There is usually time for the divulgence of personal or other information that one may not want the other to know.

WHY CAN YOU NOT GET PREGNANT?

Depending on the country you study and sometimes even on differences within a country, the causes of infertility do vary. However, the most recent figures for the UK suggest that the following are the principal reasons why couples do not conceive.

■ Problems of sperm function (low numbers, poor motility, inadequate penetration of cervical mucus or low fertilisation capacity) account for twenty-five per cent of cases and contribute the most to defined causes of failing to conceive.

■ Abnormal ovulatory function is the next most frequent cause, contributing to about twenty per cent of cases.

■ In about fifteen per cent of cases, the woman's fallopian tubes will be blocked or severely damaged to the extent that fertility will be impaired.

■ In terms of other defined causes, cervical mucus disorders and endometriosis contribute to infertility in less than ten per cent of cases.

■ Complete absence of sperm at ejaculation is very rare and may be due to a blockage or the failure of production, and is found in no more than one to two per cent of cases.

■ In a sizeable proportion of cases, no defined cause of infertility will be found and these couples will have more than one cause for their infertility.

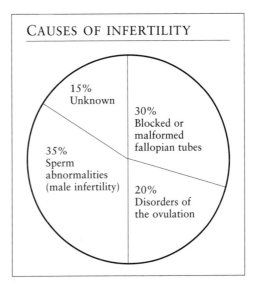

CAUSES OF INFERTILITY

15% Unknown

30% Blocked or malformed fallopian tubes

35% Sperm abnormalities (male infertility)

20% Disorders of the ovulation

IS THERE A 'BEST TIME' TO HAVE INTERCOURSE?

There are days of the month when you are more likely to conceive than others and this time is just before ovulation. Ovulation is the release of the egg from one of the two ovaries. The egg is picked up by the 'fingers' of the fallopian tube and it then gets wafted along, through the tube, on its way to the uterus.

If you conceive, it is because the sperm has met the egg while it is still in the fallopian tube, and has fertilised it. The fertilised egg (now called an embryo) begins to divide and divide again and again, over several days, before reaching the uterus. It then implants itself in the lining of the uterus, and starts to grow in size. This process can take up to ten days to complete.

Women produce mucus often throughout the menstrual cycle. This is a dry, sticky, thick fluid that is secreted from the cervix and vagina and different women produce different amounts. Some days before ovulation, the body starts to produce a thinner, stretchy type

of mucus rather like raw egg white. Some women are aware of feeling 'wetter' at this time of the month (importantly, however long or short your menstrual cycle is, ovulation always occurs twelve to sixteen days before your period is expected). This mucus is especially welcoming to sperm, nourishing them and helping them to swim upwards into the cervix, uterus and tubes, ready to meet up with the egg when it is released. After ovulation, the mucus changes back to the thicker type, which is less 'sperm-friendly'.

But how can you be sure of the right time? If you are having sexual intercourse every two days or so, you will hit the fertile period anyway. If you do not have intercourse as frequently as this, or if you want to be more precise, you can check your cervical mucus by inserting your fingers into your vagina, or by wiping a tissue over the entrance to the vagina. As we have seen, the 'right' time is when the mucus becomes wet and slippery, rather like egg white.

Another way of checking your ovulation time is to take your temperature after a minimum of five hours' sleep, before getting out of

OVULATION, CONCEPTION AND EMBRYO DEVELOPMENT

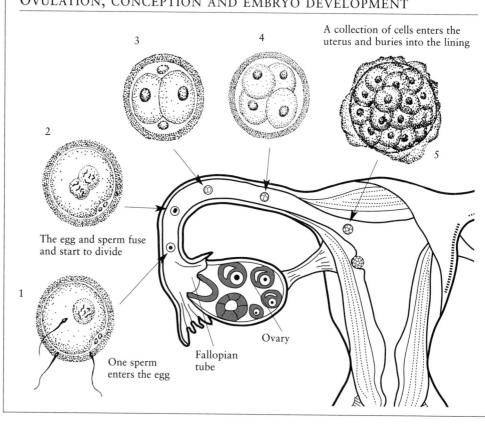

A collection of cells enters the uterus and buries into the lining

The egg and sperm fuse and start to divide

One sperm enters the egg

Fallopian tube

Ovary

Left: After fertilisation occurs an embryo forms, which implants into the uterus where it contains around 32 cells.

bed. The body temperature rises slightly after ovulation, under the influence of the hormone progesterone. Traditionally, this test has been used to check that ovulation is actually happening, with special 'fertility thermometers', marked to help you spot the small rises you are looking for. We now know that it is not a very reliable test, however, and it cannot show whether or not the egg released is a fully mature one, capable of leading to a conception. In addition, the temperature rise occurs after ovulation has occurred.

You can also buy 'ovulation kits' in chemists which predict ovulation to help you time intercourse better. With the kit, you test your urine every day for the surge in hormone that occurs around twelve to twenty-four hours before ovulation. The tests are reliable if you have a regular twenty-eight-day cycle but not if you have a longer or shorter cycle, as they are based on the twenty-eight-day cycle. They are also rather expensive and can introduce a calculated element into love-making, which some couples can find stressful. Intercourse can start to feel like a duty rather than a pleasure. It is important to continue intercourse for enjoyment and not solely for the aim of achieving pregnancy. Thus, it is better to have regular intercourse throughout the month rather than trying to predict ovulation and have intercourse only at that time.

Women are more likely to become pregnant if they are an appropriate weight for their height, so it may be worth checking that your weight falls within the desired range for your height. Ask your doctor for advice.

BASIC INVESTIGATIONS

The most common tests to establish the causes of infertility include the following ones:

■ Timed blood tests to assess ovulation. Your cycle length should determine this timing

■ A temperature chart kept over a few months; this is a method that is not particularly accurate but may be suggested by your doctor or nurse

■ Assessment to check whether the cervix, uterus and fallopian tubes are open to allow passage of the sperm, egg and fertilised egg. This assessment may be by X-ray taken after injecting dye through the cervix or by a laparoscopy (looking inside the abdomen with a tiny telescope through a small incision) to watch the dye pass out of the ends of the fallopian tubes

■ Assessment of a semen sample under a microscope to count the number, movement and normality of the sperm

■ A more sophisticated but still relatively simple test is to check that the interaction between the cervical mucus and the sperm does not impair the progress of the sperm in their journey into the uterus and onwards. This test (the postcoital test) is done around the time of ovulation and involves microscopic assessment of sperm in a specimen of cervical mucus collected up to twelve hours after intercourse.

PROBLEMS WITH OVULATION

Most women with regular periods do not have a problem with ovulation. Sometimes, women experiencing a delay in conceiving have blood tests to check on their levels of the

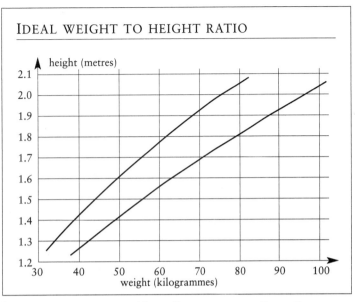

IDEAL WEIGHT TO HEIGHT RATIO

hormone progesterone. Normally, progesterone levels are high throughout the second half of the cycle that follows ovulation. If this level is low, it could indicate that ovulation is not happening. Many women have tests on day twenty-one regardless of the length of their cycle. However, this is not useful in longer cycles.

There is a wide variation in ovulation 'quality'. You need to test several cycles to be sure of a persistent problem. A real ovulation disorder usually only happens in women whose periods are very infrequent or even absent. Women in this situation need special investigations to work out the cause.

If you have problems with ovulation, there are 'fertility drugs' that you can take, in the form of tablets or injections, which stimulate the ovaries to produce more eggs each month. Research shows that this treatment works best in couples who have been trying for more than three years. If it is going to work, it will work within four to six months and there is little justification for a more prolonged course of treatment.

Above: Charts are available to determine whether you are an appropriate weight for your height.

OVULATION INDUCTION

Women can be helped to ovulate with drugs, either by tablets taken by mouth or by injections of hormones. The tablets induce mild ovulation stimulation, developing one or two follicles if the drug is used safely and as recommended. The injections are more powerful and can aid the development of one or more follicles, usually more than one. Careful observation by ultrasound and blood tests is essential for safety, lessening the risks of multiple pregnancy and ovarian hyperstimulation syndrome (see later under IVF). Success rates vary for this treatment. The most common reason to require ovulation induction is the polycystic ovarian syndrome and, in this group, pregnancy rates of fifteen to twenty per cent per cycle might be expected. Ovulation induction is discussed in more detail later in this chapter.

BLOCKED OR DAMAGED FALLOPIAN TUBES

Sometimes, the egg cannot move through the tube because the tube is blocked or damaged in some way. The 'fingers' of the tubes can be affected by inflammation or adhesions (scar tissue), perhaps after an infection or a previous pelvic operation. The tubes can become fixed, again as a result of infection or surgery, so they cannot move to pick up the egg when it is released. The surface of the ovary itself can be closed over by adhesions and that means the egg cannot get out of the ovary and into the tube.

Your doctor can arrange for a test called a hysterosalpingogram (HSG), which is an X-ray taken after a dye has been passed through the cervix to show up the outline of the inside of the uterus and the tubes. This cannot show adhesions outside the tubes and around the ovaries, however.

CAN THIS SORT OF BLOCKAGE BE TREATED?

Yes. If there is a blockage caused by adhesions, it is sometimes possible to have surgery to cut them away. But even after surgery, the problem can remain. It is also true that the lining of the tubes can be damaged permanently by infection, and the tubes just cannot work properly. Some experts now feel that most couples have a greater chance of success with IVF (in-vitro fertilisation or the 'test-tube' method), which bypasses the problem, because the sperm fertilises the egg outside the woman's body in the laboratory and the embryo is then put into the uterus. There are also other assisted conception methods, such as GIFT (gamete intrafallopian transfer), which may be tried (see page 244).

TUBAL SURGERY

Tubal surgery is an operation on the fallopian tube(s), usually for tubal fertility reasons. It was traditionally done via a laparotomy (an operation looking inside the abdomen through a cut in the skin) or with an operating microscope, but more recently, operating on the fallopian tubes via a laparoscope has gained in popularity. The main reason is because it avoids a big scar line, decreases pain after the operation and recovery time and can be done as a day procedure. Some studies have even claimed that the pregnancy rate after laparoscopic tubal surgery is as good as that from a traditional operation or microsurgery.

Laparoscopy

In this surgery, following a general anaesthetic, a laparoscope – a very narrow telescope – is inserted into the abdomen, through a small cut through the navel. This allows the doctor to check that the fallopian tubes are open and to look at the organs of the pelvis, and to check for any abnormalities. Dye is introduced into the uterus through the cervix and it can be seen travelling up the fallopian tubes and spilling through the ends.

It is not worth doing this simple operation at an early stage of investigations, however, unless it is thought that there might have been some damage done in the past. This might come from a history of infection in the pelvis, a complicated miscarriage or birth, abdominal conditions such as appendicitis, and any surgery done inside the abdomen. You may also have had a blood test that has shown chlamydia, which is an infectious disease that can cause pelvic damage.

When tubal surgery is appropriate

Tubal surgery in infertility cases is usually used in cases of isolated tubal blockage. The success rate, as measured by pregnancy, depends on the age of the woman, the extent of tubal damage and whether there are other associated factors causing the couple to be infertile, such as a low sperm count.

With the rapid advances of assisted conception (there are many different techniques now) and the high pregnancy rates associated with the procedure, tubal surgery has lost its appeal. However, there are situations where tubal surgery offers an excellent pregnancy rate and these include sterilisation reversal and microsurgical or laparoscopic clearance of adhesions in the absence of damage to the end of the tubes (the fimbriae). The advantage of tubal reconstruction over IVF is that there is the possibility of the woman conceiving more than once after the surgical procedure and also the avoidance of IVF with its associated risk of ovarian hyperstimulation and multiple pregnancy.

PROBLEMS WITH SPERM PRODUCTION

The first and most basic test on sperm is to look at them in a sample of semen. The man produces the sample, which is then studied in the laboratory. The number of sperm is then counted to check there is the quantity that might be expected in that volume of semen. However, just counting is not enough to come up with a diagnosis of a problem, except in situations where there are hardly any sperm or even none at all. Some men with normal sperm counts are infertile, and some with low counts are fertile. How the sperm actually work is just as important. They have to be able to escape from the semen, penetrate cervical mucus, and survive there for twenty-four hours or more. So the appearance and structure of the sperm, and their movements, are also studied.

TESTS FOR SPERM FUNCTIONING

One test is the postcoital test or PCT. Up to twelve hours after sexual intercourse, the woman goes to the clinic and a sample of her cervical mucus is taken from high up in her vagina (rather like the smear test). The sample will be looked at to see what the sperm are doing. This test is very encouraging if the test is positive (i.e. sperm are moving forward through the mucus) but less so if not. Positive tests are linked to strong likelihood of conception. Sperm and mucus can also be collected separately, and the way they react together can be looked at in the laboratory and compared to normal controls (a crossed penetration test).

TREATMENT FOR SPERM PROBLEMS

A very few men have no sperm at all and some have very few. Others have sperm that simply do not work very well. Unfortunately, there is as yet no effective treatment to help any of these problems. Assisted conception may be successful or ICSI (see page 247) may be used. Alternatively, donor insemination can be used. This means that the sperm of an anony-mous donor are collected and injected into the woman's cervical canal. This test is not available in all units as there is debate as to its value.

UNEXPLAINED INFERTILITY

It is difficult for many couples to come to terms with infertility, especially when relatives and friends around you appear to conceive readily. It is even more difficult to understand when, after extensive investigations, doctors may be unable to offer any explanation for the problem. Fertility is not an all or nothing matter, and even apparently normal fertile couples may take several months or even years to become pregnant. Even couples who have had one child may experience this problem, and probably one in six couples has some difficulty in trying to conceive.

A problem arises in deciding how long you should wait before considering further investigations and treatment. No two couples are the same and thus it is unwise to make too general a rule. However, it is very important to take age into consideration. As women and, to a much lesser extent, men become older, fertility decreases and problems during pregnancy, such as miscarriage, increase. The age gap between older couples and their prospective children may also present problems in later years. Thus it is sensible for older couples to seek help earlier than younger couples who may be reassured by normal investigations to continue longer to try to become pregnant without further aid.

Before considering infertility as 'unex-plained', it is important to establish that the woman is producing eggs, that the man is producing sufficient numbers of sperm, and that the sperm are able to meet the eggs. Following initial normal investigations, couples may be regarded as having unexplained fertility although later, in some cases, the cause for infertility may be established.

HOW LONG SHOULD YOU TRY?

Sometimes, fertility problems cannot be treated. In some cases, they cannot even be explained. The statistics show that couples who have been trying for two to three years, with no explanation for the delay, still have a good chance of conception. After three years, however, the chances of a natural conception start to fall, and the best hope lies with IVF and other similar methods of assisted conception, as long as your tests have shown that your eggs and your sperm are functioning well enough.

You can get help and information from the organisations offering support to couples who are experiencing fertility problems. Counselling can help you to decide what treatments to go for, or when would be the right time to opt out of medical help.

COMPLEX TREATMENTS FOR INFERTILITY

IVF

IVF is a treatment by which the eggs are fertilised in the laboratory and the embryos are then introduced directly into the womb of the mother. The eggs may be removed from the ovaries during the normal menstrual cycle or drugs may be given to increase the number of eggs produced. IVF is a helpful treatment for couples with unexplained fertility, both as a diagnostic procedure by establishing whether the eggs can be fertilised by the partner's sperm, but more importantly as a means of achieving pregnancy.

The first baby to be born as a result of IVF was in 1978. Following the pioneering work of Patrick Steptoe, a gynaecologist, and Robert Edwards, a scientist, the birth of Louise Brown heralded a new era in the management on infertility. The initial indications for IVF were limited to infertility resulting from tubal damage. Over the next few years however, it became clear that many other infertility problems responded well to IVF. It was therefore introduced on a widespread basis as a treatment for most types of infertility. The only exception to this success was with sperm disorders, where success rates with IVF continued to be less than those for other forms of infertility.

IN VITRO FERTILISATION AND EMBRYO FREEZING

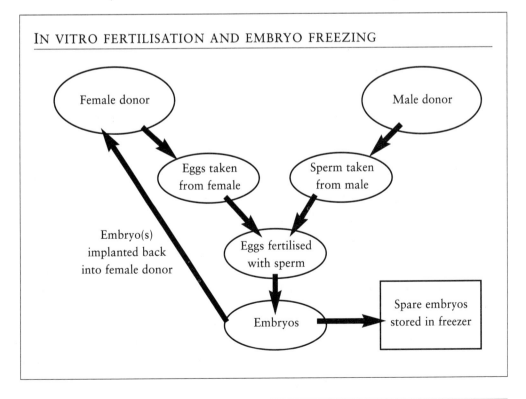

Over the years since 1978, a number of advances have improved the success rate from an IVF cycle. These include:

■ **The introduction of drugs that suppress the normal activity of the pituitary gland** (gonadotrophin releasing hormone (GnRH) agonists) and, particularly, the unwanted release of hormones, which can impair egg development

■ **Successful cryopreservation**: the ability to freeze-store embryos and thereby increase the likelihood of pregnancy from any attempt at IVF (or indeed GIFT)

■ **Better stimulating drugs** have been developed which have given rise to higher egg numbers being harvested, better quality eggs and higher pregnancy rates.

REASONS FOR USING IVF

IVF is the only appropriate treatment for women who have severely damaged fallopian tubes. It is not uncommon for this damage to lead to the collection of fluid within one or both fallopian tubes. The correct name for this condition is a hydrosalpinx. We have known for some considerable time that the presence of a hydrosalpinx reduces the chance of pregnancy from IVF treatment. Only recently have surgeons felt able to recommend removal of that tube or, in effect, sterilisation of that tube before going ahead with IVF treatment, because of some research work carried out in Scandinavia which supports this treatment approach. Apart from severe sperm disorders, IVF can be used for all the other forms of infertility although it is not the sole treatment for them. Other options would include GIFT or IUI (see later in this chapter).

SUCCESS RATES

Success rates vary considerably from centre to centre and indeed there is always some inter-nal variation within a centre from year to year. Poor results in one year will almost always be matched by good results on the following year. If you are looking at an individual centre, they should provide you with success rates appropriate to your age and the sort of treatment that you are likely to be having. In addition further information can be obtained from the Human Fertilisation and Embryology Authority. They publish live-birth rates per treatment cycle, that is to say the 'take home baby' rate. Over the past seven or eight years, there has been little or no change in the success rates from IVF, with an average live-birth rate per treatment cycle of fifteen per cent. This means that some centres will offer treatment cycle rates higher than this and obviously some will be lower. Choosing a clinic will depend on your accessibility to that clinic, the price they charge and success rates amongst other things.

PROCESS OF TREATMENT

GETTING ENOUGH EGGS TO MAKE THE PROCEDURE WORTHWHILE

When the first IVF pregnancy was conceived, it was done with the use of natural cycles, using no drugs whatsoever. It became clear that this was an inefficient and incredibly labour intensive way to carry out IVF, with very poor success rates and so a number of changes happened. First of all, drugs called gonadotrophins were given to women to increase the number of eggs growing in each cycle and then in later years, as mentioned earlier, GnRH agonists were introduced to prevent the premature release of these eggs. Treatment with GnRH agonists is now almost routine. The treatment is started seven to ten days before the woman's period is due, in the cycle prior to the planned treatment. Once the period comes, then the woman's own hormone control is significantly reduced and the growth of follicles containing the eggs in her ovaries is controlled by the injection that she will be given. These injections contain hormones called gonadotrophins which stimulate the ovaries. These hormones are given every day for an average of twelve to fourteen days and then, once the follicles are of sufficient size, a second injection is given. This latter injection mimics the normal trigger to egg release (ovulation) and collection occurs within thirty-six hours of the injection.

RECOVERY OF EGGS

Initially, most egg collections were undertaken by laparoscopy but they are now almost invariably done as vaginal operations under direct ultrasound control. A needle is passed into each follicle and the fluid and the egg it contains are removed. The eggs are then passed to the scientific staff waiting to look after the eggs. After egg collection, the eggs will be mixed with sperm that has been specially prepared to remove any abnormal sperm or debris from the fluid in which the sperm are contained. Once the appropriate amount of sperm is added to the egg culture area, the eggs are placed into an incubator overnight to allow fertilisation to occur.

EMBRYO REPLACEMENT

Evidence of successful fertilisation should be visible on the following morning and, if it has occurred, the embryos will be transferred back to the woman's uterus using a small fine catheter on the second or third day after egg collection. Once this is carried out, the woman can get up and go home without any undue delay. There maybe some additional injections or other medication to support the lining of the uterus during the following two weeks but

no other active treatment steps are undertaken during this time. Success is indicated by the failure to arrive of the next period and a pregnancy test should be positive by the second or third day after the missed period, or fifteen or sixteen days after egg collection. Success rates are calculated on 'continuing' pregnancy and live birth rates.

RISKS AND COMPLICATIONS OF TREATMENT

Like any medical intervention, there are risks associated with this treatment but thankfully they are very uncommon. These include:

■ The cancellation of treatment because of a failure to respond to the drug stimulation adequately

■ Rare side effects from the hormone treatments provided

■ Some vaginal bleeding following the egg collection

■ Occasional technical difficulties at the time of embryo transfer, sometimes due to a diffi-

Below: A needle is passed into the follicle guided by an ultrasound probe, and the egg is removed.

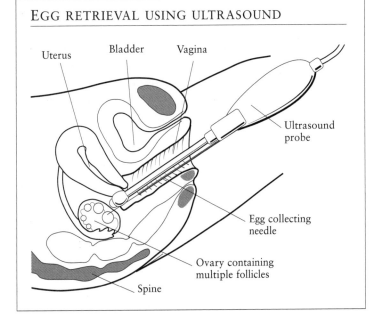

EGG RETRIEVAL USING ULTRASOUND

Uterus

Bladder

Vagina

Ultrasound probe

Egg collecting needle

Ovary containing multiple follicles

Spine

culty in passing the catheter through the cervix into the uterus.

Two significant complications of assisted conception are multiple pregnancy and the ovarian hyperstimulation syndrome (OHSS). Multiple pregnancy – the occurrence of twins, triplets or even more – is quite likely to occur in IVF treatment as, in general, more than one embryo will be returned to the uterine cavity. There has been considerable discussion about the wisdom of replacement of three embryos but certainly there are some women in whom this option has been the appropriate treatment. Since replacing three embryos gives a multiple pregnancy likelihood of close to thirty per cent whereas replacing two reduces that to under ten per cent, and the likelihood is that only a twin pregnancy will occur if at all, the recommendation is that only two are replaced. Naturally, some small reduction in overall pregnancy rates will occur.

The majority of people who develop OHSS will have some lower abdominal discomfort bloating and mild nausea. A small proportion (less than five per cent) will have more severe symptoms with more marked swelling and pain, some vomiting and perhaps some shortness of breath or a reduction in the amount of urine being passed. Development of any of these symptoms requires medical review and may even require admission to hospital. The condition occurs because the ovaries enlarge after IVF treatment and is more likely to occur when women have had large numbers of eggs collected or are known to have the polycystic ovarian syndrome. Treatment usually involved adequate pain relief and the appropriate fluid replacement.

REGULATION OF TREATMENT
We cannot discuss IVF without the mention of the Human Fertilisation and Embryology

Authority, a regulatory body which was set up following the passing of the legislation in 1990. This Authority has a licensing and regulatory role on the practice of all assisted conception techniques, donor insemination and the manipulation of embryos for transfer as well as any research undertaken in an IVF setting. Inspectors from the authority visit centres, ensure that practice is of the highest standard and perform a very valuable and useful role in this regard. The funding for their function comes from a levy which is taken off every patient's treatment cycle. While the HFEA enforce the standard regulations laid down in law, different clinics may put into practice other more stringent regulations on their own individual practice of assisted conception.

GIFT
Gamete intrafallopian transfer (GIFT) is used to help couples conceive by placing the sperm and eggs (gametes) together in the fallopian tube. Fertilisation of the eggs occurs naturally within the tube and the embryo passes into the uterus, hopefully to implant. It is a successful form of assisted conception provided it is used for the correct medical reasons. The three basic essentials for conception are:
■ Normal sperm production in the man
■ Normal egg production and release in the woman
■ Normal fallopian tubes.

As GIFT involves taking eggs from the woman and sperm from the male and placing them in the fallopian tube, it is essential for all these three factors to be entirely normal before this technique is undertaken.

You should have regular ovulatory cycles and normal hormone levels in keeping with egg release occurring once a month. Your partner must have a totally normal sperm count with a high percentage of sperm having a normal appearance and normal motility.

The fallopian tubes must be entirely normal and healthy with no adhesions or scar tissue surrounding them. The fimbrial ends of the tubes must be normal and the tubes should not appear reddened or swollen. Ideally, there should be no past history of pelvic infection as this may damage the lining of the tube and impair fertilisation and the passage of the fertilised egg into the uterus.

WHEN IS GIFT APPROPRIATE?

It is the appropriate technique for many women when there is no apparent cause for the failure to conceive. For couples aged less than thirty-five years who have been trying without success for two years, it may be worthwhile continuing with no treatment for a further eighteen months. However, after this interval the chance of a pregnancy resulting without help is rather slim and GIFT may be the ideal choice of therapy.

GIFT is not recommended for couples in whom there is tubal damage or pelvic adhesions, nor if there is a suggestion of a low sperm count or poor sperm motility. A negative postcoital test is also a poor indicator for success. This test, together with poor sperm quality, suggests a reduced capacity for the sperm to fertilise the egg. As the GIFT technique has to assume normal fertilisation will occur in the tube, GIFT is not the best treatment option. For these couples, the IVF technique is preferred.

Women with mild endometriosis are also suitable for GIFT treatment but there must be no tubal involvement or endometriosis within the ovaries. Women who have failed to conceive following twelve treatments of artificial insemination using donor sperm are also more likely to conceive using GIFT with

donated sperm than continuing with further inseminations.

WHY DOES GIFT WORK?

In couples who fail to conceive after three or four years without any obvious abnormality, there is likely to be a more subtle cause for their continued lack of success. Some of these reasons may be:

■ **Cervical mucus which blocks the passage of sperm**

To make sperm transport easy, the mucus in the cervix becomes clear, watery and thinner just prior to ovulation. Unfortunately, in some women this fails to happen and there is low mucus production or sticky mucus which makes penetration by sperm more difficult. This problem can be identified by a simple postcoital test or, preferably, a more refined sperm/mucus crossover test

■ **Irregular or absent ovulation**

A complex hormone signal begins the final maturation of the egg and causes rupture of the follicle and release of the egg. If this signal does not happen at the right time with the developing follicle, then these stages of maturing the egg may be impaired or the follicle may be prevented from rupturing

■ **Failure of the egg to enter the fallopian tube when released by the ovary**

Following ovulation, the egg has to enter the fimbrial end of the tube. Precise hormone messages from the ovary attract the fimbria to collect the egg. If these do not occur, then the egg will fail to enter the tube.

WHAT DOES GIFT INVOLVE?

Early work confirmed that replacing only a single egg and sperm did not result in satisfactory pregnancy rates. In a similar way that IVF success increased with the replacement of two or three embryos, when two or three eggs were replaced at GIFT, much better pregnancy rates were obtained. Replacing more than three produces a high number of multiple pregnancies and is unlawful in the UK.

To obtain this number of eggs it is necessary to stimulate the ovaries using drugs. Considerable progress has been made to find safe and reliable drugs that successfully stimulate the production of a number of eggs from both ovaries. The most commonly used drugs are the GnRH agonists, which are given by injection, implant or nasal spray. Their use is followed by gonadotrophin injections. The ovarian response must be monitored closely with blood tests and ultrasound to ensure there is a satisfactory number of eggs (follicles) developing, but not an excessive response. An excess can give rise to OHSS, as discussed above.

Follicles measuring 18–22 mm in diameter usually contain mature eggs capable of fertilisation. At this stage of development, the egg recovery and GIFT procedure is performed. This is carried out under general anaesthesia using a laparoscope.

The eggs are collected from both ovaries and an embryologist selects a maximum of three mature eggs for replacement. Usually one to two hours before laparoscopic recovery, the husband is required to produce a sperm sample. This is prepared to select the best concentration of normal motile sperm. One hundred thousand sperm together with the eggs are drawn into a fine catheter and then slowly injected into the middle of the fallopian tube under direct vision.

In the majority of women, a number of surplus eggs will be obtained. These can be inseminated as with conventional IVF and the embryos can be frozen (cryopreserved). If the GIFT technique proves unsuccessful, the replacement of these stored embryos offers another chance of a pregnancy without any further drug stimulation or egg recovery being required. In the near future, it is likely that eggs alone will be able to be stored and used at a later date.

DOES GIFT WORK?

GIFT is a highly successful form of assisted conception and when performed for couples with unexplained subfertility, mild endometriosis or failed donor insemination, pregnancy rates of thirty-five, thirty and forty per cent respectively, are usually quoted following the replacement of three eggs. Of these, unfortunately, one in twenty develop in the tube and produce an ectopic pregnancy, and approximately twenty per cent will miscarry.

RISKS OF GIFT

The GIFT technique is a safe procedure. Additional health risks to women embarking upon this treatment are exceedingly low. However, the technique does involve drug therapy and a surgical procedure, both of which can potentially produce adverse effects.

The drugs used are naturally occurring hormones and have few side effects. There is some discomfort at the site of the injection and a recent review has suggested that up to 20 percent of women may have a local reaction, such as a raised sore area. More serious drug reactions are exceedingly rare.

The number of eggs produced in response to the treatment varies between women and a poor response is seen more commonly in women aged over thirty-eight, or those with a history of endometriosis or ovarian surgery. An excessive ovarian response (too many eggs) is not ideal due to the risk of OHSS, which is seen in five to ten per cent of women and can require hospitalisation in the most serious cases. A milder condition of abdominal discomfort following egg recovery is quite common. OHSS can be prevented by cancelling the GIFT procedure if there is an excessive ovarian response. If IVF and cryopreservation (freezing) facilities are available, it may be possible to perform IVF and freeze the embryos. Alternatively, the use of progesterone may reduce the likelihood of OHSS.

The risks of general anaesthesia are small and with an experienced gynaecologist, the laparoscopic procedure has a low incidence of problems.

If a pregnancy results, then there is a possibility of miscarriage, tubal or multiple pregnancy. A scan should be performed four weeks after the GIFT procedure to ensure that the pregnancy is viable and within the uterus. This scan will also identify a multiple pregnancy, likely to occur in approximately fifteen to twenty per cent of cases. Multiple pregnancy has a higher risk of miscarriage and preterm delivery.

The development of GIFT is a major advance in the treatment and management of sub-fertile couples. It is likely to remain a popular treatment option and will continue to prove successful for some couples.

INTRACYTOPLASMIC SPERM INJECTION (ICSI)

Intracytoplasmic sperm injection is a technique used in the laboratory to help fertilisation take place, whereby a single sperm is injected into the centre of an egg. The ICSI technique is an extension of IVF and is used for specific indications. It is not a replacement for IVF.

REASONS FOR ICSI

The main reason for considering ICSI is male-factor infertility, where the sperm picture is extremely poor and is unlikely to fertilise the eggs with IVF. In some men who require sur-

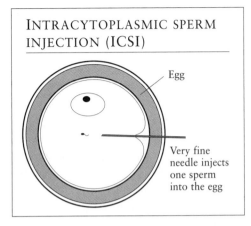

INTRACYTOPLASMIC SPERM INJECTION (ICSI)

Egg

Very fine needle injects one sperm into the egg

gical retrieval of sperm, ICSI is also necessary due to the relatively fewer number of sperm present. Finally, it is also considered for couples who have been treated with IVF who have had either very few or no eggs fertilised.

RISKS OF ICSI

Ever since the first human pregnancy was reported in 1992, many children have been born in the United Kingdom (more than 1500 in 1997–98) and many more women are pregnant using this technique. The rapid improvement in technique is reflected by higher fertilisation and pregnancy rates, in some centres surpassing conventional IVF rates. However, the procedure is not without risk. The piercing of the egg during ICSI may lead to damage, and this will be evident either during or after the procedure. These eggs cannot be used in treatment, and approximately fifteen per cent of eggs are lost in this way.

The other more obvious concern is regarding the risk of congenital and/or genetic abnormality in the babies born from this technique. In the largest ICSI group in Europe at the Brussels Free University, a follow-up study of 423 children born after ICSI was carried out. They found a total of 14 (3.3 per cent) of children with major malformations, which is not increased compared to the general population.

Men with very low sperm count are known to have an increased risk of carrying karyotype (chromosome) abnormalities. This may explain other studies that suggest that there is an increase in sex chromosome (X and/or Y chromosome) abnormalities in pregnancies conceived after ICSI. Continuing long-term studies are currently being carried out to follow-up the children born as a result of ICSI to provide more information to clinicians so that they can advise couples needing this procedure accordingly.

ICSI is an exciting procedure enabling couples who previously were unable to conceive with conventional IVF to have a genetic child of their own. However, it is important to remember that it is not a replacement for conventional IVF and should only be used when specifically indicated. With regard to the risk of the procedure producing an abnormal baby, continuing follow-up data is needed before a definitive answer is available, but to date, it would appear that at least with regards to major abnormality, this is the same as for the general population.

INTRAUTERINE INSEMINATION (IUI)

Many couples believe that they will have to resort to high-tech 'test-tube baby' techniques in order to conceive a longed-for child but there are sometimes less invasive methods that are equally effective. Intrauterine insemination (IUI) is but one.

For a woman to conceive, she must produce an egg, her partner must produce sperm in adequate numbers and quality, and the sperm must be able to travel through the woman's genital tract and fertilise the egg. Intrauterine insemination involves the placement of a 'prepared' (improved) sample of sperm into the uterine cavity at the time an egg is being released. Placing the sperm in the uterus provides a 'helping hand' and reduces the distance of, and the barriers against, sperm transport, thereby increasing the likelihood of pregnancy.

OVULATION

Prior investigations should have established that ovulation occurs or can be made to occur with fertility drugs. IUI can be done in 'natural'

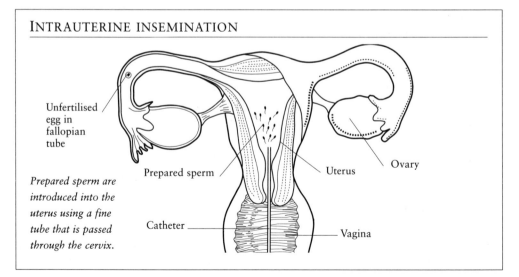

INTRAUTERINE INSEMINATION

Unfertilised egg in fallopian tube

Prepared sperm are introduced into the uterus using a fine tube that is passed through the cervix.

Prepared sperm

Catheter

Uterus

Ovary

Vagina

ovulatory cycles. However, the evidence suggests that superovulation enhances pregnancy rates. Superovulation involves the stimulation of the ovaries to produce more than one egg. This can be achieved using tablets or injections, as described above.

PROBLEMS WITH THIS APPROACH

The ovaries of some women, particularly if they are over thirty-eight years, may not respond to the initial dosage.

The ovaries may over-respond, possibly leading to far too many follicles developing which may result in the release of a large number of eggs with the potential serious risk of high multiple pregnancy more than three embryos. This must be avoided.

The other problem of over-stimulation is harm to the woman whose ovaries may become very enlarged, producing pain and sometimes excessive fluid in the abdomen (ascites). This situation generally resolves spontaneously over a period of days but is potentially very dangerous. With the dosage regime outlined above, it is extremely rare for this complication to arise with IUI.

SEMEN PREPARATION

In the past, IUI was attempted with 'neat' sperm (normally ejaculated sperm/semen) which had not been prepared. However, the results were usually poor and carried a risk of infection since there are often some bacteria even in normal sperm specimens. In addition, to ensure that a sufficient number of good sperm are inseminated, the volume of fluid was often sufficiently high to cause pain and spasm of the uterus. Over the last fifteen years, methods have been developed to 'prepare' the sperm. Primarily these techniques were aimed at IVF where a small number of normal-shaped sperm which move very well

(motile) are required to put with the egg to achieve fertilisation. These methods are now applied to the preparation of sperm for IUI.

After its production, the semen specimen is assessed under the microscope and placed with culture medium. Using a variety of laboratory techniques, the best sperm (those with high motility) are separated from the rest and also from the seminal fluid. These high-quality sperm are then mixed with culture medium and can be inseminated into the uterus. This technique allows the preparation of small volumes of good-quality sperm even from suboptimal sperm samples. Unfortunately, poor sperm samples with less than 5,000,000 sperm per sample cannot be helped by this technique.

INSEMINATION

The process of insemination is simple. The prepared semen is placed in a fine catheter (tube) which has a diameter of less than the lead of a pencil. This catheter is very flexible and has a tapered but smooth tip to avoid any damage to the lining of the womb.

The woman undergoes a speculum examination as for a smear test. The cervix is seen and the catheter inserted gently through the cervix into the uterus. Less than 0.5 ml of prepared sperm is injected and the catheter is removed. The whole process takes only five to ten minutes. There is minimal discomfort in most cases and no anaesthesia is required. About ten per cent of women will experience temporary cramping pains like those felt during a period.

An important aspect of the procedure is timing. Most sperm survive for more than twenty-four hours in the genital tract (up to seven days if the conditions are right, although more usually three to five days). They take six to twelve hours to swim into the fallopian tube. Therefore, ideally, the sperm should be inseminated within six to twelve hours of predicted ovulation. However, ovulation is not always predictable and so many fertility units undertake two inseminations twenty-four hours apart.

There is no evidence that resting after the insemination alters the outcome in any way. Therefore once the procedure is completed, you can go home.

WHO IS IUI FOR?

Infertility specialists vary in their view of IUI and its place in the treatment of infertility. Some believe that it has a major role to play whereas others think that it has only a limited application.

Given the advantage that it is relatively non-invasive compared with assisted conception techniques, it is certainly worth trying when the prerequisites are fulfilled. These are:
■ Ovulation
■ Good-quality sperm after preparation
■ Normal uterus and fallopian tubes.
For the two to fifteen per cent of couples with unexplained infertility, IUI has a ten to twenty-five per cent chance of pregnancy per cycle.

Some doctors believe that the preparation techniques for sperm can remove a high proportion of sperm antibodies from the sperm, thereby providing a specimen which is more likely to result in successful IUI.

Some doctors believe that the cervix may not produce appropriate mucus to allow sperm to penetrate the uterus. To bypass the cervix, IUI has been used to achieve success. Normally women using donor sperm to achieve conception have the sperm deposited in the upper vagina and the outer surface of the cervix. Good pregnancy rates result but some units report higher conception rates employing IUI.

GAMETE DONATION

EGG DONATION

Egg (ovum) donation offers new hope for a large number of women who previously thought they could never have children. Many of these women will have lost either ovaries or their ovarian function when they were young, possibly because of cancer, surgery, chemotherapy or radiotherapy. In a surprisingly large number of women, there is no explanation for the onset of their early menopause. As premature menopause affects one per cent of women under the age of 40, well over 100,000 women are affected in the United Kingdom alone. Egg donation is also of benefit to women who have a high risk of passing genetic disorders to their offspring, or for those who fail to respond to IVF treatment.

Types of egg donation

There are two forms of egg donation:
■ 'Known' in which the donor and the recipient know each other – for example, they are friends or relatives
■ 'Anonymous' in which the identity of the donor is not revealed to the recipient.

In anonymous donation, traditionally the source of these donated eggs were 'excess' eggs from infertile women undergoing assisted conception treatment themselves. However, with the advent and improvement of cryopreservation of human embryos, this source has been drastically curtailed. As a result, it means that the main sources of anonymously donated eggs in the United Kingdom are from altruistic volunteers and women about to undergo sterilisation.

EGG DONORS

Ideally, egg donors should be between the ages of twenty-one and thirty-five years. It is preferable that they are of proven fertility but this is not essential. A medical history and examination will be conducted to assess the donor's fitness to donate. It is the responsibility of the donor to inform the doctor of any genetic or inheritable diseases that may be present in her immediate family. All donors will be tested for HIV antibody (AIDS), hepatitis B and C, syphilis and cystic fibrosis. Two HIV tests will be carried out three months apart. Counselling is an important part of the first consultation and you will be offered this, together with an opportunity to speak to other women who have donated.

In general, donors will be prescribed three forms of medication:
- A 'down-regulation' drug which comes in either a nasal spray or a daily injection under the skin. This stops the ovaries working for themselves
- A 'fertility' drug which only comes in an injectable form, used to stimulate the ovaries to produce eggs in a controlled manner
- A 'midnight' injection given usually very late at night to allow the eggs to mature finally before collection.

The side effects of the 'down-regulation' drug include hot flushes, feelings of depression, irritability and headaches. Occasionally, women respond excessively to the 'fertility' drug injection and the procedure has to be cancelled. At the other extreme, the procedure is also cancelled if women respond poorly to the 'infertility' drug. Very rarely, despite careful monitoring, about one per cent of women will develop OHSS, described above.

Donors are free to withdraw consent to egg donation at any time before the operation, without threat of financial penalty or fear of recrimination. As to the number of times a donor can donate, the law states that no more than ten children should be born from any one donor.

DONOR INSEMINATION

This is the use of sperms from a donor to produce a pregnancy for couples who could not otherwise achieve a successful pregnancy on their own. It was previously known as AID (artificial insemination with donor sperm) but the term DI is now preferred to avoid any possible confusion with AIDS.

There are three main reasons for couples resorting to donor insemination:
- Infertility of the male partner, not treatable in other ways
- Genetic defects carried by the male partner that could entail an unacceptable risk of a child having a major abnormality
- Blood group incompatibility (usually rhesus incompatibility) producing problems of such severity that the couple is unlikely to be able to produce a live child themselves.

MALE INFERTILITY

Male infertility is by far the most common of the reasons for treatment and accounts for over ninety per cent of donor insemination treatment. About two-and-a-half per cent of all men produce no sperms at all and others have problems with sperm quality or function. Men with this problem are usually reluctant to talk about it and often conclude that they are alone in this. However, this is far from true. There have been advances in the treatment of male infertility, particularly in the use of IVF for low sperm numbers. However, there are still many types of problems where no treatment exists other than donor insemination. Thorough investigation and expert advice are essential if you are to be certain that this is an appropriate choice of treatment.

GENETIC PROBLEMS

In the genetic field, there are a number of genetic or chromosomal problems that give a high risk of a particular couple having a child with a serious abnormality. Sometimes it is possible to diagnose these abnormalities in early pregnancy so that an affected pregnancy can be terminated, and the scope of such prenatal diagnosis is expanding rapidly. If prenatal diagnosis is not available, the couple may opt for donor insemination rather than take the risk, and even where prenatal diagnosis is possible some may prefer donor insemination to the ethical and practical problems associated with prenatal diagnosis and possible termination.

BLOOD GROUP PROBLEMS

The typical blood group problem producing a request for donor insemination would involve a couple where the man is rhesus positive and the woman is rhesus negative but sensitised against rhesus positive blood. If she has high-level sensitisation (high antibody levels) and the man has a double rhesus positive genetic component, they may be in the situation of only being able to produce pregnancies so severely affected by rhesus disease that a live baby is not a possibility. This is now very uncommon because of effective measures to prevent rhesus sensitisation in nearly all cases and good treatment for those who are sensitised. However, for the few who do still have severe problems the option of DI with the sperm of a rhesus negative donor is available. Comparable situations will occur occasionally with blood groups other than rhesus.

IS DONOR INSEMINATION THE RIGHT TREATMENT?

Doctors in clinics that are licensed to provide donor insemination can only make the treatment available if it is appropriate for a couple, taking into account the nature of their problem and their emotional needs They are also required to take into consideration the needs of any child produced by treatment 'including the needs of that child for a father'. Therefore, clinics will provide donor insemination only when it is the appropriate treatment. They will also want to make some assessment of a couple's ability to offer a reasonably normal upbringing to the child, and factors such as their health or life expectancy will also be examined.

What is involved?

If you and your partner are referred for donor insemination treatment or when the decision is made within the clinic to offer it, you will be offered counselling which will involve a detailed description of the nature of the treatment and its implications. Once the staff are satisfied that the choice of treatment is appropriate and you are happy to go ahead with DI, you will be asked to sign standard consent forms.

As a woman, you will probably have had investigations done to ensure that you are ovulating and that your hormone function is satisfactory, but if this has not been done these things will be checked. You may be asked to use an ovulation prediction kit. If your cycle is very irregular, you may be put on to a fertility drug to regularise it.

When any tests that are deemed necessary are completed, a date can be selected to start insemination, timed to coincide with your ovulation. The insemination will be performed at the clinic by a doctor or a fertility nurse trained in the technique. From the records of available donors, an appropriate donor is selected to give a satisfactory match with the male partner.

The semen is removed from the liquid nitrogen store and its identity checked from the clear colour coding system of the plastic straws in which it is frozen. Once removed from the liquid nitrogen, it thaws rapidly and the thawed semen is then injected into the cervical canal (the neck of the womb). This procedure is painless and very much like having a smear test done. The whole clinic visit need take no longer than ten minutes or so. Whereas some clinics do a single insemination per cycle, others aim to do two inseminations on consecutive days.

How successful is donor insemination?

The pregnancy rate varies with the age of the woman, dropping in women over forty. The average pregnancy rate is about seven per cent per cycle of treatment, rising to seventy-five per cent after twelve cycles of treatment in women who keep on trying. However, all clinics find that a small proportion fail to conceive regardless of how long they carry on trying.

Unfortunately, achieving a pregnancy is not quite the same as having a baby, and about one in seven DI pregnancies will miscarry. However, such women will often manage to conceive again quite quickly and have a successful outcome to the pregnancy.

How are donors selected?

Donors are all volunteers who are selected and carefully screened by centres licensed by the Human Fertilisation and Embryology Authority. The majority of centres are in university cities and a high proportion of donors are students. Donors are accepted only if they have no personal or family history of inheritable disease and have no identifiable high risk factors for infections, such as hepatitis or HIV. They are then tested rigorously for transmissible infections and fertility potential. Donors are counselled to make sure they understand the full implications of their involvement.

Their physical characteristics are recorded so that samples can be matched with the partner in terms of height, eye colour, hair colour and racial origin. Donors are also invited to provide a brief 'pen portrait' of themselves which can be made available to recipients or to the child in due course. This might include their occupation and interests but would not contain details that could identify the donor subsequently. Blood groups would also be tested.

Within the clinic, a range of donor samples are available and the staff will select the sample that matches most closely the characteristics of the father. For poorly defined reasons, there is often a shortage of donors from ethnic minorities. Clinics have experienced difficulties in making appropriate matches in the past in such cases and will probably do so again in the future. Most clinics will have arrangements for making samples from the same donor available for future pregnancies for that couple.

RISKS OF DONOR INSEMINATION

For the most part, the risks of donor insemination are no different from those of getting pregnant naturally but the following points are worth considering:

■ Infection

In theory, any infection that could be transmitted by sexual intercourse could also be transmitted by donor insemination. The techniques for preserving sperms will also preserve any bacteria or viruses in the semen sample. However, donors are recruited only from low-risk groups and their semen samples are screened rigorously for hepatitis and HIV.

■ Fetal abnormality

Every couple runs a small risk of producing an abnormal child and no form of treatment can avoid that risk totally. The risk of a fetal abnormality with donor insemination is lower than that run by the general population.

Donors are selected carefully to avoid any who have a personal or family history of inheritable abnormality.

■ Miscarriage

Unfortunately, about one in five of all pregnancies in the general population miscarry and a similar risk applies to pregnancies resulting from donor insemination treatment. If this should happen to you, it is worth emphasising two points:

1 You have at least proved that you can get pregnant

2 A single miscarriage does not significantly affect your chances of your next pregnancy being successful.

■ Related parents (consanguinity)

Couples worry occasionally about the possibility of their child unwittingly marrying another child of the same donor. Statistically the likelihood of this happening in the UK at random is about once per century. When such children know of their origins, it will be possible for them to check in future through the HFEA that they are not related through a common donor father.

■ Failure to conceive

This is perhaps the most common problem that could be considered a risk of donor insemination treatment. Although pregnancy prospects are very good for those prepared to continue with treatment, if necessary for two years or more, a significant proportion may lose heart and give up treatment before succeeding. The risk of failure is higher for older women or for women with other problems affecting their fertility.

THE LEGAL SITUATION

Until the Human Fertilisation and Embryology Act of 1990, the legal position of a donor and of children conceived from donor insemination was poorly defined. The 1990 Act states that children from donor insemination are to be considered the legitimate children of the couple where that couple are married, and that the donor has no rights over or responsibilities for the child. In effect, a child from donor insemination now has the same legal status as the natural child of a married couple. When the couple are not married but jointly agree to donor insemination treatment, the child will be the legal child of both partners. The birth certificate of a child born from donor insemination will not in any way differ from that of a child conceived naturally by the same couple.

TELLING THE CHILD

In the past, couples who have undergone donor insemination have often been reluctant to talk to anyone about their problems and disinclined to tell the child about his/her origins. The secrecy surrounding donor insemination has tended to be self-perpetuating. It is difficult for the public to accept the concept as a normal part of life without being aware of 'normal' people who have been through the experience and who can talk about it openly, as happens, for instance, with adoption. There does appear to be a growing public awareness of the misery of infertility and an acceptance of the need for treatments such as donor insemination. It is to be hoped that this will remove what some may see as a stigma and will allow greater openness about donor insemination.

There is no legal requirement to tell a child born from donor insemination about his/her origin but there are strong arguments for doing so.

■ It is argued that everybody has a right to know about their origins. We all have a natural curiosity about where we came from and would be hurt to feel that those we know and trust deliberately hide such information from us.

■ It is also argued that it is very difficult for parents to live with such a secret and to keep it from their child for ever. Children will ask questions about their origins quite naturally and they are very good at sensing disquiet in their parents.

■ There is now a chance of a child finding out through the HFEA, which keeps a central register of all children conceived during donor insemination treatment with the express intention of giving children born in this way information about their genetic origin at the age of eighteen if they should enquire.

■ If the child finds out that he/she was conceived by donor insemination when the parents were trying to conceal that fact, it can lead to a breakdown of trust and a major crisis in the parent-child relationship. If there is any possibility of the child finding out, then it is probably better for the parents to tell the child. If this is done when the child is relatively young, he or she can grow up naturally with the idea.

There is no need for anyone other than the clinic staff and the HFEA staff to know about your donor insemination treatment or pregnancy. Your own doctor will be told only with your permission and he will be encouraged not to enter any information in the child's medical records concerning donor insemination.

Whether you choose to tell your family and friends about your donor insemination treatment is up to you, but it is worth bearing in mind that it makes it very much easier in the long run if you are open with them.

STERILISATION REVERSALS

Microsurgery for reversal of tubal sterilisation can be associated with excellent results if only a small segment of the tube has been damaged. The expected pregnancy rate depends on the site of the join (anastomosis), the length of the tube remaining, and the length of time between sterilisation and reversal, varying from twenty-eight to ninety per cent in the best cases where the inner third of the tube has been preserved, the length of the remaining tube is greater than four centimetres and the time interval is less than five years.

ADVANTAGES

■ The obvious advantage of tubal reversals is that with only one treatment, the woman can conceive more than once.

■ Another advantage is the avoidance of IVF (which is the only viable alternative to sterilisation reversal) and its associated risks of hyperstimulation and multiple pregnancy.

DISADVANTAGES

■ The theoretical increase risk of ectopic (tubal) pregnancies.

■ The waiting time after the operation before embarking on IVF if the operation is not successful. This waiting time may be critical, especially in older women, as the success of IVF is highly dependent on the age of the woman and falls with increasing age.

COUNSELLING

All women undergoing a surgical procedure for sterilisation should be counselled about the nature of the operation, its alternatives, efficacy, safety and complications. It is important to present alternatives and review suitability for that particular woman. It should be emphasised to the patient that tubal sterilisation is not intended to be reversible but cannot be guaranteed to be without failure. The possibility of ectopic pregnancy should also be mentioned.

REASONS FOR REGRET

There are several reasons for sterilisation that may lead women to regret having been sterilised at a later date. These include:

■ Being sterilised at a young age, less than twenty-five years old

■ Sterilisation at an apparently convenient time, e.g. after a caesarean section or immediately after a difficult labour and/or delivery

■ A relationship crisis at the time of sterilisation and a new partner. Women who were pressurised to be sterilised have a higher incidence of psychological problems compared to women who were well informed about alternatives and had sufficient time and opportunity to make their own decision.

These factors should be taken to account when counselling a woman about sterilisation as any change of mind after the operation will mean either tubal surgery or IVF.

FUTURE PROGRESS IN INFERTILITY TREATMENTS

It is always interesting to speculate on the future. It is likely that IVF treatment will become more successful over time. Part of what may contribute to this will be the role of an intervention called assisted hatching. This is carried out using laser treatment to the external surface of the developing embryo to increases its chances of implanting. It appears to be of most benefit in a small subgroup, women over the age of thirty-eight years.

Gonadotrophin releasing hormone blockers (antagonists) are likely to be introduced into wide spread clinical practice within the next couple of years. They should make the patient's treatment more user-friendly and reduce the amount of drug stimulation required to achieve the same effect as is currently achieved.

Better methods of freezing embryos will result in a higher overall pregnancy rate from an individual cycle of treatment and this will in the long term improve pregnancy rates. Considerable enthusiasm in the media in the autumn of 1999 gave rise to much unfounded hope for treatments based upon egg cryopreservation. This is obviously a critically important treatment for couples who are undergoing chemotherapy for cancers but, as yet, all such treatments should be regarded as experimental and to have no proven success record in humans. Obviously, this may change with time and with advances in treatment. This is not to say that such treatments should not be considered but rather that they must be understood to be in the developmental stage rather than clearly established as treatment options.

Another important feature will be the need to reduce multiple pregnancy rates which will be achieved to some extent by the reduction in embryos transferred to women although this practice should not be introduced on a wide spread basis without ensuring that the individual patients needs are taken into account, while taking note of current guidelines from the Royal College of Obstetricians and Gynaecologists and any future changes in legislation put in place by the Human Fertilisation and Embryology Authority.

Chapter thirteen

LOSING A BABY

Losing a baby is always a terrible experience regardless of the stage in your pregnancy at which it occurs. Most parents-to-be look forward with great excitement to meeting the new person who will become such a large part of their lives and to lose a baby without ever having had the chance to know him or her is a shattering blow that parents, and their families, find very hard to bear. If this happens to you, you will need plenty of understanding and support from everyone around you – your partner, family, friends and health professionals.

EARLY PREGNANCY LOSS

Miscarriage is the loss of a pregnancy before the baby is able to survive outside the mother's womb. This usually means before the pregnancy has reached twenty-four weeks. It is the commonest complication of pregnancy as approximately fifteen per cent of all pregnancies end this way, and twenty-five per cent of women who become pregnant will experience at least one miscarriage.

SYMPTOMS OF MISCARRIAGE

Most miscarriages occur within the first twelve weeks of pregnancy. However, occasionally the pregnancy can be lost at a later stage, which is termed 'late' or 'mid-trimester' miscarriage. Often, a miscarriage is heralded by vaginal bleeding, which can be heavy and associated with cramp-like abdominal pain. For this reason, bleeding or pain in early pregnancy should be discussed with your GP in the first instance. In later pregnancy, the miscarriage may begin with pain, bleeding or the waters breaking. If this occurs, medical help should be sought from either your GP or your maternity unit.

A pregnancy can be lost with no bleeding or pain. In this case, the embryo or fetus dies inside the womb and may not be discovered until a routine antenatal visit. There may have been a gradual loss of the usual symptoms of pregnancy, such as breast tenderness or sickness, but these symptoms can last for days after a pregnancy dies, due to the high levels of circulating pregnancy hormones. Why some women expel the pregnancy spontaneously and some women do not is not understood. The causes of the miscarriage appear to be the same for both types of miscarriage.

WHAT CAUSES MISCARRIAGE?

There is no obvious cause for the vast majority of miscarriages. A great number of factors have been claimed to cause miscarriage. Emotional stress or worry and working with VDUs (visual display units) are commonly cited but there is little evidence to support these or any of the other claims. In fact, numerous studies have shown that working in front of a VDU screen has no known harmful effects, either in terms of miscarriage or causing abnormalities in the baby.

The majority of fetuses that miscarry would not have developed into a healthy baby, the problem usually starting at the time of fertilisation right at the very beginning of pregnancy. Indeed, in many cases the problem lies with the egg and occurs even before pregnancy begins. Much less frequently, there are also problems with the sperm, and thus most miscarriages are due to chromosomal aberrations in the embryos that prevented them from developing properly. A problem in the very early stages of pregnancy is difficult for doctors to detect but it is recognised by the mother's body which then initiates a miscarriage. In view of this it is rare for the cause of a miscarriage to be found, and because it is very likely that a subsequent pregnancy will proceed normally, doctors do not usually perform extensive investigations except where three or more consecutive miscarriages have occurred.

Women who have suffered three or more miscarriages are best cared for in a specialist recurrent miscarriage unit. Recurrent pregnancy loss affects one per cent of women (see below).

CHROMOSOMES AND MISCARRIAGE

More than fifty per cent of all early miscarriages are caused by chromosomal (genetic) abnormalities in the fetus. It is important to understand that nearly all the chromosomal defects seen in sporadic miscarriages arise out of the blue. For those who have had a miscarriage caused by a trisomy (where the cells of

the baby contain three copies of one chromosome instead of the usual two), there is a slightly higher risk of suffering another miscarriage for the same reasons, and the doctor will probably discuss an amniocentesis or other type of prenatal test in a future pregnancy. Certainly the risk for this condition is related to increasing maternal age.

In three to five per cent of couples with a history of recurrent miscarriage one or both partners carries a chromosomal abnormality (parental balanced translocation) which causes no obvious abnormality in that parent. However, when the chromosome affected is passed on at fertilisation an abnormal (unbalanced) fetus develops. The abnormality is discovered when the couple present with repeated miscarriages at which time their own chromosomes are tested. If an abnormality is discovered referral will then be made to a genetic counsellor who can advise about the chances of a future successful pregnancy.

YOUR EMOTIONS

Many women feel guilty after a miscarriage, worrying whether there was anything they could have done to prevent it. A common concern is that having sex caused the miscarriage, but there is no evidence to suggest that sex in early pregnancy is harmful. Once the bleeding has started, if a miscarriage is going to occur, it will happen no matter what you did. Even staying in bed cannot prevent it from happening so you should not feel guilty.

Everybody is different so no two people will cope with a miscarriage in exactly the same way. Even though the baby has been lost at a very early stage, it is natural to feel upset. After a miscarriage you may go through the same grief reactions as you would for a normal bereavement. It can be hard to accept that such deep feelings can occur for something that you never saw or even felt move but it is quite normal and you shouldn't try to suppress it.

You may experience various changes of mood and this too is part of the grieving process. These changes may often be unpredictable and of varying duration and are partly due to the changes in your hormone levels as your body readjusts to its non-pregnant state. At first you may feel very shocked and unable to believe what has happened. Briefly, you may also feel relieved once the physical trauma of the miscarriage, which can be quite frightening, is over.

Some people feel they need company and the moral support of family and friends while others may need solitude and prefer to be alone. Sometimes you may feel angry, either with your doctor, your partner, pregnant women, yourself or the world in general for letting this happen to you. A common thought is 'Why me?'

It may seem important for you to find a cause and blame something or someone for the miscarriage. You may blame yourself for causing it and feel guilty for what you have lost for your partner. You may feel a failure as a woman and lose self-confidence. If it's your first pregnancy, you may feel that your body has let you down. This can be a vicious circle as failing to cope with the emotions that miscarriage has brought may lead to failure to cope with your job and everyday tasks, and thereby may increase any loss of self-confidence. With the loss of your baby and your future plans, you may feel depressed at various times.

It is important to understand that all these reactions to your loss are normal and other women will have felt the same as you do before getting over it. Knowing this should be reassuring but if you feel that you cannot cope you should not be afraid to see your doctor and discuss the situation.

The initial deep sadness will usually pass during the following few weeks, but it may be months before it fully resolves. In the long term, you may never fully forget your miscarriage and it may remain an important part of your life, affecting you and the way you view things. There are, of course, particular times in the future when you may feel more upset, such as the date the baby would have been born or the anniversary of the miscarriage. Such reactions are natural and as time passes these occasions will become less distressing.

HELPING YOURSELF TO GET OVER IT

It is important that you give yourself time and do whatever you want to do. If you feel like crying, then cry; don't be ashamed and don't blame yourself. It is often helpful to talk to people who have been through the same experience, or who are involved in health care. There may be a counselling service set up at your local hospital, or health visitors may be available. Alternatively, specialist support organisations may be useful.

Meeting other people again may seem like a big hurdle, but there are things you can do to make this easier. Take your time and make sure you are ready before you try. If people knew you were pregnant, it may be helpful to ensure that they know in advance about your miscarriage; for example, before you return to work. This will avoid you being asked how your pregnancy is going, which would be upsetting and embarrassing for both of you.

People will react to the knowledge in different ways: some may be very sympathetic and understanding while others may be less able to deal with other people's emotions and may be less forthcoming or even ignore what has happened. It will soon be obvious who you can talk to and share your feelings with, knowing they will not be surprised or embarrassed if you are upset or cry at this time.

YOUR PARTNER

Some men will feel the loss just as much as women and will show this. However, many men may not feel the same sorrow, partly because they have not experienced physically the changes of pregnancy. Not having felt or seen any of these changes at an early stage sometimes makes it difficult for them to realise what they have lost. At the time of your miscarriage your partner may have been so worried about you that he has not felt deeply yet the loss of your baby. Or your partner may be just as upset as you but without actually showing it as he may feel that he must appear strong in order to support you. Therefore it is important that you talk to each other about how you both feel.

YOUR FAMILY

Your sadness is likely to affect all your family. Children may sense grief or may be frightened by your emotions, but it is important that they do not feel excluded and you probably need to tell them honestly in some way.

Grandparents may also grieve over the loss of a potential grandchild.

PHYSICAL RECOVERY

From a medical point of view, recovery from miscarriage is usually very rapid, and the body soon returns to normal. In many cases, early miscarriage will be 'complete', and all the tissue will come away naturally. If this does not occur, or if there is heavy or prolonged bleeding, an operation may be advised to remove this tissue. This operation is called 'evacuation of retained products of conception' or 'ERPC'. Sometimes this procedure is referred to as a 'D and C' (dilatation and curettage, or a 'scrape') and is usually performed under a light general anaesthetic. Most women are able to return home from hospital the day of, or day after the operation. It is best to take things easy for the first few days at home, but return to your normal level of activity as and when you feel able.

It is likely that bleeding will continue for some days. Women vary in how much bleeding they have, what it looks like and how long it lasts. it may be red or brownish in colour and there may be some small blood clots at first. It should gradually lessen and after two weeks it usually stops completely. If there is a sudden increase in the amount of bleeding, it is important to see a doctor for advice. If at any time the loss becomes unusually smelly this could be a sign of infection and which will require treatment. Using tampons is not advisable as inserting a tampon may introduce an infection so sanitary towels can be used until the loss stops.

In some hospitals, drugs may be used to induce the uterus to empty fully after a miscarriage. Sometimes, the developing baby will die but the afterbirth remains, so it is necessary to use an anti-progesterone drug (mifepristone), following by a prostaglandin to make the uterus contract. This usually works quickly, but is may take some days before the bleeding completely stops.

The first period after miscarriage will usually occur within six weeks. It is safe to use tampons at this time. Periods will return to their previous pattern, although it may take a few cycles for this to happen.

YOUR SIX-WEEK CHECK

This may be done at the hospital or at your own doctor's surgery. This is the opportunity for the doctor to ensure that you have recovered physically and are coping emotionally. This is also the time for you to ask any questions you may have about what has happened. If you had an ERPC, the doctor will have a report on the results any tests that were done on the tissues that were removed. However, this testing is not done as a routine in most hospitals.

GETTING PREGNANT AGAIN

It is best not to have intercourse until the bleeding has stopped completely after a miscarriage, but it is safe to do so if you wish. However, many women and their partners find that they have less interest in sex and this can last for a long time: several months even, and is perfectly normal. Don't worry; your interest will return.

You may feel that you want to get pregnant again as soon as possible, but for several reasons it is better to wait for two or three months before trying again. This is an important breathing space because:

■ It allows your body to recover
■ It allows you to get in the best possible physical and emotional shape for the next pregnancy
■ You can help your recovery by stopping smoking, drinking less alcohol, eating a sensible diet, taking exercise and talking about your plans and concerns for your next pregnancy.

It is possible to get pregnant very soon after a miscarriage (even before your next period) and therefore if you do choose to wait for two or three months some form of contraception will be needed. You can discuss what is a sensible method with your doctor.

WILL IT HAPPEN AGAIN?

The chance of having a successful pregnancy next time is very high. Even if you have had two or three miscarriages and feel despondent, the chances of success are strongly in your favour. As soon as you think you are pregnant again, arrange to see your doctor so that you can be referred to the hospital clinic at an early stage and a scan can be arranged. Once a pregnancy has been confirmed by scan, the chances of it continuing successfully are very high and this is very reassuring at a time when you will be understandably anxious.

RECURRENT MISCARRIAGE

This refers to the occurrence of three or more consecutive miscarriages. Less than three consecutive miscarriages, or a number of miscarriages separated by successful pregnancies, are termed 'sporadic miscarriages'. Although the chances of a woman experiencing a sporadic miscarriage are high, recurrent miscarriage is a condition that affects only one per cent of women.

CAUSES OF RECURRENT MISCARRIAGE

These can be divided into six broad groups:
- Genetic
- Anatomical
- Immune
- Endocrine (hormonal)
- Infective
- Unexplained.

GENETIC CAUSES

An abnormality in the chromosomes of one of the parents is present in approximately three to five per cent of couples who experience recurrent miscarriage. Chromosomes carry the genetic makeup of an individual. The baby inherits half of its chromosomes from the mother and the other half from the father. Although the abnormality, which is usually a 'balanced translocation', may have no noticeable effects in the parent, when passed on to the baby it may become 'unbalanced' and cause severe abnormalities, many of which are incompatible with survival. A simple blood test can detect these abnormalities in the parents who should be advised to consult a clinical geneticist, who can calculate the chances of recurrence of the particular abnormality in future pregnancies.

By contrast, at least half of all sporadic miscarriages are caused by genetic abnormalities in the baby which occur randomly (out of the blue) and are not inherited from the parents.

ANATOMICAL CAUSES

These fall into two main categories: cervical incompetence and congenital abnormalities of the uterus.
- Cervical incompetence is a condition in which a weakness of the neck of the womb results in a characteristically painless miscarriage, occurring after the pregnancy has reached fourteen weeks. This condition is rare and in the past has been over-diagnosed. It is possible to insert a stitch into the cervix during pregnancy, in an attempt to prevent miscarriage reoccurring from this cause.
- It has been suggested that as many as ten per cent of women with a history of recurrent miscarriage are born with an abnormally shaped uterus. However, the proportion of women without a history of miscarriage who have such abnormalities is unknown, and it seems likely that most women with uterine abnormalities have successful pregnancies. These abnormalities can be diagnosed by ultrasound scan, X-ray tests using special contrast dyes (hysterosalpingogram), or by looking directly at the inside of the uterus with a telescopic camera called a hysteroscope. In some cases, it is possible to correct uterine defects by surgery but whether this improves the chances of a future successful pregnancy is unproven.

IMMUNE CAUSES

Antiphospholipid antibodies are a group of antibodies which cause recurrent miscarriage by the formation of small blood clots in the placental blood vessels, thereby compromising the blood supply to the baby. As many as fifteen per cent of women with a history of recurrent miscarriage have these antibodies in their blood. Recent research has shown that the miscarriage rate in these women is very high – ninety per cent. However, when these antiphospholipid antibodies are identified before pregnancy the women can be offered treatment with aspirin and heparin during their next pregnancy. The live take-home baby rate with this treatment increases dramatically from ten to seventy per cent.

ENDOCRINE (HORMONAL) CAUSES

It has long been presumed that hormonal abnormalities are an important cause of early pregnancy loss, but the exact mechanisms are still not understood. Well-controlled diabetes and thyroid disorders are not a cause of recurrent miscarriage. Polycystic ovaries are present in more than fifty per cent of recurrent miscarriage sufferers, but why this condition is so common in these women is not understood. It has been suggested that the high levels of luteinising hormone (LH) found in women with polycystic ovaries is the reason for the higher risk of miscarriage. However, in a recent clinical trial, the suppression of high LH levels with drug treatment did not significantly improve the miscarriage rate, and therefore the role of raised LH levels in miscarriage is unclear. The use of hormone pessaries and hCG injections during the early stages of pregnancy is of no proven benefit. Further research is urgently needed in this important area.

INFECTIONS

Infections, such as rubella, toxoplasmosis, cytomegalovirus and listeria, can lead to sporadic miscarriage. They have not been positively associated with recurrent miscarriage. Other infections, such as bacterial vaginosis, as a potential cause of late miscarriages continue to be investigated.

UNEXPLAINED CAUSES

Even after careful investigation no obvious cause is found in approximately fifty per cent of women who present to their doctor with recurrent miscarriage. It is important to emphasise that these women with no specific underlying cause can be reassured that the outlook is far from bleak. In fact, it has been shown that such women have a seventy-five per cent chance of a successful pregnancy next time around when cared for in a dedicated early pregnancy clinic.

ECTOPIC PREGNANCY

In a normal pregnancy the embryo implants within the cavity of the womb (uterus). An ectopic pregnancy is the term used to describe a pregnancy that implants outside the womb. The most common place for this to happen is somewhere along the fallopian tube (in ninety-five per cent of cases), but other possible sites include the ovary, the cervix and, very rarely, in the abdominal cavity itself.

Ectopic pregnancies occur in half a per cent (one in 200) of all conceptions. Ectopic pregnancy carries the risk of considerable internal bleeding and, if unrecognised or untreated, can lead to the death of the mother.

There are some factors that make an ectopic pregnancy more likely, and these include the following:
■ In women who have already suffered an ectopic pregnancy the risk of a further ectopic pregnancy increases to ten to twenty per cent
■ Any previous event that results in damage to the fallopian tubes, such as pelvic infection and abdominal or pelvic surgery, increases the risk of ectopic pregnancy
■ Ectopic pregnancies occur more frequently in women undergoing fertility treatments, such as in vitro fertilisation (IVF), secondary to previous tubal damage

■ The rate of ectopic pregnancy has risen sharply during the last fifteen years reflecting the increase in pelvic infections caused by *Chlamydia trachomatis* – a sexually transmitted infection

■ Ectopic pregnancy is not prevented by an intrauterine contraceptive device and may be more common in some women taking the progestogen-only pill, although the progestogen-releasing intrauterine system ('Mirena') does not seem to have any increased risk of ectopic pregnancy. Most women who have an ectopic pregnancy are not using any contraception.

SYMPTOMS OF ECTOPIC PREGNANCY

The symptoms of an ectopic pregnancy are very variable but usually occur after a missed period or a light scanty bleed and are accompanied by a positive pregnancy test and lower abdominal pain which almost always starts before any vaginal bleeding has occurred. This pain may become severe, suggesting that the fallopian tube is being stretched and/or internal bleeding has started. Abnormal vaginal bleeding, in the form of a brown discharge or a light period, is common.

Sometimes these symptoms appear to settle down and then restart a few days later as the ectopic enlarges in size. Heavy internal bleeding (haemorrhage) is often accompanied by feeling faint and pain which is felt in the shoulder tip. The abdominal pain is usually more widespread and severe at this stage.

TREATMENT

It is important that the diagnosis of ectopic pregnancy is made promptly by an experienced doctor. The symptoms you are experiencing, the physical findings on examination and the results of the pregnancy test may not

---

ECTOPIC PREGNANCY SITES

A pregnancy outside the uterus may implant in a number of sites.

1 Tubal (95% of all ectopic pregnacies)
2 Cornual
3 Ovarian
4 Abdominal (very rare)
5 Cervical

REMOVAL OF ECTOPIC PREGNANCY

Ectopic pregnancy

A tubal ectopic pregnancy can be removed either with or without the tube, in a simple operation.

Removal of fallopian tube

---

be clear-cut and an ultrasound scan is often performed. This will demonstrate that there is no pregnancy sac within the uterine cavity, although the uterine lining may be thickened, and if internal bleeding has occurred, a pool of fluid may be seen in the bottom of the pelvis behind the uterus.

The diagnosis can be confirmed at an operation called a laparoscopy, which is carried out under general anaesthetic and involves the insertion of a small telescope through the umbilicus, enabling a view of the internal pelvic organs.

The ectopic pregnancy will be treated surgically, either by removing the fallopian tube containing the pregnancy or by removing just the ectopic pregnancy. Many hospitals have now developed the surgical expertise to deal with ectopic pregnancies with 'keyhole' techniques. However, if an open operation is required, the scar will be a 'bikini line' one.

Occasionally it may be possible to treat the ectopic medically at the time of laparoscopy by injecting a drug (methrotrexate) which stops the pregnancy growing.

Some women may experience a grief reaction after an ectopic pregnancy similar to that experienced after miscarriage, or a loss in later pregnancy. This is sometimes forgotten by both staff and women in general, since the pregnancy is usually lost prior to eight weeks' gestation.

STILLBIRTH AND NEONATAL DEATH

Stillbirth is defined as the death of a baby in the womb after the twenty-fourth week of pregnancy. The baby may die before labour starts but, just occasionally, the baby dies during labour itself. If the baby has died before labour begins the mother may suspect this because she no longer feels any movements. Her suspicion is then confirmed at the hospital, usually by ultrasound scan.

LABOUR

If your baby has died, then you would eventually go into labour quite naturally, but this may mean a wait of several days or more. Some couples want the delivery to take place as soon as possible. Others feel that they want to spend a night or two at home before going into the hospital for the delivery. Talking over the options with your midwife or doctor is important, so that you can reach the right decision for you.

If your labour is induced, instead of waiting for it to happen by itself, it can be done with tablets, with vaginal pessaries or a drip. Pain relief is available as you need it. The baby is usually born normally as it is in happier circumstances, and it is hardly ever advisable to do a caesarean section.

WHAT ABOUT WHEN THE BABY IS BORN?

If you wish, you can see, touch, hold and name your baby. The midwife will help you decide what is right for you. Many parents find it helpful at the time, and afterwards, to have seen their baby and to have shown their love and care. However, the decision is yours and you do not need to feel that you must hold your baby simply because the staff expect it. They will respect your choice. You may also change your mind about what you want to do or your partner may wish to see the baby even if you do not.

You will be in your own room and not in a ward with other people. You may want to be alone with your partner and your baby, without staff present. The midwives and doctors will be happy for you to do this so long as there is no medical problem – for example, provided that the afterbirth has been delivered and there is no problem with bleeding. You can dress or be helped to dress your baby in clothes from home or in clothes provided by the hospital.

Your baby may need to be weighed and measured and this may mean taking him/her away from you for a short time. You can take pictures of your baby or the staff will do this for you. You may want a lock of your baby's hair and to have a hand print or footprint. Again, the staff will help to arrange this for you if you wish.

You can have your baby with you for as long as you wish, and you can ask to have your baby back with you if he/she has been taken away. Close relatives and friends can be invited to see and hold the baby too. Normally your hospital stay will be quite short unless there are other complications.

NEONATAL DEATH

This means that the baby has died at some point in the first few days after birth. Sometimes a baby is born so small or early or poorly that it is known from the start that there is very little hope of survival. Some babies are born alive but only survive a few hours or less.

If it is known that your baby is dying, you can take the opportunity to help him/her leave the world with your love. You can hold and cuddle your baby and say goodbye peacefully. After your baby's death, you can stay together as long as you want and see the baby again later if you wish.

CAUSES OF DEATH

What causes a baby to die? Sometimes the causes of stillbirth and neonatal death are clear. For example, with a stillbirth there may have been an abruption; when the placenta has separated from the wall of the uterus and this has cut off the baby's oxygen supply. In both stillbirth and neonatal death, the baby may have had an abnormality which made survival impossible. Perhaps the baby has been too small or weak to survive for long outside the womb.

However, in many cases it is just not clear why the baby has died. Sometimes tests can give the answer and the results may help the doctors to give the best possible care in a future pregnancy.

HOW ARE THE TESTS DONE?

After a stillbirth, the doctor will examine the baby to look for signs of the cause of death and will ask the parents for permission to take a small sample of skin or blood from the baby. This can be sent to the laboratory for analysis to see if an abnormality in the baby's chromosomes (which carry the genetic material) has led to the baby's death.

Whenever a baby has died, the parents are asked if a post-mortem examination can be done by a doctor who specialises in problems of this sort. It can be very useful in finding out the cause of the baby's death. The cuts made in the baby's skin to allow the examination will be carefully closed at the time of the post mortem, if you chose to have this examination performed. If you wish, you can take your time deciding whether or not you want this done. In the meantime, you can give permission for simpler tests and examinations to be carried out.

Blood tests will be taken to check for possible causes of stillbirth, such as diabetes or infection. Swabs will also be taken from the vagina as sometimes infection, which is not apparent to the mother, can affect the baby.

If the baby died because labour began much too soon, then it is possible that there might be a weakness in the cervix (the neck of the womb) or an abnormality in the womb. The doctors may arrange tests to check for this as well.

WHAT HAPPENS NEXT?

When a baby dies after twenty-four weeks of pregnancy, a funeral has to take place. Many parents now wish to make their own arrangements for this. The hospital chaplain can advise all parents and can help them come to a decision. For those who do not feel able to organise a funeral, the chaplain can make the arrangements instead.

For babies born before twenty-four weeks, there is no legal obligation to arrange a funeral. However, one can still be arranged if the parents wish. In some areas, there are regulations preventing very small babies being buried in single graves or having a funeral – the chaplain will know what applies in your area.

Your hospital may have a book of remembrance where you can enter the baby's name and other details. There may be room for some more writing – a poem, for example.

WHEN YOU RETURN HOME

Returning home after the death of a baby is very difficult and painful. Sometimes you may be able to take your baby home with you instead of leaving him/her at the hospital until the funeral. Some parents prefer not to do this but it is your choice.

There are bound to be many things at home that act as reminders of the future the parents were expecting to share with their new baby. You may want to ask a member of the family to visit and to tidy away any baby things before you get back.

It's likely that many mothers will begin to produce milk in the days after the baby's birth. Tablets can help reduce this and the midwife will advise on dealing with the discomfort of full breasts.

It is normal to feel a wide range of emotions after the death of a baby – and that's true for your family and friends as well. Nearly all women whose babies have died, at whatever stage of pregnancy or afterwards, and for whatever reason will at times feel very angry with themselves and with other people and they may feel guilty too. If you are the mother of a baby who has died, you may feel that if you had done something differently or not done something then your baby would still be with you. Or perhaps you feel angry with your partner or with the midwives or doctors. You need to be able to talk to someone about how you feel. Share your grief with others. They may have their own reasons for sadness. Grandparents have lost a grandchild they would have loved and cherished. Your own brothers and sisters have lost a little niece or nephew who might have played a special role in their lives.

Making the effort to go out and about can be hard. The world will seem full of healthy babies, mothers pushing prams or pregnant women. Your own close family or friends may have their own babies, which will mean that your own loss is even harder to bear. If it is your first baby you may worry that you will never be able to have children of your own in the future. This is not usually the case.

It is important to realise that these feelings are normal and that they may last for a while. However, the feelings of pain and the sense of loss should become less intense as time goes by. You can seek help from a counsellor if needed; see your doctor or contact a specialist organisation, such as SANDS (see Useful Addresses).

COPING WITH OTHER PEOPLE'S REACTIONS

Meeting friends and family can be hard. The people you see may feel uncomfortable and just not know what to say. They may even avoid you, just because they are frightened of saying something that could upset you. People who don't know what's happened may ask you how the baby is, or where the baby is – and that is bound to be deeply distressing.

There is no easy way of coping in these situations. However, it does help to talk to someone who can offer support and understanding. Relatives and friends should try to be available to listen and to share any memories. Most parents have given their baby a name, and those close to you should try to refer to the baby by this.

If you have other children they are likely to feel confused and upset too. Sometimes siblings blame themselves for the death of the baby – especially if they haven't been too sure how to feel about a new brother or sister. Young toddlers are bound to feel distressed at

your own sadness. You may need to explain why you are sad, in ways that your child can accept, although may children will not be able to understand how final death is or why it has happened to such a tiny baby.

MEDICAL FOLLOW-UP

You will receive an appointment from the hospital where your baby was born after about two months. You can take this opportunity to find out the results of any tests that were carried out and to discuss what these may mean. You may see any obstetrician or a paediatrician or a specially trained nurse, depending on when and why the baby died. The obstetrician has specialist knowledge of why pregnancy and childbirth may go wrong; the paediatrician knows about problems after birth that might have caused your baby to die.

Going back to hospital is likely to be painful, and most parents prefer to go as a couple or with a friend or relative for support. It's a good idea to make a list of all the questions you may want to ask. It is unlikely that anything you have done or not done will have contributed to the baby's death, but you may need to hear this 'officially' from the doctor to feel reassured.

The doctor will discuss the results of the tests you have had and whether they make any difference to your future pregnancies. In many cases of stillbirth no cause for the baby's death will be found. Even if this is so, the doctor will usually want to plan special care for the future. If a specific cause is found, then plans for the future can be more focused. Sometimes if there is a major risk of the same problem happening again, specialised genetic counselling will be offered to help you plan whether you wish further pregnancies and what tests you might need in them.

THINKING ABOUT ANOTHER BABY

There are no rules about if and when parents should try for another baby. As long as there are no medical problems, you yourselves are the best judge of whether to try straight away or leave it for a while. It's normal to be especially anxious during another pregnancy, particularly at the stage when the last baby died. If you feel this way, tell the midwife and doctor how you feel – nobody will think that you are making an unnecessary fuss, and the extra care and reassurance you get may help a lot.

You will never forget or replace the baby you lost, but most mothers who have a stillbirth or neonatal death do go on to have healthy pregnancies and to deliver healthy babies at a later date.

On purely physical grounds, doctors usually advise parents who are keen to try and conceive again to wait until the woman has had two or three normal periods and is back into a normal cycle. On an emotional level, many professionals feel that parents benefit emotionally if they wait for longer, at least six months or possibly a full year before embarking on another pregnancy.

Chapter fourteen

THE MENOPAUSE

The menopause as a landmark in a woman's' life has been recognised throughout history. The menopause is viewed by different women in different ways; their views being influenced by the culture of the society in which they live, as well as a woman's own personal experience, expectations and personality. For many women, the menopause is viewed as a very positive experience, signifying the cessation periods, relief from the constant fear of unwanted pregnancy and elevation to the status of respected elder in society, with all the associated privileges. For other women, particularly in contemporary western society which places such emphasis on youth and beauty, the menopause may be viewed negatively, with fear for loss of femininity, loss of attractiveness to the opposite sex and loss of fertility. In these women there may be an associated loss of both self-esteem and self confidence, resulting in depression. An individual woman's perception of the menopause is an important factor in determining the way in which she will approach and deal with any post-menopausal symptoms.

Traditionally, the last spontaneous period has been regarded as the marker of the change of life and coincides with the ovaries ceasing their reproductive function. Ovulation no longer occurs regularly and the production of the sex hormones (oestradiol and progesterone) decreases. However, for many women the levels of oestrogen have been variable for some years before the periods eventually stop. Therefore, symptoms of the menopause can occur during this phase of change and prior to the last menstrual period.

In Roman times, the average life expectancy of a women was twenty-five years. This had increased to forty years by the Elizabethan age but remained unchanged until 1900. Since then, with improvements in nutrition and a reduction in maternal mortality associated with childbirth, there has been a progressive rise in life expectancy, such that if a women reaches the menopause today, she may reasonably expect to live until the age of eighty. This means that she will spend thirty years or almost one-third of her life in the post menopause. In the UK today, there are an estimated 10,000,000 postmenopausal women. By the time they reach the menopause, about fifteen to twenty per cent of British women will already have had a hys-

Below: Life expectancy has risen over the past century from 40 years to 80 years.

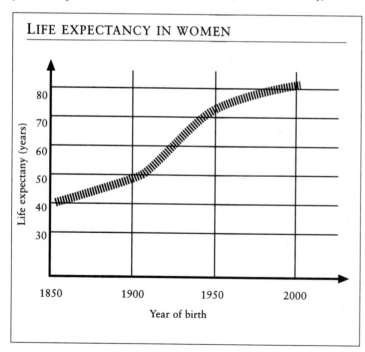

LIFE EXPECTANCY IN WOMEN

Life expectancy (years) / Year of birth

terectomy. Since after this operation there are no periods, it is less easy for a woman to be sure when she has become menopausal unless symptoms occur.

WHY DOES THE MENOPAUSE HAPPEN?

All the eggs that a woman will ever have are formed in the ovaries whilst she is still inside her mother's womb. Women do not continue to produce new eggs after birth, the maximum being present in the unborn baby unlike males who continue to produce sperm into old age. The numbers decline with age until only a few remain. These tend to fail to respond to the pituitary hormone stimulation (see Chapter 1), resulting in irregular ovulation. The climacteric is the period of progressive ovarian failure and lasts about five years until the time of the last menstrual period.

Although the ovaries stop producing eggs after the menopause, they do not completely stop the production of all hormones. Small amounts of oestrogen continue to be made for many years. In addition, they continue to produce testosterone (the male hormone) which is converted in the body fat to oestrogen. The adrenal glands (which lie above the kidneys) also produce male hormones. The type of oestrogen produced by the postmenopausal woman differs from that produced by the premenopausal woman and generally has weaker effects on reproductive tissues.

DIAGNOSIS OF THE MENOPAUSE

Diagnosis of the menopause is always retrospective and can only be confirmed by the absence of periods for twelve months. If a fifty year old women has not had a period for

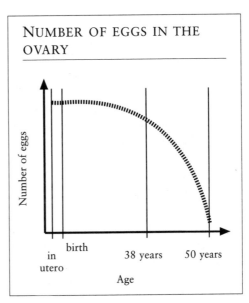

NUMBER OF EGGS IN THE OVARY

Left: Women are born with all the eggs they will produce. Numbers decline with age.

more than three months she has a greater than fifty per cent change of being menopausal.

Unfortunately, there is no clinical or blood test to confirm the menopause since women will occasionally have bursts of ovarian activity after many years. Such women experience a 'period-like bleed' preceded by typical premenstrual symptoms.

FACTORS AFFECTING THE TIMING

The average age of a women at the menopause is 50.7 years, but five per cent of women will reach the menopause by the age of forty-five, and one per cent by the age of forty. The age of the menopause is not influenced by the following:

- Age of first period
- Total number of lifetime pregnancies
- Total number of pregnancies
- Marital status
- Weight or height
- Use of the oral contraceptive pill or hormone replacement therapy.

The only feature known to definitely affect the time of the menopause is that smokers are likely to achieve the menopause one or two years earlier than those who do not smoke. Also, early menopause may run in families or may be due to previous operations involving the ovary and some treatments for cancers.

CONDITIONS WHICH IMPROVE WITH THE MENOPAUSE

Any condition that is dependent on the presence of oestrogen is likely to be improved at the time of the menopause. Obvious examples of this are endometriosis and uterine fibroids whose growth is dependent on oestrogen and which will normally regress when oestrogen is withdrawn.

Other symptoms occur because of the cyclical nature of oestrogen production during the cycle, such as premenstrual syndrome and some women also note menstrually related headaches and other symptoms which again are relieved at the time of the menopause.

It does not necessarily mean that these symptoms will recur when taking hormone replacement therapy, but this is discussed in more depth further on in this chapter.

EARLY POSTMENOPAUSAL SYMPTOMS

Many women do not experience any significant menopausal symptoms. However, for those who do experience the symptoms, there are certain factors that influence their severity. Symptoms most commonly experienced during the early part of the menopause include the following.

PERIOD PROBLEMS
Periods may change in character, becoming progressively light and infrequent in some women or frequent and heavy in others.

HOT FLUSHES AND NIGHT SWEATS
These may begin up to five years before the menopause, and persist for a further five years – a small number of women even get flushes and sweats in their late sixties. These are due to instability of blood vessels and are known as vasomotor symptoms and are usually self-limiting.

PSYCHOLOGICAL SYMPTOMS
A relatively common problem in the menopause and premenopausal years is a range of minor psychological symptoms which may be due to the hormonal changes. These include:
- Tiredness
- Poor concentration and memory
- Lack of confidence
- A loss of interest in sex
- A mild degree of depression.

These symptoms result in a loss of a sense of well-being. Despite a general misconception that menopausal women are more likely to become depressed, there is no conclusive evidence to support this belief.

The menopause is not associated with any increase in blood pressure, weight or blood sugar levels. However, it is noted that there is an increase in cholesterol level in the blood.

VULVAL AND VAGINAL SYMPTOMS
These include vaginal dryness and loss of lubrication. These symptoms tend to start in the early part of the menopause but are likely to gradually worsen as the menopause proceeds and oestrogen levels fall.

Five to ten years following the menopause

many women will begin to notice changes in the vulva and vagina. There is a progressive loss of fat below the skin leading to shrinkage in the size of the labia. The skin becomes thinner, more susceptible to local trauma, such as abrasion from underwear and less able to withstand infections. This may in extreme cases result in almost constant soreness and even bleeding. This 'urogenital atrophy' is a very common problem of the menopause and can cause a great deal of distress.

These symptoms occur because of lack of oestrogen which keeps the tissue of the vulva and vagina healthy. The tissue tends to thin and therefore it bleeds very easily and is also prone to infection. It tends to worsen as the menopause proceeds and in women in their late 70s and 80s the vagina can become very narrow and bleed very easily on touching. Urinary symptoms may also be a result of urogenital atrophy with an increased predisposition to infection and pain on passing urine (dysuria). Stress incontinence (see page 71) is not due to the menopause and, although prolapse may become worse in women who are low in oestrogen (hypo-oestrogenic), it is not thought to be the underlying cause. Vaginal dryness is a very common symptom and is frequently complained about by the older woman.

OSTEOPOROSIS

This is a problem which occurs in both men and women with age, although the problem tends to be worse in women since their bones are less dense than men's, and also bone density is adversely affected by lack of oestrogen. It shows itself in fractures of wrist, vertebrae and hips which are much more common in women than in men and particularly in their seventies and eighties. Osteoporosis is a very important public health problem and is discussed on page 282.

ALZHEIMER'S DISEASE

There is now information suggesting that Alzheimer's disease and dementia may be affected by the menopause and lack of oestrogen. This is an area of intense research interest and more information will become available in the future.

CARDIOVASCULAR DISEASE

The risk of heart attack and stroke increases with age. There are data to suggest that this may be related to oestrogen deprivation although other factors such as smoking may be of more importance.

Oestrogen may confer a protective effect against developing cardiovascular disease. Not only does it reduce the risk of the arteries hardening (atheroma), but it also causes many arteries to dilate which improves the blood supply to various organs, including the heart and the brain. Atheroma are the fatty plaques which form in blood vessels and gradually reduce the space along which the blood can pass. Finally, these vessels block off completely leading to death of the tissue, which in the case of the heart is the muscle beyond.

The use of hormone replacement therapy appears to reduce the risk of heart attack when used for a number of years. This is due to the above factors as well as the effects on the fat circulating in the blood. Studies in this field are difficult to interpret because many of the women who take HRT tend to be healthier than those who do not, which obviously complicates the picture.

The beneficial effects of oestrogen must be balanced against its effects on blood clotting, which can be a concern in the first months, particularly for women in their seventies who are starting HRT for the first time (see below).

HORMONE REPLACEMENT THERAPY (HRT)

This is the use of low-dose natural hormones to replace the female hormones that are no longer made by the women's ovaries. HRT is very effective in relieving the symptoms of the climacteric and post-menopause. It is likely that symptoms associated with a lack of oestrogen will respond to administration of hormone replacement therapy, as will be discussed below. This means that one of the purposes of taking HRT, apart from symptom relief, could be prevention of diseases such as osteoporosis, cardiovascular disease and Alzheimer's disease. This obviously has important public health implications.

There are very few absolute contraindications to HRT and for a majority of women the advantages associated with the use of HRT greatly outweigh any disadvantages. HRT is a form of drug treatment which is designed to counteract the effects of the reduced oestrogen hormone levels that women experience at and after the menopause. It consists of oestrogen, the principal female sex hormone, as well as a second hormone, known as progestogen. This is added for part or all of the monthly cycle and is similar to the female hormone progesterone. It is only needed in women who have not had a hysterectomy.

SHORT-TERM EFFECTS OF MENOPAUSE

Oestrogen is very effective in relieving vasomotor symptoms (hot flushes) and may also improve psychological symptoms in some women although these symptoms are less consistently helped by HRT. Some women with psychological difficulties at this time in life experience a noticeable improvement in their problem when given HRT and when HRT is stopped these symptoms may or may not return.

Both flushes and the psychological symptoms tend to be self-limiting and eventually resolve, sometimes after a number of years. The other common symptoms are less short-lived because they are due to the effect of the reduced oestrogen levels on the skin of the pelvis and on the organs of the pelvis, most of which are stimulated by oestrogen and shrink or become thin without this hormone, as described above. HRT will usually resolve such symptoms but they are likely to return after the HRT is stopped.

WAYS OF TAKING HRT

There are increasing number of ways to take HRT, and different women will suit different methods. For those women who have weighed up the pros and cons and have decided that they wish to take HRT, it may be a process of trial and error to find the right preparation. Similarly, there is no single correct dose of HRT that suits everyone. Women who are still having menopausal symptoms whilst taking HRT, for example hot flushes and night sweats, may need to increase the amount of oestrogen that they are taking.

TABLETS
In the UK, the majority of women chose to take HRT in tablet form. Those who have had a hysterectomy need to take only oestrogen

tablets, and these are usually prescribed on a daily basis. For the majority of women who have not had a hysterectomy, progestogens must also be taken in order to prevent overgrowth of the lining of the womb (the endometrium).

Progestogens can be taken in a cyclical (intermittent) or continuous regime. Cyclical progestogens should be taken for at least twelve days out of each month in order to protect the endometrium. Some women find the side-effects of progestogens troublesome. These may include bloating, breast tenderness and mood changes. In addition, many women do not wish to have regular monthly bleeds in their fifties, sixties and later. For this reason, newer HRT regimes aim to avoid menstrual type bleeding. These are known as 'continuous combined' or 'no bleed' HRT. Unfortunately, not all women avoid bleeding with these regimens. This type of HRT seems to be most effective in women who are at least one year into the menopause. Even then, many will get some bleeding in the first months, though this has often settled by the end of one year.

PATCHES, CREAMS AND GELS

When oestrogen is taken by mouth in the form of a tablet, a high dose must be given as blood from the gut passes to the liver where nutrients and drugs are processed. A proportion of the oestrogen will be active in the body and the remainder passes through the kidneys into the urine. When oestrogen is given via a patch, cream or gel, it passes straight into the blood stream and the dose of hormone reaching the liver is less. This may be important when considering the effects that HRT has on the production of substances such as fats or clotting factors, which are produced by the liver.

HRT skin patches also have the advantage that they only need to be changed twice

weekly. In some women, certain HRT patches can cause skin irritation or become detached. Patches are available which contain oestrogen and a progestogen, so are suitable for those with and without a uterus.

HRT is also available as a cream or gel, to rub on the skin.

IMPLANTS

Oestrogen, (but not progestogen) can be given as an implantable pellet which is placed under the skin as a minor operation or at the time of hysterectomy. The implant has the advantage that it only needs to be replaced every six months, but women who had not had a hysterectomy will also need to take progestogens as tablets or patches in order to prevent overgrowth of the womb lining (endometrium). Progestogens are not available as implants, although some women have successfully taken protective progestogen as the hormone-releasing intrauterine system (The Mirena) inserted in a similar way to the intrauterine contraceptive device. A further potential problem with implants is that with prolonged use some women find that their menopausal symptoms return sooner than the due date for their next

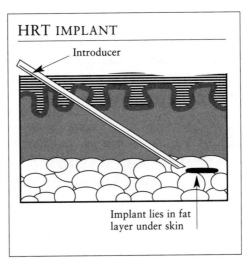

HRT IMPLANT

Introducer

Implant lies in fat layer under skin

Left: The hormone implant is placed in the fatty tissue under the skin.

implant, and before their oestrogen levels have fallen. This is a phenomenon known as tachyphylaxis. Many doctors would advise waiting until high oestrogen levels fall before inserting another oestrogen implant, since the long-term impact of prolonged high levels of oestrogen is unknown.

The long-lasting action of implants can produce a problem if a women wishes to stop implant therapy for any reason. Since the implant can continue to be active for up to two years after insertion, it is vital that those who have not had a hysterectomy continue to take cyclical progestogen every month for at least two years after the last implant or until taking the progestogen no longer produces a withdrawal bleed.

The hormone testosterone may also be given as an implant. This hormone may act to improve sex drive (libido) in some post-menopausal women, but the studies on this hormone are inconclusive.

Very occasionally there may be some inflammation or infection around the implant which soon settles down. There may also be a chemical reaction to the testosterone pellet which occurs many weeks after the implantation and the testosterone pellet then works its way to the surface where it can be removed easily. This is not produced by infection or careless implantation and antibiotic therapy will not help. The local swelling will either settle down or the pellet will be rejected.

TOPICAL HRT

For women who are particularly troubled by vulval and vaginal symptoms of the menopause, such as vulval soreness and vaginal dryness, HRT can be given directly onto the genitals as a cream, tablet or jelly. This produces an effect locally on the vulva and vagina but has little effect on the rest of the

body, which is suitable for some women.

PERIMENOPAUSAL HRT

For some women the perimenopause, the time when the ovaries are gradually ceasing to function and hormonal levels may be fluctuating, can be a difficult time. Heavy and irregular menstrual bleeding is also more common during this time and HRT may be of help in relieving menopausal symptoms and regulating bleeding. However, the amount of hormone in HRT may not be enough to achieve this, and more potent treatments such as the oral contraceptive pill, or daily progestogens may be required.

Rarely, heavy and irregular bleeding in the perimenopause may be a sign of excessive endometrial thickening, polyps or even cancer of the uterus and will need to be investigated by your doctor. Irregular bleeding can also come from the cervix, and all women are encouraged to attend for regular cervical smears as part of the national prevention programme for cervical cancer.

DISADVANTAGES OF HRT

Some women do not like taking long term medication when not actually ill. In addition, there are associated risk and side effects. For those further into the menopause then the 'continuous combined' regimens can be used. Regular 'periods' are avoided although irregular bleeding is common particularly in early months.

HAVING TO TAKE DRUGS LONG-TERM

If you are troubled by some of the symptoms mentioned above, then you may well feel better by taking HRT. Once your symptoms have been relieved you must decide how long to continue on it. While you stay on it, your symptom relief is likely to continue; if HRT is taken over several years, you will gain some of the longer-term health benefits. Since you cannot be sure if your symptoms will return if you stop treatment, your decision will be influenced by your personal philosophy about taking drugs for five or more years to prevent conditions that can be devastating but which may never happen to you. The decision to take HRT might be easier if you have reason to believe that you are at increased risk of osteoporosis, heart attack or stroke. However, we know that it is extremely difficult to predict with accuracy who is at risk from these problems.

COMMON SYMPTOMS CAUSED BY HRT

For those who have not had a hysterectomy and may still be having some irregular periods, it is advisable to take HRT of the type which usually induces periods. The continuing of periods for several years is a real disadvantage of HRT for many women, particularly when the intensity of the periods cannot be predicted before you have tried HRT. Generally the proportion who have troublesome periods is lower than with natural periods and they do tend to become lighter as the months pass. The small percentage who have no bleeding on HRT should not worry, it simply means that the HRT is not stimulating the uterine lining enough to induce a bleed at the end of the cycle

Another relative common effect of HRT is the occurrence of symptoms while taking the progestogen in the final part of the cycle. This effect is variable and for many women is not a problem, but some are distressed by symptoms similar to the premenstrual syndrome (PMS). These can include abdominal bloating, breast fullness and effects on mood. If this problem arises, a change of HRT preparation may solve it. If you were troubled by premenstrual syndrome before the menopause, HRT will not necessarily reproduce the problem.

Weight gain on HRT is generally not a problem. There can be a mild degree of fluid retention which may cause a minimal weight gain of a couple of pounds, but troublesome weight gain is a rare side-effect.

Other symptoms may occur for the first time when HRT is started. These may include:
■ Headache or migraine
■ Fluid retention, which may be perceived as weight gain
■ Skin rashes (more common in women who take HRT in the form of a skin patch)
■ Painful breasts.

Often these difficulties are intermittent and respond to a change in therapy.

RISKS OF USING HRT

OESTROGEN-RELATED RISKS

There is a very small risk of having a blood clot in a vein and, in some women, taking oestrogen this possibility is increased very slightly. Thrombosis (blood clot) can have serious and potentially fatal consequences in a tiny number of cases. If you have previously had thrombosis, many general practitioners will seek specialist advice before starting you on HRT.

This risk is lower than that associated with the oral contraception pill because HRT contains lower doses of different kinds of oestrogen than the contraceptive pill.

BLOOD PRESSURE

HRT has no significant effect on blood pressure although some studies have shown that high blood pressure improves on HRT; therefore, high blood pressure does not mean that you cannot take HRT.

CANCER RISK

Discussion of the cancer risk of HRT used to focus on the risk of cancer of the lining of the uterus (the endometrium). In the 1970s, it was discovered that American women who had taken HRT in the form of oestrogen on its own were at increased risk of this form of cancer. It was realised that oestrogen was stimulating the endometrium in the same way as it does in the menstrual cycle. In the menstrual cycle, however, the hormone progesterone is produced after ovulation and acts to oppose the oestrogen stimulation of the endometrium in the latter half of the cycle. For more than a decade, since the late 1970s therefore, HRT treatment has included additional progestogen for part of the monthly cycle. Progestogen is a hormone similar to a natural progesterone but is more potent in its protective effect on the endometrium.

The other form of cancer risk which has been of concern is breast cancer, now known to be the commonest female cancer. Many factors in life affect the risk that a women might develop breast cancer, some of which can lead to an increase in risk. For instance, a women whose mother or sister had breast cancer or who had her first child relatively late in life can have a risk which is increased by fifty to one hundred per cent. When the HRT is used for a very long time, such as fifteen to twenty years, then it appears that the risk of breast cancer may be increased by three in 500 women.

For less than ten years of HRT, it is likely that the risk of breast cancer is not significantly increased. All women over fifty years of age are advised to take part in the National Breast Cancer Screening Programme. This involves a mammography screen every three years which should detect early breast cancers which are more responsive to treatment.

RISKS OF HRT IN WOMEN WHO HAVE KNOWN PROBLEMS

Most health problems remain unaffected by HRT, but there are some that have the potential to be affected. There are very few conditions that would prevent a women being able to use HRT, but it may only be after specialist advice that the treatment can be given. Menopause clinics can provide that advice. The potential problem conditions can be summarised as follows:

- Conditions in which the disease may be worsened by using HRT. Examples include porphyria (a metabolic imbalance) and possibly otosclerosis (formation of new bone in the ear, which can cause progressive deafness)
- Conditions where the oestrogen in HRT might stimulate the recurrence of an oestrogen-sensitive cancer which has already been treated. Examples include endometrial cancer and breast cancer
- Conditions where the disease affects the breakdown of the HRT hormones. Examples include forms of chronic liver disease.

Seeking advice

You should contact your doctor if you are on HRT and have any of the following symptoms:

- If you bleed irregularly several days before the end of the pack. This might indicate that the drugs are not fully effective and although your doctor may not need to change anything immediately, he or she may wish to alter your treatment. Irregular bleeding without any pattern requires referral to a gynaecologist
- If you feel a discrete breast lump. The

breasts are more active in HRT users and the lump may not be an abnormality, but it should be checked.

Finally, the majority of women who use HRT obtain relief from distressing symptoms and do not experience problems with the treatment.

If you wish to continue to take HRT for a number of years so that you may gain the benefits for long-term health, you must have confidence that the treatment is safe and you should have access to advice if problems develop. If you have any doubts about using HRT, contact your doctor.

ALTERNATIVES TO HRT

SELECTIVE OESTROGEN RECEPTOR MODULATORS

This is a new group of drugs currently under development which may be useful in treating women with osteoporosis. For oestrogen to have an effect on a tissue it must bind with a receptor (an analogy for this would be a lock-and-key mechanism. When the binding has occurred then changes occur within the genetic material of the cell which leads to the production of substances which affect the action of that cell. Different types of oestrogen receptor are found in differing proportions in the various tissues which are oestrogen-sensitive, such as bone, breast and uterus. The new group of drugs are known as selective oestrogen receptive modulators (SERMs) and they are similar to oestrogen in some ways but not in others, e.g. a well-known SERM, tamoxifen, used in the prevention and treatment of breast cancer is an anti-oestrogen in the breast but has oestrogen effects in the uterus and in bone. This can lead to undesirable side-effects such as vaginal bleeding and abnormalities in the endometrium itself.

A new SERM has recently been developed called raloxifene. This has oestrogenic effects on bone and is thus useful in the prevention and treatment of osteoporosis. The evidence so far suggests that it is anti-oestrogenic on the breast and maybe very important in preventing development of breast cancer. It also is anti-oestrogenic in the uterus and its use is not associated with abnormal vaginal bleeding. Unfortunately, it is not effective in treating postmenopausal symptoms and, therefore, is unlikely to be very useful in perimenopausal women who have hot flushing, but it is probable that it will be an appropriate therapy for those with osteoporosis in later life. Other new agents are being developed and it is likely that more 'designer oestrogens' will come on to the market.

PHYTO-OESTROGENS

These are naturally occurring foods with oestrogen-like biological activity. The use of certain plants in traditional medicine and folklore may be ascribed to their oestrogenic properties. For example, hops were believed by the German clergy in the middle ages to lower libido. Also, infertility may occur in sheep fed too much clover since it is rich in oestrogenic steroids. Phyto-oestrogens occur in a number of plants or their seeds. Soya bean and soya sprout are the best known and when eaten in the diet are taken in through the gut and passed to the liver where they are extensively modified before circulating round the body.

Legumes and beans are rich in phyto-oestrogens but second-generation soya foods can be made by adding soya ingredients to a wide variety of manufactured foods, e.g. Tofu, yoghurt and soya noodle. Linseed oil is a rich source and wholegrain cereals, vegetables, fruit and seeds contain some phyto-oestrogens. Although, they are up to 10,000 times less potent than oestrogens produced by the body, they may have some effects if consumed in sufficient quantities. The quantity of phyto-estrogens in the diet varies considerably from population to population but are known to be particularly high in the east in countries such as Japan, Taiwan and Korea. This may explain why women living in these countries are supposed to have fewer menopausal symptoms.

There is some evidence that phyto-oestrogens may suppress the growth of certain types of breast-cancer cells when grown in the laboratory. Recent evidence suggests that they may reduce hot flushes in some women and help relieve vaginal dryness.

Asian countries have a lower incidence of heart disease and this may be related partly to their diet and phyto-oestrogen consumption. The phyto-oestrogens lower lipids and cholesterol in the blood, which is beneficial, and may thus decrease the hardening of the arteries which leads to heart disease and strokes. As yet, there is a not much information about the possibility of a role in the treatment of osteoporosis although what there is looks promising.

Phyto-oestrogens are available in the health food shops and phyto-oestrogen-enriched bread, milk and other produce are being sold as being good for menopausal women. Caution must be exercised as little is known about their effects within the body. Hormone replacement therapy has been extensively studied and the good and bad effects are well known. This is not true of phyto-oestrogens. It is also more difficult to be certain of how much is being taken in. It is possible that quite a lot of food or milk must be eaten to achieve an effect which, also, may be associated with weight gain. Capsules are becoming available although, so far, there is little standardisation or control. It is likely that these will be very useful in the future, particularly for women who prefer a more natural means of hormone replacement and further information is awaited with interest.

CONTRACEPTION FOR PERIMENOPAUSAL WOMEN

Hormone replacement therapy is not contraceptive. Women are advised to continue to use contraception:

■ For two years after the menopause if the menopause occurred before the age of fifty years

■ For one year after the menopause if the menopause occurred after the age of fifty years.

Fertility is significantly reduced in women over the age of forty-five years. Although contraception is still necessary, methods that may be associated with unacceptably high failure rates in young women are likely to be highly reliable in this group of women

SUGGESTED CONTRACEPTION FOR PERIMENOPAUSAL WOMEN

The following methods of contraception can be considered by perimenopausal women:

■ **Barrier methods:** Vaginal creams, including oestrogen creams and lubricants, may damage the latex of condoms and caps/diaphragms

■ **Intrauterine contraceptive device:** If inserted after the age of forty years, this will afford protection until the menopause. However, it should be removed twelve months after the last period

■ **Hormone releasing intrauterine system (Mirena):** This system contains the hormone levonorgestrel and it is associated with a reduction in menstrual blood loss and may be particularly appropriate for use in a perimenopausal women who is experiencing heavy periods

■ **Sterilisation:** This is becoming an increasing popular choice.

IMPROVING HEALTH AND WELL-BEING GENERALLY

Any woman's experience of the menopause will be influenced by her general state of health and well-being. For example, the average age of the menopause is three years earlier in smokers than in non-smokers. Furthermore, smoking itself increases the risks of osteoporosis and of heat disease. Preparation for a healthy menopause starts in earlier life. Adequate weight bearing exercise and calcium in the diet will contribute to the development of healthy bones throughout life. A diet that is low in fat will reduce the risk of cardiovascular disease. Strong muscles will help to avoid falls and thus help prevent fractures in later life. HRT is not a panacea, and getting the most out of life at any age will be enhanced by a healthy lifestyle, a good diet and a positive attitude.

IMPROVING HEALTH

Exercise: In menopausal women, there is some evidence that exercise may reduce the severity of hot flushes. Walking for an extra five hours a week will help to reduce blood pressure where it is slightly raised and also helps to reduce blood cholesterol. It may also lead to weight reduction and possibly also reduce chances of developing adult-onset diabetes. Moderate, regular exercise of low intensity, such as walking for 30–60 minutes a day, will improve muscle strength, joint stability and flexibility and will help to reduce the incidence of falls.

Incontinence: This is common in postmenopausal women and may be improved by pelvic floor exercises (see Chapter Two).

Smoking: Smokers have an earlier menopause (by an average of one-and-a-half to two years) and a higher incidence of brittle bones (osteoporosis). Stopping smoking will improve your health.

Weight: being overweight is associated with high blood pressure, increased cholesterol and diabetes, as well as with heart disease. However, being underweight may increase the likelihood of osteoporosis and bone fractures.

OSTEOPOROSIS

Osteoporosis is a bone disorder that results in low bone mass and a deterioration of the bone structure leading to an increase in bone brittleness and, consequently, an increase in fracture risk after relatively minor trauma. These fractures can occur almost anywhere in the body but the most common sites are the hip, lumbar spine and wrist. Osteoporosis is a painless disease and only when a fracture occurs does pain develop, although two-thirds of all fractures of the spine are painless and the only evident symptom may be loss of height.

Osteoporosis is sometimes referred to as the silent epidemic as most women who suffer from it may not even be aware that they are affected until their bones become fragile and fracture. However, most women do not have to have their post-menopausal years blighted by this disease, which is, to a great extent, preventable. Modern effective treatments now exist that can help prevent or delay any deterioration in bone mass density and alleviate any associated problems.

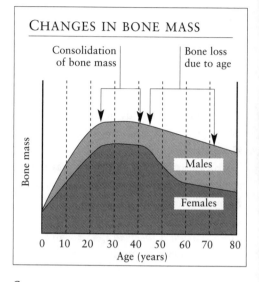

CHANGES IN BONE MASS

SYMPTOMS OF OSTEOPOROSIS

As already stated, most women do not notice the onset of osteoporosis often until many years after their menopause, which accelerates bone loss. The bones of people who suffer from osteoporosis lose some of the calcium

Right:
Osteoporosis occurs particularly in the spine, hip joints and wrists, where it leads to fractures.

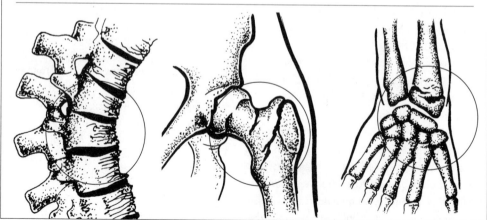

OSTEOPOROSIS

content that keeps them strong, and eventually become brittle. This results in fractures, commonly of the spine, wrists and hips.

■ In general, the bones of the spine fracture in such a way that the back becomes curved and in severe cases this is known as a 'dowager's hump'.

■ Wrist fractures, known as Colles fractures, occur after a fall on the outstretched hand and require hospital treatment for plaster cast application and realignment of the break.

■ The most important clinical site for osteoporotic fracture is the hip because mortality is highest in women who suffer this type of fracture. Classically, hip fractures occur when women fall backwards onto their buttocks, and thus loss of balance and muscle build are important contributors to this type of fracture. One in five women who fracture their hip will die within a year and approximately twenty per cent never return home to an independent existence and require long-term care in a nursing home. The average age of women who sustain hip fracture is eighty years.

In the UK there are currently 60,000 hip fractures, 50,000 wrist fractures, and at least 40,000 spinal fractures annually, which cost in the region of £750,000,000, while in the United States, costs exceed $10 billion. The frequency of these fractures is likely to increase with time as the population ages and life expectancy improves.

WHO IS MORE LIKELY TO SUFFER FROM OSTEOPOROSIS?

The maximum level of bone mass is reached by the age of sixteen in girls and eighteen in boys, and it is generally believed that attainment of optimal peak bone mass is important

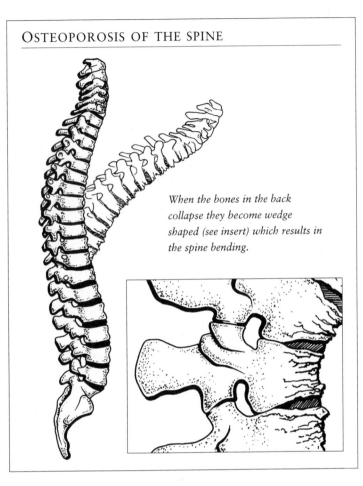

OSTEOPOROSIS OF THE SPINE

When the bones in the back collapse they become wedge shaped (see insert) which results in the spine bending.

in reducing the risk of osteoporosis development in later life. Males reach a higher peak bone mass because bone formation continues over a longer period of time. In both men and women, small increases in bone density occur in the forearm and skull up until the third decade of life.

The risk of developing osteoporosis thus appears to be higher in women compared to men – seventy-five per cent of osteoporotic fractures occur in women – and there is also a geographic variation with the highest incidence of osteoporosis in Asia. In North America and Northern Europe, particularly Scandinavia, the lifetime risk of osteoporotic fracture risk in post-menopausal women is at least thirty per cent. Black men and women very rarely get osteoporosis because they obtain a higher peak bone mass than white people.

Genetic factors are also important in the process of osteoporosis development. Approximately eighty per cent of the diversity of bone mass is attributable to hereditary factors although this influence occurs mainly at the spine rather than at the hip or wrist.

During the period of time just before the menopause – the perimenopausal period – bone thinning begins and this is likely to be due to a reduction in circulating hormones produced by the ovary. After the menopause, bone loss accelerates and as much as five per cent of trabecular (the inner substance of bone) and one-and-a-half per cent of cortical bone (the outer covering) is lost annually. However, after five to ten years, this rate slows to less than one per cent per annum. This reduction in bone mass seen at the menopause is related to a decrease in ovarian function and, consistent with this, a similar loss of bone density is seen in women who undergo a premature menopause, i.e. under the age of forty. Other factors that increase the risk of osteoporosis development are listed below.

RISK FACTORS FOR DEVELOPING OSTEOPOROSIS

- Post-menopausal state
- Low peak bone mass
- Premature menopause – under the age of forty
- Family history of osteoporosis
- Prolonged episodes of period cessation, as in women athletes and anorexia nervosa
- Not having any children
- Chronic use of oral steroids, long-term heparin therapy

- Overactive thyroid/parathyroid conditions
- Bone disorders, such as multiple myeloma (cancer of the bone marrow), secondary bone cancers
- Chronic liver disease
- Chronic immobilisation
- High alcohol intake
- Cigarette smoking
- Having a hysterectomy
- Low intake of calcium in the diet
- Having a low level of exercise.

HOW IS OSTEOPOROSIS DIAGNOSED?

The best way to diagnose osteoporosis is with a bone density measurement using DEXA (dual energy X-ray absorptiometry). This machine takes approximately fifteen minutes to assess bone density and delivers minimal radiation. For osteoporosis to be diagnosed, the bone density measurement, usually at the spine and hip, should be 2.5 or more standard deviations below the young adult reference mean.

In general, osteoporosis begins at the lower end of the spine and measurements at this point are a good reflection of bone content in the rest of the skeleton. Furthermore, because of the high content of trabecular bone in the spine, fractures usually occur at this part of the body before the hip.

The risk of future fracture risk may be assessed, approximately, if a DEXA scan is done around about the time of menopause. However, a follow-up scan may need to be done one to two years later as women lose bone at very different rates.

Plain X-rays can be used to diagnose osteoporosis but thirty per cent of bone loss must have occurred already before X-rays show up osteoporotic bones and detection with this method is successful.

PREVENTING OSTEOPOROSIS

By the time an osteoporotic fracture occurs a considerable amount of bone has already been lost – at least fifty per cent – and therefore prevention is likely to be more effective than treating established disease.

ACHIEVING MAXIMUM BONE MASS

In early adolescent life, adequate calcium supplementation and exercise are advised to promote maximum achievement of bone mass. Calcium intake during a girl's teenage years should be between 1200 and 1600 mg daily. Excessive exercise, especially in long-distance female runners, and girls with anorexia nervosa, can cause a resultant fall in oestrogen levels which has a deleterious effect on the skeleton. Oestrogen supplementation in these women is essential and this can be in the form of the combined contraceptive pill.

BEFORE MENOPAUSE

Regular exercise can play an important part in keeping your bones healthy and strong. During the time leading up to the menopause, and afterwards, weight-bearing exercises, such as weight-training in the gym, walking and jogging rather than swimming, may improve bone mass at the hip but they do not seem to affect bone density at the spine. Menopausal women are advised to consume 1000 mg of calcium a day. This can be achieved with three servings of dairy products, plus the extra calcium contained in a normal, well-balanced diet, or from a dietary supplement of 600–1000 mg a day.

Other lifestyle habits, such as smoking and excessive alcohol intake, should be discouraged as these increase the risk of developing osteoporosis. Therefore, as a woman, you should not exceed more than fourteen units of alcohol in a week. One unit is equivalent to a single measure of spirits, a glass of wine or half a pint of beer or lager.

HORMONE REPLACEMENT THERAPY (HRT)

Hormone replacement therapy (HRT) prevents bone loss at all sites in the body and reduces the risk of osteoporosis development and subsequent fracture. HRT consists of oestrogen and, if the woman has not had a hysterectomy, a progestogen. Both of these hormones are produced by the ovary in a woman's reproductive years, and the use of progestogens in HRT formulations is to protect the lining of the uterus (endometrium) from excessive stimulation by the oestrogen component. Several studies have shown that HRT reduces the risk of all osteoporotic fractures by thirty to fifty per cent with an exposure of three to ten years. Unfortunately, if HRT is stopped, then bone loss resumes at the pre-treatment rate for that particular individual. Since the vast majority of fractures occur after the age of seventy, continuous treatment after the menopause would seem to be more appropriate. However, there are concerns that this may increase the risk of breast cancer development, as discussed earlier in this chapter.

CALCIUM AND VITAMIN D

The role of calcium supplements and Vitamin D is controversial but some studies suggest that calcium may improve bone mass by a small amount but this is much less than the improvements seen with HRT usage. Their use is probably most effective in elderly women in nursing homes and there is evidence to suggest that hip fracture rates can be reduced by twenty-five per cent in this group of women. The National Institutes of Health suggest that calcium intake for women aged fifty and above should be in the region of 1500 mg daily.

You can increase your calcium consumption by including calcium-rich foods in your everyday diet. These include the following:

■ Milk, yogurt, cheese and dairy products
■ Broccoli, spinach, watercress and green leafy vegetables
■ Canned fish, containing edible fish bones, such as sardines and pilchards
■ Most nuts and seeds, especially sesame seeds, Brazil nuts and almonds
■ Dried fruit, such as prunes, apricots and figs
■ White and brown bread is made with flour fortified with calcium in the UK
■ Some mineral waters and tap water in hard-water areas contain reasonable amounts of calcium
■ Vegans can obtain calcium from soya milk and soya bean curd
■ Beans, e.g. baked beans and red kidney beans.

WHEN YOU NEED EXTRA CALCIUM

At certain times of a woman's life, it is important that she has extra calcium in her diet or, at least, an adequate calcium intake.

■ **In childhood:** Calcium is needed by children for building strong, healthy bones, making them better equipped to withstand bone loss in their later lives.

■ **In adolescence:** Teenagers need plenty of calcium as this is the peak time for their bone development when thirty-seven per cent of the adult skeleton is formed.

■ **In pregnancy:** Expectant mothers need cal-

cium in their diet to build the bones of their unborn child. If they do not get sufficient calcium from their diet, the baby will take their own supplies.

■ **In later life:** Elderly people absorb calcium less efficiently and need to eat a diet containing calcium-rich foods. They may also need calcium supplements.

■ **Slimmers:** People following a low-fat slimming diet must ensure that get adequate calcium and do not stop eating all dairy products. Skimmed milk and low-fat yogurt are fortified with calcium and they can continue to eat green vegetables, beans and calcium-fortified bread.

TREATMENT FOR OSTEOPOROSIS

Treatment is aimed at slowing down further bone loss and, to some extent, increasing bone mass in the skeleton.

■ Oestrogen replacement (HRT) is the therapy of choice because it has additional advantages with respect to protection against the development of coronary heart disease. Women should have regular DEXA scans to ensure that they are responding to treatment and, because bone changes are slow, these should be done after a year of therapy. Bone density has been shown to increase by up to ten per cent in post-menopausal women with osteoporosis treated with a year of HRT.

■ Other agents in use include a group of drugs called the bisphosphonates, and examples of these are alendronate and etidronate. These drugs work on the bone in such a way as to reduce the activity of bone-eating cells (osteoclasts) and thus improve bone content in the body by up to seven per cent. Currently, there is no convincing evidence to suggest that HRT and bisphosphonates act together in a superior way, and thus treatment should be with one or the other agent.

■ Women who have developed osteoporosis from chronic steroid use should be maintained on the lowest possible dose of steroids to control their steroid dependent disease – for example, asthma, rheumatoid arthritis or inflammatory bowel diseases.

■ In addition to giving bone conserving drugs, women should also receive adequate pain relief as well as calcium and Vitamin D supplements.

■ Physiotherapy and appropriate orthopaedic advice should be given in individual cases.

REDUCING ACCIDENTS

If your bones are brittle and are susceptible to fractures, there are some things that you can do to prevent the likelihood of falls and accidents. Most accidents occur in the home and thus it is a good idea to check the following:

■ Ensure that there are no curled or frayed carpet edges

■ Make sure that steps and stairs are well lit

■ Watch out for trailing flexes and electric wires

■ It is a good idea to fit a hand rail to the wall side of steep steps and stairways

■ Avoid rugs on highly polished floors – fitted carpets are safer and softer, cushioning your impact if you fall

■ Put a non-slip bath mat in your bath and fit a hand rail to the side of the bath if necessary

■ A walk-in shower may be preferable to a bath.

In addition, by doing regular exercise – say, walking for approximately twenty minutes three times a week – you can improve your balance and co-ordination and thereby help avoid falls.

COMPLEMENTARY THERAPIES

Many women feel that they do not wish to rely on healthcare professionals or on 'conventional' providers in order to maintain their physical and mental wellbeing, and they may wish to adapt their lifestyles in order to maximise their health or seek advice from complementary therapists.

Complementary medicine covers a wide range of practices from traditional Chinese medicine to more recent and exotic forms such as colour therapy and psychic healing. Use of these therapies is increasingly popular among women in the UK, although the majority of these services are only available privately. These 'alternative' treatments include non-prescribed vitamins, herbal medicines, evening primrose, homoeopathic remedies and aromatherapies. There is evidence that one of the reasons that people turn to alternatives is because they are dissatisfied with their relationship with their doctors, who are unable to help their particular problem.

Evidence for the effectiveness of most complementary treatments and the risks associated with them is limited. Most herbal products are unlicensed and therefore no medicinal claims can be made for them. Licensed medical products require evidence of quality, safety and efficacy and their development and marketing is closely regulated. Herbal medicines supplied by herbalists are exempt from licensing. Despite this, herbal medicine is perceived by the general public as being safer than 'conventional' medicine and as having fewer side effects.

EVENING PRIMROSE OIL

Despite abundant popular claims, there is no evidence that evening primrose oil has any benefit over placebo (dummy tablets) for menopausal hot flushes.

PROGESTERONE CREAM

A compound similar to the female hormone progesterone can be derived from the Mexican wild yam or soya. This has been available as a gel or cream for several years.

Absorption of these hormone preparations through the skin is not very effective, and these products are not sufficient to replace progesterone in HRT. This means that women who still have a uterus who are taking HRT should not rely on progesterone creams or gels to protect the uterine lining (endometrium) from overgrowth (hyperplasia), a condition which may lead to endometrial cancer. Wild yam creams do not contain progesterone and there are no studies which show that this product is useful for menopausal women.

HOMOEOPATHIC REMEDIES

These are extremely weak dilutions of medicines that treat 'like with like'. As the preparations are so dilute, they are generally con-

---

HERBAL REMEDIES

There are several popular herbs prescribed for menopausal symptoms. These should only be recommended by qualified naturopaths. There are currently no studies which support the claims of herbal treatments for menopausal symptoms.

Black cohost	No evidence for a role in the treatment of menopausal symptoms.
Flavonoids (found in plants, tea and red wine)	These are anti-oxidants, and may contribute to the reduced risk of heart disease in red-wine drinkers.
Dong quai (Chinese angelica)	Not to be used with aspirian or anti-coagulants. Not more effective than placebo in menopausal sytmptoms.
Licorice	No evidence for its use as a treatment for menopausal symptoms. May raise blood pressure.
Panax ginseng	Recommended to increase energy levels, but no evidence for this.
Hops	Closely related to maijuana. Recommended for water retention and insomnia. No clinical trials.
Hypericum (St John's wort)	Some evidence of efficacy in depression.

sidered non-toxic and free of side effects. Homoeopathy views menopause as a long-term imbalance requiring treatment. Common remedies for menopausal symptoms include lachesis (derived from snake venom), alchemilla (derived from the wild flower anemone pulsatilla) and sepia (derived from cuttlefish). There is a lack of knowledge about the way homoeopathic remedies work and there are no studies showing that these drugs are more effective that placebo (dummy) treatment.

TRADITIONAL CHINESE MEDICINE

There are currently studies examining the effect of traditional Chinese herbal remedies and menopausal symptoms, but no specific recommendations can be made as yet.

ACUPUNCTURE

The method of acupuncture seems to be the release of morphine-like drugs into the brain. There is a small amount of evidence that acupuncture may be of benefit in the treatment of hot flushes.

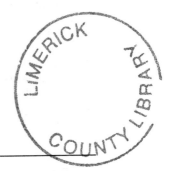

USEFUL ADDRESSES

ADOPTION

British Agencies for Adoption and Fostering (BAAF)
Skyline House
200 Union Street
London
SE1 0LX
Tel. 020 7593 2000
Fax. 020 7593 2001
Email: mail@baaf.org.uk
Website: www.baaf.org.uk

**National Organisation for Counselling Adoptees and Parents
(NORCOP)**
112 Church Road
Wheatley
Oxfordshire
OX3 3LU
Helpline: 01865 875000
Fax: 01865 875686

ANTENATAL SCREENING

Leeds Antenatal Screening Service
26 Clarendon Road
Leeds
LS2 9NZ
Tel. 0113 234 4013
Fax. 0113 233 6774
Email: i.k.sehmi@leeds.ac.uk
Website: www.leeds.ac.uk/lass/

ASTHMA

National Asthma Campaign
Providence House
Providence Place
London
N1 0NT
Tel. 020 7226 2260
Helpline: 0845 7010203
Website: www.asthma.org.uk

BEREAVEMENT

The Child Bereavement Trust
Brindley House
4 Burks Road
Beaconsfield
Bucks.
HP9 1PB
Tel. 01494 678088
E mail:
enquiries@childbereavement.
org.uk

Stillborn and Neonatal Death Society (SANDS)
28 Portland Place
London
W1N 4DE
Tel. 020 7436 7940
Email:
support@uk-sands.org.uk
Website: www.uk-sands.org.uk

BREASTFEEDING

The Breastfeeding Network
(independent support
and information about
breastfeeding)
PO Box 11126
Paisley
Scotland
PA2 8YB
Helpline: 0870 900 8787
Email:
broadfoot@btinternet.com

La Leche League
Box BM 3424
London

WC1N 3XX
Tel. 020 7242 1278

National Childbirth Trust
Alexander House
Oldham Terrace
Acton
London
W3 6NH
Tel. 020 8992 8637
Website: www.nct-online.org

CANCER

Breast Cancer Care
Kiln House
210 New Kings Road
London
SW6 4NZ
Tel. 020 7384 2984
Helpline: 0808 800 6000
Fax: 020 7384 3387
Email:
bcc@breast cancercare.org.uk
Website:
www.breastcancercare.org.uk

**Cancer, you are not alone
(CYANA)**
31 Church Road
Manor Park
London
E12 6AD
Tel. 020 8553 5366
Helpline: 020 8553 5366

**British Association of Cancer United Patients
(Cancer Bacup)**
3 Bath Place
Rivington Street
London
EC2A 3DR
Tel. 020 7613 2121

Website:
www.cancerbacup.org.uk

Cancer Link
17 Britannia Street
London
WC1X 9JN
Tel. 020 7833 2451

CAESAREAN BIRTH

Caesarean Support Network
55 Cooil Drive
Douglas
Isle of Man
IM2 2HF
Tel. 01624 661269

National Childbirth Trust
(see under Breastfeeding
opposite)

Continence
Continence Foundation
307 Hatton Square
16 Baldwins Gardens
London
EC1N 7RJ
Tel. 020 7404 6875
Helpline: 020 7831 9831
Email:
continence.foundation@dial.ti
pex.com
Website: www.continence-
foundation.org.uk

DIABETES

British Diabetic Association
10 Queen Anne Street
London
W1M OBD
Tel. 020 7323 1531; 020
Helping: 020 7636 6112
Fax: 020 7637 3664
Email: bda@diabetes.org.uk
Website: www.diabetes.org.uk

EATING DISORDERS

Eating Disorders Association
1st Floor
Wensum House
103 Prince of Wales Road
Norwich
NR1 1DW
Adult Helpline: 01603 621414
Youth Helpline: 01603 765050
Recorded Information:
0906 302 0012
Email: eda@netcom.co.uk
Website:
www.gurney.org.uk/eda/

ECTOPIC PREGNANCY

Ectopic Pregnancy Support Network
c/o Miscarriage Association
Clayton Hospital
Northgate
Wakefield
West Yorkshire
WF1 3JS
Website: www.the-ma.org.uk

ECZEMA

National Eczema Society
163 Eversholt Street
London
NW1 1BU
Tel. 020 7388 4097
Helpline: 020 7388 3444
Website: www.eczema.org

ENDOMETRIOSIS

National Endometriosis Society
50 Westminster Palace
Gardens
1–7 Artillery Row
London
SW1P 1RL

Tel. 020 7222 2781
Helpline: 020 7222 2776
Email:
Endonifo@compuserve.com
Website: www.Endo.org.uk

FAMILY PLANNING

Family Planning Association
2 Pentonville Road
Islington
London
N1 9FP
Tel. 020 7837 5432
Website: www.fpa.org.uk

British Pregnancy Advisory Service
Austy Manor
Wootton Walwen
Solihull
West Midlands
B95 6BX
Tel. 01564 793225

Brook Advisory Centre
165 Grays Inn Road
London
W1P 6BE
Tel. 020 7708 1234
Helpline: 020 7617 8000

Marie Stopes International
108 Whitfield Street
London
W1P 6BE
Tel. 020 7388 2585
Fax: 020 7388 3409
Website:
www.mariestopes.org.uk

Margaret Pyke Centre
73 Charlotte Street
London
W1P 1LB
Tel. 020 7753 3600
Fax: 020 7530 3646

FERTILITY

Issue – The National Fertility Association
114 Litchfield Street
Walsall
West Midlands
WS1 1SZ
Tel. 01922 722 888
Email: webmaster@issue.co.uk
Website: www.issue.co.uk

CHILD: The National Infertility Support Network
Charter House
3 St Leonards Road
Bexhill-on-Sea
East Sussex
TN40 1JA
Tel. 01424 732361
Email: office@child.org.uk
Website: www.child.org.uk

Human Fertilisation and Embryology Authority
Paxton House
30 Artillery Lane
London
E1 7LS
Tel. 020 7377 5077
Website: www.hfea.gov.uk

FOSTERING

National Foster Care Association
Leonard House
5–7 Marshalsea Road
London
SE1 1EP
Helpline: 020 7620 2100

Family Care
21 Castle Street
Edinburgh
EH2 3DN
Helpline: 0131 225 6441
Fax: 0131 225 6441
Email: birthlink@charity.v3.com

HIV AND AIDS

Positively Women
347-349 City Road
London
EC1V 1LR
Tel. 020 7713 0444
Helpline: 020 7713 0222
Email:
poswomen@dircom.co.uk

Avert
4 Brighton Road
Horsham
West Sussex
RH13 5BA
Tel. 01403 210202
Fax: 01403 211001
Email: avert@dial.pipex.com
Website: www.avert.org.uk

Foundation for AIDS Counselling Treatment and Support (FACTS)
Between 23–25 Weston Park
Crouch End
London
N8 9SY
Tel. 020 8348 9195
Fax: 020 8340 5864

National AIDS Helpline
1st Floor
Cavern Court
8 Mathew Street
Liverpool
L2 6RE
Helpline: 0800 567 123

HOME BIRTH

International Home Birth Movement
The Manor
Standlake
Witney
Oxford
OX8 7RH
Tel. 01865 300266/300154

HOMOEOPATHY

Faculty of Homeopathy
15 Clerkenwell Close
London
EC1R OAA
Tel. 020 7566 7800
Email:
info@trusthomeopathy.org.uk
Website:
www.trusthomeopathy.org.uk

MENOPAUSE, HRT

Women's Health Concern Publications
Wellwood
North Farm Road
Tunbridge Wells
TN2 3DR
Tel. 020 8780 3007

Amarant Trust
11-13 Charterhouse
Buildings
London
EC1N 7AN
Helpline: 0891 660620

MISCARRIAGE

Miscarriage Association
Clayton Hospital
Northgate
Wakefield
West Yorkshire
WF1 3JS
Website:
www.the-ma.org.uk

St Mary's Recurrent Miscarriage Clinic
Samaritan Hospital
Marylebone Road
London
NW1 5YE
Tel. 020 7258 085

MULTIPLE BIRTHS

Multiple Birth Foundation
Queen Charlotte's and
Chelsea Hospital
Goldhawk Road
London
W6 OXG
Tel. 020 8383 3510
Email: mbf@ic.ac.uk
Website:
www.multiplebirths.org.uk

**Twins and Multiple Birth
Association (TAMBA)**
Harnott House
309 Chester Road
Little Sutton
Ellesmere Port
CH66 1QQ
Tel. 0870 121 4000;
0151 348 0020
Email:
tamba@information4u.com
Website: www.tamba.org.uk

**UK Twin to Twin
Transfusion Syndrome
Association**
Tel. 020 8581 7359/0895
846688
Email:
correenukt2t@aol.com
Website:
www.twin2twin.org

NATURAL FAMILY PLANNING

**Fertility Awareness and
Natural Family Planning
Service**
Clitherow House
1 Blythe Mews
London
W14 ONW
Tel. 020 7371 1341
Fax: 020 7371 4921
Email: jknight@fertilityuk.org

OSTEOPOROSIS

**National Osteoporosis
Society**
PO Box 10
Radstock
Bath
BA3 3YB
General enquiries:
01761 471771)
Medical enquiries:
01761 472721
Email: info@nos.org.uk
Website: www.nos.org.uk

POSTNATAL DEPRESSION

**Association for Postnatal
Illness**
25 Jerdan Place
London
SW6 1BE
Tel. 020 7386 0868

PRE-ECLAMPSIA

**Action on Pre-eclampsia
(APEC)**
31-33 College Road
Harrow
MIDDLESEX
HA1 1EJ
Tel. 020 8863 3271
Helpline: 020 8427 4217
Fax: 020 8424 0653
Email: enquiries@apec.org.uk
Website: www.apec.org.uk

PREGNANCY AND BIRTH

Active Birth Centre
25 Bickerton Road
London
N19 5JT
Tel. 020 7482 5554
Email:
info@activebirthcentre.com

**British Pregnancy Advisory
Service**
(see under Family Planning
on page 291)

National Childbirth Trust
(see under Breastfeeding on
page 290)

BLISS
89 Albert Embankment
London
SE1 7TP
Tel: 020 7820 9471

PREMATURE BABIES

BLISS
89 Albert Embankment
London
SE1 7TP
Tel: 020 7820 9471

PREMENSTRUAL SYNDROME (PMS)

**National Association for
Pre-Menstrual Syndrome
(NAPS)**
No 7
Swift Court
High Street
Seale
Kent
TN15 OEG
Tel. 01732 760011
Helping: 01732 760012
Email:
contact@pms.org.uk
Website: www.pms.org.uk

PMS Help
PO Box 83
Hereford
HR4 8YB
Tel. 01432 760993

Pre-Menstrual Society
PO Box 429
Addlestone
Surrey
KT15 1DZ
Tel. 01932 872 560

SEXUAL HEALTH

Family Planning Association
(see under Family Planning
on page 291)

**Institute of Psychosexual
Medicine**
11 Chandos Street
Cavendish Square
London
W1M 9DE
Tel. 020 7580 0631
Email: ipm@telinco.co.uk
Website: www.ipm.org.uk

SEXUALLY
TRANSMITTED
DISEASES

Family Planning Association
(see under Family Planning
on page 291)

Herpes Association
41 North Road
London
N7 9DD
Tel. 020 7609 9061

SPECIAL NEEDS

**Association for Spina
Bifida and Hydrocephalus
(ASBAH)**
Asbah House
42 Park Road
Peterborough
PE1 2UQ
Tel. 01733 555988
Email:
postmaster@asbah.demon.co.uk

Website:
www.asbah.demon.co.uk
Birth Defects Foundation
Martindale
Hawks Green
Cannock
Staffordshire
WS11 2XN
Helping: 08700 707020
Email:
enquiries@birthdefects.co.uk
Website:
www.birthdefects.co.uk

British Diabetic Association
10 Queen Anne Street
London
W1M 0BD
Tel. 020 7323 1531

**Cleft Lip and Palate
Association**
134 Buckingham Palace
Road
London
SW1 9SA
Tel. 020 7827 8110
Website:
www.clapa.mcmail.com

Cystic Fibrosis Trust
11 London Road
Bromley
Kent
BR1 1BY
Tel. 020 8464 7211; out-of-
hours 020 8464 0623
Website: www.cftrust.org.uk

**Down's Syndrome
Association**
155 Mitcham Road
London
SW17 9PG
Tel. 020 682 4001
Email:
info@downs-syndrome.org.uk
Website:
www.downs-syndrome.org.uk

Genetic Interest Group
Unit 4D, Leeroy House
436 Essex Road
N1 3QP
Tel. 020 7704 3141
Email: mail@gig.org.uk
Website: www.gig.org.uk

WATER BIRTH

**Birthworks (National
Birthing Tub Hire)**
Unit 9
Fiddlebridge Lane
Hatfield
Herts
AL10 0SP
Tel. 01707 880333
Fax: 01707 880333
Email:
Birthworks@birthworks.co.uk
Website:
www.birthworks.co.uk

ACKNOWLEDGEMENTS

This book is based on the texts of a series of patient information leaflets, written by Fellows and Members of the Royal College of Obstetricians and Gynaecologists, some of which have been separately published. The idea of the book was conceived as a way of providing women with more comprehensive information than would have been available in a leaflet. Further text was written by Mary Ann Lumsden and Martha Hickey.

OTHER ACKNOWLEDGEMENTS
Valerie Alasia, Beverley Lawrence Beech, Toni Belfield, Meg Goodman, Louise Pengelley, ME Setchell (members of the Royal College of Obstetricians and Gynaecologists Consumers' Forum), for their reading of the draft manuscript and many helpful suggestions; Jane Cunning, midwifery sister at The Queen Mother's Hospital, Glasgow, for reading and commenting on the text of the pregnancy and birth chapters; Peter Bowen-Simpkins, for reading and commenting on the draft manuscript.

GLOSSARY

Abortion
Medical term used for termination of a pregnancy, whether miscarriage or induced.

Adenomyosis
The presence of endometrium in the muscle of the uterus.

AIDS
Acquired Immune Deficiency Syndrome.

Alphafetoprotein (AFP)
A protein in the mother's blood measured in pregnancy in order to screen for spina bifida.

Amenorrhoea
The absence of menstrual periods.

Amniocentesis
The removal and examination of a sample of amniotic fluid, which is the fluid within the uterus (or womb) in which the fetus lives.

Amniotic fluid (Liquor)
The water around the fetus in the uterus (womb).

Anorexia nervosa
A condition of extreme thinness associated with amenorrhoea and osteoporosis.

Antibodies
Produced by the body in response to foreign substances or organisms.

Atopic
Tendency in a person to develop an allergic response to particular substances (allergens) in the environment. These allergens may be breathed in, may be eaten or, rarely, touched. Asthma is only one of the possible manifestations of allergy; others include watering eyes, a runny nose, an itchy throat and eczema.

Augmentation of labour
Use of a drug (oxytocin) given by a drip into a vein in the arm or hand to strengthen contractions and speed up labour.

Bacterial vaginosis
A common vaginal infection in pregnancy and in non-pregnancy.

Bartholin's cyst
Benign (non-cancerous) cyst caused by blockage of a gland at the back of the vagina. The resulting swelling is regular and varies in size from pea-sized to egg-sized. It becomes very painful when infected.

Biopsy
A small piece of tissue taken from the body for examination in the laboratory.

Bronchus
The breathing tube that carries air into and out of the lungs.

Caesarean section
The abdominal delivery of a baby by operation involving cutting into the uterus (womb) and extracting the baby under anaesthetic.

Carcinoma
A medical word for cancer.

Cardiovascular disease
Heart attacks and strokes.

Cervical smear
A test to detect abnormal cells present on the cervix which are pre-cancerous.

Cervix
The neck of the uterus (womb).

Chemotherapy
Drug treatment for malignant disease (cancer).

Chromosomes
Long strands of genetic material which are housed in the nucleus of the body cells. They contain the code for the different genes which make up an individual, and store, copy and pass on this genetic information.

CIN
Cervical Intraepithelial Neoplasia — a condition affecting the outer and inner lining of the cervix within the so-called transformation zone, which has the potential to develop into cancer.

Climacteric
The years leading up to the menopause. Its average length is four years.

Colposcope
A binocular instrument for examining the cervix under magnification.

Cone biopsy
An operation to remove a cone-shaped piece of tissue from the cervix.

Contraceptive
A device or drug which stops pregnancy occurring.

Crohn's disease
A disease of unknown cause, symptoms of diarrhoea with blood and mucus accompanied by weight loss. It affects the bowel.

Cryosurgery
A method of destroying CIN by freezing the tissue.

Cyst
A fluid-filled swelling which can be benign or cancerous. Ovarian cysts may be very large.

Cytology
The study of cells under a microscope.

Cytomegalovirus (CMV)
A common viral infection which may not cause symptoms in the mother but can cause problems for an unborn child.

Dilatation and curettage (D and C)
Scraping away of the womb lining, performed by widening the cervix, which also removes any pregnancy tissue that may remain after miscarriage.

Doppler sonic-aid
A small, hand-held instrument for listening to the unborn baby's heart beats.

Down syndrome
The most common chromosomal anomaly that used to be known as 'Mongolism'. It can be diagnosed antenatally.

Duct ectasia
Inflammation of the breast ducts which may be due to a blocked duct.

Dysmenorrhoea
A term for the cramping pain associated with periods.

Dyspareunia
Painful sexual intercourse.

Ectopic pregnancy
A pregnancy which implants outside the womb, not forming in the cavity of the uterus, but usually in one of the two tubes. It can be dangerous and must be treated in hospital.

Electro-coagulation diathermy
A method of destroying CIN by vaporising tissue.

Electronic fetal monitoring
Use of an electronic monitor to record the baby's heart rate and contractions on the same paper trace.

Endometrial ablation
An operation in which the lining of the womb is destroyed by heat, electric current or laser.

Endometrial biopsy
Insertion of a thin tube into the womb to obtain a sample of the lining of the womb.

Endometrial resection
An operation in which the womb lining is removed in thin strips using a hot wire loop (diathermy).

Endometriosis
A condition in which the endometrium grows elsewhere in the body.

Endometrium
The lining of the uterus (womb) which is shed during a menstrual period.

Epidural
Form of pain relief given by an injection of anaesthetic drugs in the back around the spinal nerves.

Episiotomy
A small cut made by a doctor or midwife to the vagina and vulva to widen the vaginal outlet aimed at preventing uncontrolled tearing during childbirth.

Epithelial hyperplasia
An overgrowth of the lining of the ducts and lobules of the female breast.

Fetal alcohol syndrome
The term used to describe

the syndrome (a collection of symptoms and medical findings which have a common cause) caused by the action of the mother's alcohol intake affecting the baby before birth.

Fetal blood sampling
The taking of a drop of the baby's blood from the scalp during labour to measure the acidity of fetal blood.

Fetal distress
Term used to describe a condition in which the baby is likely to be short of oxygen.

Fetal heart rate
The number of the unborn baby's heart beats per minute.

Fetal scalp electrode
Usually a small curved needle attached to the skin of the baby's head, which is used to pick up the baby's heart beat.

Fetal stethoscope
A short, hand-held, trumpet-shaped instrument used to listen to the baby's heart beats through the abdomen.

Fetus
The early, developing baby.

Fibroadenoma
A small mobile lump which may occur in the breast and often disappears of its own accord.

Fibroid
A benign (non-cancerous) growth in the wall of the womb.

Forceps
Spoon-shaped metal instruments placed on either side of the baby's head and used to help delivery of the baby.

Genito-urinary medicine
Sexually transmitted diseases.

GIFT
Gamete intrafallopian transfer. Sperm and eggs are placed together in the fallopian tube. Fertilisation occurs naturally.

GnRH
Gonadotrophin-releasing hormone controls the release of the hormones FSH and LH (gonadotrophins) from the pituitary gland.

Granulation tissue
A raised area on the vagina which is red and bleeds easily, caused by overgrowth of the healing process after infection of irritation from suture (stitching) material.

Herpes
A viral infection causing painful blisters on the vulva.

Hirsutism
The presence of excessive coarse body hair on a woman, especially on the chin, upper lip, chest, thighs and lower abdomen.

HIV
Human Immunodeficiency Virus.

HIV status
Whether HIV antibody is

positive or negative.

Hormones
Chemicals that one organ in the body uses to control another.

HRT
Hormone replacement therapy. Prescribed to women around or after menopause to replace the body's falling supply of female sex hormones.

Human papillomavirus (HPV)
Some subtypes of this virus cause genital warts and others are associated with cervical cancer.

Hysterectomy
The removal of the uterus (womb), usually including the cervix.

Hysteroscope
A thin telescope used to inspect the womb lining.
Hysteroscopy
Investigation of the womb using a hysteroscope.

ICSI
Intracytoplasmic sperm injection. A single sperm is injected within the egg to facilitate fertilisation.

Immune system
The body's defence mechanism against infection.

Inclusion cyst
Skin trapped below the usual skin surface will produce a cyst. Often associated with tears during childbirth or after episiotomy.

Induction of labour
Starting labour with drugs (such as prostaglandin or oxytocin) or breaking the waters.

Infertility
The inability to achieve pregnancy.

Inhaler
A device which, when correctly used, delivers small doses of medicine directly into the bronchi.

Irritable bowel syndrome
Overactivity of the bowel muscle leading to symptoms of abdominal pain in different areas of the abdomen, alternating loose bowels and constipation, often accompanied by a feeling of incomplete emptying after opening the bowels.

IUCD (or IUD)
Intrauterine contraceptive device/coil.

IUI
Intrauterine insemination. The semen containing the sperm is placed straight into the cavity of the uterus via the cervix.

IVF
In vitro fertilisation. The sperm and egg are mixed together in a test tube and the resulting embryo re-implanted into the mother's womb.

Laparoscopy
Operation carried out with an instrument that is inserted through the abdomen to enable the surgeon to see the whole pelvic area.

Laparotomy
The traditional method of performing abdominal or pelvic surgery through an abdominal incision.

Liquor
(see Amniotic fluid)

Lochia
The term given to normal blood loss from the womb after childbearing.

Mammogram
An X-ray of each breast to show the tissues and detect any abnormalities.

Mass
A firm lump found on examination.

Mastalgia
Pain in the breast.

Mastectomy
Surgical removal of the breast.

Meconium
Stool from the baby's bowel.

Membranes
A thin bag which surrounds the fetus and liquor inside the uterus.

Menarche
The starting of a girl's periods.

Menopause
The stage when ovaries cease to produce hormones, which results in the periods stopping.

Menorrhagia
A term for periods that are heavier than is acceptable to a woman.

Menstruation
The shedding of the lining of the uterus, usually once a month, often called the menstrual period.

Mifepristone
An anti-hormone used in the medical termination of pregnancy.

Miscarriage
The loss of a pregnancy before the baby is able to survive outside the mother's womb, usually before the pregnancy has reached twenty-four weeks.

Molar pregnancy
An abnormal pregnancy due to a problem in the placenta (afterbirth). There is usually no recognisable fetus, and it can cause bleeding from the vagina. Usually the pregnancy has to be terminated or the womb emptied by surgical means.

Myomectomy
An operation to remove fibroids from the wall of the womb.

Myometrium
The muscle wall of the uterus.

Neonatal death
The death of a baby in the first few days after birth.

Nodule
Lump or swelling.

Oestradiol
A natural oestrogen produced by the ovary before the menopause.

Oestrogen
A group of female hormones that include oestradiol.

Oligomenorrhoea
Infrequent menstruation, or periods.

Osteoporosis
A decrease in bone density and strength which predisposes to fractures.

Ovulation
The regular release of eggs from the ovary.

Oxytocin
A natural hormone, produced from the pituitary gland. Synthetic forms are used to stimulate labour.

Palpable
A palpable lump in the breast is one that can be felt by you or your doctor. Lumps that are too small to be felt are called impalpable.

Peritoneum
The lining which covers all the contents of the abdomen and pelvis, including the tubes, womb and the supporting ligaments.

Pessary
A dissolving tablet containing medicine that is inserted into the vagina.

Phytoestrogens
These are natural plant estrogens found in soy-containing foods which may be useful in treating menopausal symptoms.

Pituitary gland
A small gland at the base of the brain that releases a variety of vital hormones involved in sexual reproduction.

Placenta
Also known as the afterbirth. An organ attached to the inner wall of the uterus of a pregnant woman, providing transfer of oxygen and nutrients to the fetus and waste products back to the mother. It is connected to the fetus by the umbilical cord.

Placenta praevia
Where the placenta (afterbirth) lies over the cervix and causes bleeding in pregnancy.

Placental abruption
Where the placenta separates from the uterine wall causing bleeding and pain in later pregnancy.

Polyp
A small benign (non-cancerous) swelling of the lining of an organ, e.g. womb or gut.

Polycystic ovary syndrome
A condition where the ovaries contain multiple small cysts.

Pre-eclampsia
A complication of pregnancy involving abnormally raised blood pressure which, in severe cases, is associated with protein in the urine.

Premenstrual syndrome (PMS)
A group of physical and psychological symptoms that start between two and fourteen days before menstruation and are relieved with, or soon after, the onset of menstruation. Mood changes and swings are the most prominent features.

Preterm labour
Where labour starts prior to the 37th week of pregnancy.

Primary postpartum haemorrhage
Bleeding from the birth canal in excess of half a litre or excessive bleeding which lasts more than twenty-four hours after the baby is born.

Progesterone
A natural hormone secreted by the ovary that plays an important part in the control of periods. It is produced as a result of ovulation.

Progestogen
A synthetic substance that has a similar effect to progesterone. It prevents over-stimulation of the uterus by oestrogens.

Prolactin
A hormone released by the pituitary gland. This hormone is always present in small amounts but increases when a woman is breast feeding to stimulate milk production.

Prolapse
The descent of the female pelvic organs through the pelvic floor. The uterus and/or vaginal walls, having lost their supports in the pelvis, are allowed to drop when standing or straining.

Prostaglandin
A natural hormone in a woman's body concerned in the constriction of blood vessels and the womb wall. Synthetic prostaglandins are used to cause contraction of the muscle of the womb and start labour.

Puberty
The term used to describe the changes in body, mind and emotions that both girls and boys undergo between the ages of ten and eighteen years. During puberty, the child is slowly transformed into a young adult.

Puerperium
The postnatal period which starts with the delivery of the baby and is completed when the mother is fully recovered from the birth. This may be some weeks.

Rectum
The part of the bowel that lies behind the vagina and leads to the anus.

Rubella
The medical term for German measles.

Salpingitis
Swelling, redness and pain in the fallopian tubes due to infection.

Sebaceous cyst
Cyst containing the greasy fluid that keeps skin moist. Blockage leads to a cyst in the skin.

Second stage of labour
The time after the cervix is fully open when the baby is pushed out.

Secondary postpartum haemorrhage
Maternal bleeding between twenty-four hours after the birth of the baby and the sixth week after childbirth. This is often due to infection.

SERMs
Selective oestrogen receptor modulators. These are new drugs which have some properties of oestrogen and are used in the prevention and treatment of osteoporosis.

Sphincter muscle
A muscle encircling the outlets to the body which controls continence.

Spina bifida
A common condition where the spinal cord does not form properly. It can be diagnosed by ultrasound and a blood test during pregnancy.

Stillbirth
The death of a baby in the womb after the twenty-fourth week of pregnancy.

Suturing
Repairing a tear or cut with stitches.

Telemetry
Radio transmission of signals such as the baby's heart rate.

Testosterone
The 'male sex hormone' which is produced by the ovaries as well as the testes.

Thrombosis
A blood clot occurring in a deep vein (deep vein thrombosis).

Thrush
The common name for an infection caused by a yeast-like fungus known as *Candida albicans*.

Toxoplasmosis
An infection which may be picked up from cats that can cause problems in pregnancy.

Transducer
Small instruments held onto the abdomen by a belt to record the baby's heart beat and contractions.

Trimester
There are three trimesters in pregnancy, each of approximately thirteen weeks.

Ultrasound
High frequency sound waves used to detect shapes and movements inside the uterus.

Urge incontinence
Where urine leaks from the bladder, frequently due to instability of the bladder muscles.

Umbilical cord
The blood vessels passing between the placenta and the fetus.

Uterine catheter
A small tube which goes into the cervix and past the baby's head to measure the pressure of contractions from inside the uterus.

Uterosacral ligaments
Fibrous tissue and smooth muscle fibres that extend backward from the uterus (womb) to the sacrum.

Uterus
Also known as the womb. The organ where the baby grows.

Ventouse
A suction device which is attached to the baby's head to help delivery.

Vulva
The area of skin around the opening of the vagina.

INDEX

Hyperplasia 288
Hyperprolactinaemia 107
Hyperstimulation 255
Hypoprolactinaemia 24
Hypothalamus 19
Hysterectomy 30, 31, 35–41, 45, 48, 62, 107, 128, 284
Hysterosalpingogram (HSG) 238, 262
Hysteroscopic endometrial ablation 32
Hysteroscopy 27, 28, 45, 57

I

Incontinence 70–74, 281
Induction of labour 149, 216
Infertility 29, 60, 128, 234–256
    unexplained 240
    treatments for 241–256
Inflammatory bowel disease 287
Insemination, artificial 249
    with donor sperm (DI) 251
Insomnia 147, 288
Interferential therapy 72
Intracytoplasmic sperm injection (ICSI) 240, 247–248
Intrauterine devices (IUDs) 27, 28, 42, 83, 119–122, 125
Intrauterine insemination (IUI) 242, 248–250
Intrauterine system (IUS) 118
In-vitro fertilisation (IVF) 60, 173, 238, 239, 240, 241–244, 251, 263
Iron 158

tablets 27, 30, 151, 173, 214
Irritable bowel syndrome 58, 113

K

Kidney disease 182–184
Kidney stones 58
Kidney transplant 185
Knee rolling 232

L

Labia 67, 100
Labour 11, 149, 155, 176, 187, 202–224, 265
    delays in 219
    induction of 149, 176, 203, 216
    monitoring in 206, 217
    pain relief in 176, 207–209
    positions during 210
    premature 173, 214
    preterm 214–215
    stages of 203
Lachesis 289
Laparoscope 36
Laparoscopic hysterectomy 36
Laparoscopy 43, 61, 66, 123, 237, 238, 246, 265
Laparotomy 61
Laxatives 21
Licorice 289
Ligaments, softened 146
Listeriosis 158, 263
Lochia 225, 232
Loop diathermy excision 82
Luteinising hormone 14, 52, 263

M

Mammography 77
Marathon runners 21
Mastectomy 93
Masturbation 105, 109
Meconium 149
Menarche 13, 16
Menopause 13, 17, 29, 34, 53, 65, 66, 70, 85, 97, 107, 110, 270–289
    premature 24
Menorrhagia 23, 25, 45
Menstrual cycle 12, 13–14, 23, 26, 54
    irregular 23
Menstrual pain 55
Menstruation 15, 16, 46, 59
Microwave coagulation 32
Migraines 148, 277
Mini-pill 24
Mirena 31, 264, 275, 281
Miscarriage 27, 29, 154, 160, 164, 168, 254, 257–260
    recurrent 258, 261–263
    sporadic 261
Mons 12
Multiple births 215
Multiple pregnancy 173, 238, 244, 255
Muscle cramps 147
Myomectomy 30

N

NSAIDs 30
Nappy changing 228
National Childbirth Trust 202, 208
Natural family planning 122